PELVIC PAIN MANAGEMENT

PELVIC PAIN MANAGEMENT

EDITED BY

ASSIA T. VALOVSKA, MD
Director, Pelvic Pain Center
Brigham and Women's Hospital
Instructor in Anesthesia and Pain Management
Harvard Medical School
Boston, Massachusetts

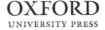
OXFORD
UNIVERSITY PRESS

OXFORD

UNIVERSITY PRESS

Oxford University Press is a department of the University of Oxford. It furthers
the University's objective of excellence in research, scholarship, and education
by publishing worldwide. Oxford is a registered trade mark of Oxford University
Press in the UK and certain other countries.

Published in the United States of America by Oxford University Press
198 Madison Avenue, New York, NY 10016, United States of America.

© Oxford University Press 2016

Library of Congress Cataloging-in-Publication Data
Pelvic pain management / edited by Assia T. Valovska.
p. ; cm.
Includes bibliographical references and index.
ISBN 978–0–19–939303–9 (alk. paper)
I. Valovska, Assia T., editor.
[DNLM: 1. Pelvic Pain—therapy. 2. Chronic Pain—therapy.
3. Physical Therapy Modalities. WP 155]
RD549
617.5′5—dc23
2015036946

1 3 5 7 9 8 6 4 2

Printed by Webcom, Canada

CONTENTS

PREFACE

This book was inspired by my patients and written by leading experts in the field of pelvic pain. The demand to understand pelvic pain is driven by the perplexity of their suffering. Over the years working as a pain physician, I realized that I need knowledge that was not taught in medical school or during the pain fellowship; even my teachers were struggling to treat these patients.

Pelvic pain is a complex disease. The abundance of organs, nerves, vessels, and muscles in the abdomen and pelvis ensure that the clinical picture is confusing, misleading, and often presented with poorly defined symptoms. Involvement of distant organs as well as the musculo-skeletal system further adds to the diagnostic dilemma.

Pelvic pain touches every aspect of the patient's life—physically, emotionally, socially, professionally and sexually. The exhausting experience is a cause for low self-esteem, depression, anxiety, which further worsen the pain.

Misunderstanding the complicated aspects and challenges of treating pelvic pain are the emerging reason for delayed or improper diagnosis.

Usually, the patients are evaluated by physicians across multiple specialties—gynecology, urology, gastroenterology, surgery, and more. Not uncommonly, these people are subjected to invasive procedures that do not provide pain relief. The procedural ineffectiveness and the increasing demand for opioids prompt a last-resort referral to the pain clinic. The lack of interdisciplinary care coordination and management is a common cause for failed treatment.

The emerging need for comprehensive education across the specialties about the complexity of pelvic pain causes, pathology, evaluation, and treatment strategies is the driving force behind this book. The goal is to provide the healthcare practitioner with background knowledge as well skills to diagnose the origins of pelvic pain, to perform a proper physical examination, and to develop a treatment plan with emphasis on multidisciplinary management.

Assia T. Valovska, MD
Boston, Massachusetts

ACKNOWLEDGMENTS

I am eternally thankful to my patients for making me who I am. My determination to never give up the fight is fuelled by your resilience.

My deep appreciation for my colleagues from the Pain Management Center at Brigham and Women's Hospital, Boston, MA—big thank you for your support and understanding.

What would I do without the nursing team "Tenderloin" on "Pearl Thursday"? Your tireless work and deep compassion lighten my days. I consider you my biggest friends and supporters. Thank you for putting up with my long hours. Keep wearing those pearls!

To my husband: You are always next to me, lending a shoulder to lean on. I love you dearly for that.

To my beautiful daughters and budding physicians: Thank you for growing smart and strong. Study hard, the rest is going to come on its own!

To mom and dad: Thank you for tirelessly helping me achieve my dreams.

Assia T. Valovska, MD

CONTRIBUTORS

Chris R. Abrecht, MD
Resident
Department of Anesthesiology, Perioperative,
  and Pain Medicine
Brigham and Women's Hospital
Boston, Massachusetts

Tanya E. Anim, MD
Assistant Clinical Professor
Family Medicine Residency Program
University of Florida
Gainesville, Florida

**Lila Bartkowski-Abbate, PT, DPT, MS,
  OCS, WCS, PRPC**
New Dimensions Physical Therapy, PLLC
Manhasset, New York

Raheel Bengali, MD
Fellow, Interventional Pain Management
Harvard Medical School
Brigham and Women's Hospital
Boston, Massachusetts

Lesley E. Bobb, MD
Resident
Department of Anesthesiology, Perioperative,
  and Pain Management
Brigham and Women's Hospital
Boston, Massachusetts

Mario E. Castellanos, MD, FACOG
Creighton University School of Medicine
Assistant of Obstetrics and Gynecology
St. Joseph's Hospital and Medical Center
Division of Gynecologic Surgery
Phoenix, Arizona

Sybil G. Dessie, MD
Division of Urogynecology
Mid-Atlantic Permanent Medical Group
Upper Marlboro, Maryland

Adam R. Duke, MD
Fellow
Department of Obstetrics and Gynecology
Division of Minimally Invasive Gynecologic
  Surgery
University of Tennessee College of Medicine
Chattanooga, Tennessee

Eman Elkadry, MD
Clinical Instructor
Harvard Medical School
Fellowship Director, Female Pelvic Medicine
  and Reconstructive Surgery
Department of OB/GYN
Mount Auburn Hospital
Boston, Massachusetts

Emmanuel A. Ghormoz
Temple University School of Medicine
Philadelphia, Pennsylvania

Karina Gritsenko, MD
Co-Director Resident Rotations: Acute Pain,
  Regional, Chronic Pain
Co-Associate Regional Fellowship Director
Assistant Professor of Anesthesiology, Family &
  Social Medicine, and Physical Medicine and
  Rehabilitation
Montefiore Medical Center/Albert Einstein
  College of Medicine
Bronx, New York

Ana Lucía Herrera-Betancourt, MD, FACOG
Advanced Laparoscopy and Pelvic Pain
  Unit—Algia
Clínica Comfamiliar
Pereira, Colombia

Michael Hibner, MD, PhD, FACOG, FACS
Creighton University School of Medicine
Professor of Obstetrics and Gynecology
St. Joseph's Hospital and Medical Center
Division of Gynecologic Surgery
Phoenix, Arizona

Alin Ionescu, MD
Division of Advanced and Minimally Invasive
  Gynecology
Department of Graduate Medical Education
Florida Hospital
Orlando, Florida

Mohammed Issa, MD
Harvard Medical School
Clinical Instructor
Brigham and Women's Hospital Departments
  of Anesthesiology and Psychiatry
Boston, Massachusetts

Nii-Kabu Kabutey, MD
Department of Vascular and Endovascular
  Surgery
University of California, Irvine
UC Irvine Medical Center
Irvine, California

Yury Khelemsky, MD
Assistant Professor
Program Director, Pain Medicine Fellowship
Department of Anesthesiology
Division of Pain Medicine
Icahn School of Medicine at Mount Sinai
New York, New York

Ducksoo Kim, MD
Professor of Radiology
Boston University School of Medicine
Boston Medical Center
Director of Cardiovascular and Interventional
  Radiology
Boston VA HealthCare
Boston, Massachusetts

Vesela Kovacheva, MD, PhD
Instructor in Anesthesia
Harvard Medical School
Attending Anesthesiologist
Department of Anesthesiology, Perioperative
  and Pain Medicine
Brigham and Women's Hospital
Boston, Massachusetts

Georgine Lamvu, MD, MPH
Gynecologic Surgery and Pain Specialist
Department of Surgery, Veterans
  Administration (VA) Medical Center
University of Central Florida
Orlando, Florida

Gillian Lieberman, MD
Director of Radiologic Education
Harvard Medical School
Beth Israel Deaconess Medical Center
Boston, Massachusetts

Courtney S. Lim, MD
Clinical Assistant Professor
Department of Obstetrics and Gynecology
University of Michigan
Ann Arbor, Michigan

Jason Litt, MD
Fellow, Pain Medicine
Department of Anesthesiology
Division of Pain Medicine
Icahn School of Medicine at Mount Sinai
New York, New York

Jorge Darío López-Isanoa, MD
Advanced Laparoscopy and Pelvic Pain
  Unit—Algia
Clínica Comfamiliar
Pereira, Colombia

José Duván López-Jaramillo, MD
Advanced Laparoscopy and Pelvic Pain
  Unit—Algia
Clínica Comfamiliar
Pereira, Colombia

Nichole Mahnert, MD
Kaiser Permanente Northern California
Associate Physician
Obstetrics and Gynecology
Walnut Creek, California

Michele L. Matthews, PharmD, CPE, BCACP
Associate Professor of Pharmacy Practice
Massachusetts College of Pharmacy and Health
    Sciences University
Advanced Pharmacist Practitioner in Pain
    Management
Brigham and Women's Hospital
Boston, Massachusetts

Adeoti Oshinowo, MD, MPH
Gynecology Specialists of Garland
Baylor Medical Center
Garland, Texas

María del Pilar Pardo-Bustamante, MD
Advanced Laparoscopy and Pelvic Pain
    Unit—Algia
Clínica Comfamiliar
Pereira, Colombia

Mona K. Patel, MD
Interventional Pain Fellow
Department of Anesthesiology, Pain and
    Perioperative Medicine
Brigham and Women's Hospital
Boston, Massachusetts

Michel A. Pontari, MD
Temple University School of Medicine
Philadelphia, Pennsylvania

Stephanie Prendergast, MPT
Pelvic Health and Rehabilitation Center
Los Angeles, California

Neeraj Rastogi, MD
Department of Vascular and Interventional
    Radiology
University of Massachusetts Medical School
Worcester, Massachusetts

Louis Saddic, MD, PhD
Department of Anesthesiology
Pain and Perioperative Medicine
Brigham and Women's Hospital
Boston, Massachusetts

Bethany Skinner, MD
Department of Obstetrics and Gynecology
University of Michigan
Ann Arbor, Michigan

Jonathan Snitzer, MD
Fellow, Pain Medicine
Department of Anesthesiology
Division of Pain Medicine
Icahn School of Medicine at Mount Sinai
New York, New York

Amy Stein, MPT, DPT, BCB-PMD, IF
Owner/Founder
Beyond Basics Physical Therapy, LLC
New York, New York

Richard D. Urman, MD
Associate Professor of Anesthesia
Harvard Medical School
Brigham and Women's Hospital
Boston, Massachusetts

Juan Diego Villegas-Echeverri, MD, FACOG
Advanced Laparoscopy and Pelvic Pain
    Unit—Algia
Clínica Comfamiliar
Pereira, Colombia

Karen Wang, MD
Instructor
Associate Director MIGS
Fellowship Director
Brigham and Women's Hospital
Boston, Massachusetts

Alison M. Weisheipl, MD
Instructor in Anesthesia and Pain Management
Department of Anesthesiology, Perioperative
    and Pain Medicine
Harvard Medical School
Brigham and Women's Hospital
Boston, Massachusetts

Adham Zayed, MD
Fellow, Pain Medicine
Department of Anesthesiology
Division of Pain Medicine
Icahn School of Medicine at Mount Sinai
New York, New York

Pelvic Pain Management

An Introduction

LOUIS SADDIC, RICHARD D. URMAN, AND ASSIA T. VALOVSKA

Chronic pelvic pain is a ubiquitous condition that affects both men and women. Despite its familiarity, there is no uniform definition of this disease, which has obstructed research efforts to accurately describe its epidemiology, pathology, and successful management. The inconsistency of its definition has been described by many groups who cite large variations in many components, including the duration of symptoms, location of pain, exclusion of cyclic pain, and many more.[23,25,28,32,38] A widely cited definition that encompasses both men and woman comes from the International Association for the Study of Pain. It states that "Chronic pelvic pain is chronic or persistent pain perceived in structures related to the pelvis of either men or woman that is often associated with negative cognitive, behavioral, sexual and emotional consequences as well as with symptoms suggestive of lower urinary tract, sexual, bowel, pelvic floor or gynecological dysfunction."[28] Although this statement is fairly generalized, it is well suited for this text, which attempts to describe a fairly comprehensive collection of conditions associated with chronic pelvic pain. That being said, the conclusions stated in research studies need to be carefully analyzed in the context of their specific inclusion and exclusion criteria.

Sub-categorizing chronic pelvic pain has also been a subject of widespread debate. A common strategy is to distinguish chronic pelvic pain associated with a known pathology (such as malignancy) from cases without such association (collectively referred to as "chronic pelvic pain syndromes").[23,28,32,38] Further subdivisions have also been described but are far beyond the scope of this text. We simply highlight this distinction because of its prevalence in the literature and because it may have significant implications for determining pathophysiology and management. Even more so, care must be taken to ensure that the diagnosis of chronic pelvic pain syndromes is a diagnosis of exclusion.[23,28]

Like many chronic pain disorders, accurately describing the prevalence of chronic pelvic pain can be challenging. As mentioned above, part of this challenge is due to variations in how this condition is defined. Despite these differences, high prevalence rates are consistently cited.[1,3,4,5,11,34] For example, based on an updated review published in 2014, the estimated global prevalence of chronic pelvic pain in woman ranged between 5.7–26.6%, which is comparable to the prevalence of asthma at 4.3–8.6% and one-month prevalence of lower back pain at 20.3–26.1%.[34] Unfortunately, it is well known that there can be significant delay between onset of symptoms and diagnosis,[34] and many reports have shown that up to 50% of women fail to be diagnosed, even after many years of follow-up.[3,5,11,34] Even more so, of the women diagnosed in the primary care setting, only 40% receive secondary or tertiary referral, which is surprising given the concrete evidence that supports the essential role of multimodal and specialized therapy in the successful management of these patients.[18,34] Furthermore, many women with chronic pelvic pain also have coexisting symptoms of depression and anxiety, and sadly, many patients also report a history of sexual and/or physical abuse.[11,18,34] Frequently, these issues lead to absence from work, and among the women who do receive treatment, there is recurrent use of medical resources and thus high healthcare costs.[11,14,34,38] In the United States, for example, it has been estimated that chronic pelvic pain in woman costs the economy over $3 billion.[38]

Similarly in men, a recent analysis of five comparable studies of male chronic pelvic pain syndrome/chronic prostatitis demonstrated a prevalence of 2.2–9.7%, with a median of 8.2%.[20]

The mechanisms of chronic pelvic pain are complex and poorly understood. Nevertheless, studies have shown that chronic pelvic pain involves changes not only in the peripheral nervous system, but in the central nervous system as well.[23,28,25,29] A popular model for the development of chronic pain syndromes describes an initial functional insult in the periphery, such as inflammation, that due to some underlying genetic or environmental factors, induces self-perpetuating changes in both the peripheral and central nervous systems which translate into chronic pain.[23,28,29]

In the periphery, repeated stimulation of nociceptors can lead to peripheral sensitization.[23,29] This process can be exacerbated by the release of tissue-derived local inflammatory substances such as prostaglandins and histamine. Activated C fibers also produce substance P, calcitonin gene-related peptide (CGRP), and other factors that not only sensitize surrounding nociceptors, but also lead to increased vascular permeability and further inflammation via a process referred to as "neurogenic inflammation."[29] Even more commonly, hormones such as estradiol have also been shown to contribute to sensitization in many types of chronic pelvic pain, especially endometriosis. Once sensitized, these neurons can at times develop the ability to signal even after the initial stimulus has been removed.[26,29,37]

Animal and human studies have also demonstrated important anatomical and development changes that occur in the periphery throughout the progression of chronic pelvic pain. In a rat model of endometriosis, ectopic endometrial growths were shown to develop their own perivascular sympathetic and sensory innervation.[10] These findings matched results from human studies. For example, one group reported that the percentage of woman with hyperalgesia is higher in cohorts of women with deeply infiltrating endometriotic lesions in highly innervated areas compared to those with lesions elsewhere.[13] These results underscore the dynamic changes that occur in certain disease states, which probably contribute significantly to the prevalence and severity of pain.

As with most chronic pain syndromes, there is an abundant body of evidence to support the necessary role of the central nervous system in the formation of chronic pelvic pain.[23,28,29,33,36] "Central sensitization" is the process whereby there is an enhanced response of neurons in the central nervous system that leads to hyperexcitability. The mechanisms of this phenomenon have been well studied, and its development in chronic pelvic pain is probably partly due to both responses from the periphery and maladaptive changes within the central nervous system itself.[29,33] This may help explain why some patients with endometriosis obtain relief after surgical or medical ablation, while others do not.[2,8,9,15] In a sense, patients in the latter category have pain that becomes more or less independent of peripheral stimulation.[29,36]

In addition to the derangements of pain that occur at the site of insult, there is commonly a collection of sensory and functional disturbances that develop in nearby organs. For example, an insult in the bladder may lead to irritable bowel syndrome or dysmenorrhea. This visceral–visceral crosstalk is likely to be a complicated version of sensitization, which can also extend locally from viscera to somatic tissue, or even globally from pelvic viscera to viscera in other parts of the body.[23,33]

Evidence of central changes can be found throughout the literature. Neuroimaging with functional magnetic resonance imaging (fMRI) and positron emission tomography (PET) has been used to demonstrate alterations in the activity in certain regions of the brain in women with chronic pelvic pain.[12,36] For example, patients with a history of dysmenorrhea who were not experiencing menstrual pain had increased activity of the entorhinal cortex compared to controls, following noxious stimulation.[30] Some studies have also reported gross changes in brain volume in patients suffering from chronic pelvic pain,[22,31,36] and others have described alterations in the hypothalamic-pituitary-adrenal (HPA) axis.[21,24,36] Endogenous pain inhibitory mechanisms have recently received a great deal of attention with regard to their contribution to chronic pelvic pain. Unfortunately, many of these studies have conflicting outcomes; therefore, more investigation is required to fully understand their role in chronic pelvic pain.[17,12,36] As we begin to learn more about the central changes that take place in the development of chronic pelvic pain, we may increase our repertoire of treatment mechanisms designed to target the central nervous system.

Given the complexity of chronic pelvic pain, it is not surprising that the evaluation of patients with this disease can be time-consuming and challenging for the healthcare provider. In addition to the physical complaints, these conditions are almost always associated with psychological and social impairment and often are coupled with more than one chronic pain condition.[23,25,26,32,38] The physician must remain compassionate, reassuring, and open-minded when evaluating each patient, as these factors contribute to patient satisfaction, which ultimately affects the quality of management.[7,32,36] The International Pelvic Pain Society provides a detailed template for the history and physical assessment of patients with pelvic pain.[19] Although this document is targeted for female patients, it can be adapted for the evaluation of men with pelvic pain.

The history of chronic pelvic pain should begin with the identification of its onset, location, duration, chronology, quality, severity, any radiation, and any provoking or alleviating factors. Special attention should be given to pain associated with sex, defecation, urination, and the menstrual period. Developing a pain map and having the patient keep a pain log are essential, as the elements of chronic pain tend to morph over time. A detailed social history including substance, physical, and sexual abuse should be obtained, as the high prevalence of these conditions in patients with chronic pelvic pain is well established. A psychological assessment including mood, coping mechanisms, and the patient's own theory about the cause of their pain should be elicited. The history should also include other medical comorbidities, past surgeries, and a detailed description of past and current therapies used to treat chronic pelvic pain. A review of systems can be beneficial to elicit coexisting chronic pain syndromes outside the pelvis.[7,25,26,38] Research has also shed light on the important genetic components of chronic pelvic pain. For example, a recent twin study estimated the heritability of female chronic pelvic pain to 46%. Genome-wide association studies of common causes of chronic pelvic pain can also be used to identify common genetic variants.[39] In the future, genetic sequencing studies may play a large role in the screening of high-risk patients for the development of chronic pelvic pain. Therefore, a thorough family history should be obtained.

Physical examination of patients with chronic pelvic pain can be difficult for many reasons, including severity of pain, history of sexual abuse, and coexisting psychological conditions.[7,26] Patience and sensitivity must be applied to maximize patient comfort. Special attention should be given to the back, pelvis and pelvic floor muscles, and abdomen. In men, this includes a thorough assessment of the penis, testicles, rectum, and prostate. In women, this includes an extensive pelvic examination involving the external genitalia and reproductive organs.[23,25,38]

Laboratory testing is not routinely performed in the initial assessment of chronic pelvic pain. Some clinicians do favor basic testing, which can include a complete blood count, urinalysis, inflammatory markers, pregnancy test, and sexually transmitted infection screening. Other tests, such as prostate-specific antigen (PSA) and CA-125, should be tailored to specific clinical findings.[7,25,38]

Nerve blocks and intramuscular injections such as trigger-point injections can be not only therapeutic, but diagnostic as well. Sometimes repeated blocks are necessary to observe a clinical effect.[35] Clinical suspicion for nerve entrapment or muscle spasm should guide intervention, and these procedures should only be performed by physicians trained in non-invasive pain management techniques.

The role of imaging in the evaluation of pelvic pain is controversial. Routine use of computed tomography (CT) and MRI is discouraged; however, specific imaging modalities can be used to confirm suspected pathology, such as pelvic ultrasound to identify an ovarian cyst, pelvic venography for pelvic congestion syndrome, or cystoscopy for interstitial cystitis.[6,25,38]

One of the most hotly debated forms of evaluation is the use of laparoscopy. Chronic pelvic pain is the primary indication for up to 40% of laparoscopies. Benefits include both diagnostic and therapeutic potential.[2,8,25,26,38] Advances in laparoscopic techniques, including laparoscopic pain mapping whereby tissues are probed under local anesthesia and patients are able to report the presence and severity of pain, have been successful for select patient populations.[16,27] Disadvantages to laparoscopy include its cost, complications of surgery, and the risk of negative findings. With respect to endometriosis, countless studies have demonstrated that the degree of pathology does not correlate with the severity of pain, pain sometimes persists despite ablation, and the lack of physical evidence of disease does not exclude microscopic lesions.

A complete workup of chronic pelvic pain should be initiated prior to laparoscopy, and in many circumstances, such as with endometriosis, medical management can be tried prior to surgery.[8,25,26,38]

As alluded to previously, the standard of care for the evaluation and treatment of patients with chronic pelvic pain includes a multidisciplinary approach. This consists of consultations by physicians such as gynecologists, urologists, and gastroenterologists dedicated to treating the functional sources of pain, and psychologists and physiotherapists specialized in treating the emotional and physical impairments associated with the disease. Interventional pain physicians should play a central role in coordinating this care team. These specialists are trained in the assessment and management of both functional chronic pain and chronic pain syndromes; they are skilled in diagnostic and therapeutic interventional pain procedures; they are leaders in laboratory and clinical research on chronic pelvic pain; and their history of collaboration and exposure to other medical specialties provides them with the unique ability to orchestrate a team of diverse consulting physicians. Furthermore, in situations where resources are limited and multiple specialists cannot be recruited, pain medicine physicians are best equipped to provide comprehensive care.

REFERENCES

1. Grace VM. Problems of communication, diagnosis, and treatment experienced by women using the New Zealand health services for chronic pelvic pain: A quantitative analysis. *Health Care Women Int.* 1995;16(6):521–535.
2. Howard FM. The role of laparoscopy in the evaluation of chronic pelvic pain: pitfalls with a negative laparoscopy. *J Am Assoc Gynecol Laparosc.* 1996;4(1):85–94.
3. Mathias SD, Kuppermann M, Liberman RF, Lipschutz RC, Steege JF. Chronic pelvic pain: prevalence, health-related quality of life, and economic correlates. *Obstet Gynecol.* 1996;87(3):321–327.
4. Zondervan K, Yudkin PL, Vessey MP, Dawes MG, Barlow DH, Kennedy SH. Prevalence and incidence of chronic pelvic pain in primary care: evidence from a national practice database. *Br J Obstet Gynaecol.* 1999;106(11):1149–1155.
5. Zondervan K, Yudkin PL, Vessey MP, Dawes MG, Barlow DH, Kennedy SH. Patterns of diagnosis and referral in women consulting for chronic pelvic pain in UK primary care. *Br J Obstet Gynaecol.* 1999;106(11):1156–1161.
6. Cody R, Ascher S. Diagnostic value of radiological tests in chronic pelvic pain. *Baillieres Best Pract Res Clin Obstet Gynaecol.* 2000;14(13):433–466.
7. Gambone JC, Mittman BS, Munro MG, Scialli AR, Winkel CA. Consensus statement for the management of chronic pelvic pain and endometriosis: proceedings of an expert-panel consensus process. *Fertil Steril.* 2002;78(5):961–972.
8. Howard FM. The role of laparoscopy in the chronic pelvic pain patient. *Clin Obstet Gynecol.* 2003;46(4).
9. Swank DJ, Swank-Bordewijk SCG, Hop WCJ, et al. Laparoscopic adhesiolysis in patients with chronic abdominal pain: a blinded randomised controlled multi-centre trial. *Lancet.* 2003;361(9365):1247–1251.
10. Berkley KJ, Dmitrieva N, Curtis KS, Papka RE. Innervation of ectopic endometrium in a rat model of endometriosis. *Proc Natl Acad Sci U S A.* 2004;101(30):11094–11098.
11. Grace VM, Zondervan KT. Chronic pelvic pain in New Zealand: prevalence, pain severity, diagnoses and use of the health services. *ANZJPH.* 2004;28(4):369–375.
12. Wilder-Smith CH, Schindler D, Lovblad K, Redmond SM, Nirkko A. Brain functional magnetic resonance imaging of rectal pain and activation of endogenous inhibitory mechanisms in irritable bowel syndrome patient subgroups and healthy controls. *Gut.* 2004;53(11):1595–1601.
13. Berkley KJ, Rapkin AJ, Papka RE. The pains of endometriosis. *Science.* 2005;308(5728):1587–1589.
14. Grace V, Zondervan K. Chronic pelvic pain in women in New Zealand: comparative well-being, comorbidity, and impact on work and other activities. *Health Care Women Int.* 2006;27(7):585–599.
15. Lamvu G, Williams R, Zolnoun D, et al. Long-term outcomes after surgical and nonsurgical management of chronic pelvic pain: one year after evaluation in a pelvic pain specialty clinic. *Am J Obstet Gynecol.* 2006;195(2):591–598.
16. Swanton A, Iyer L, Reginald PW. Diagnosis, treatment and follow up of women undergoing conscious pain mapping for chronic pelvic pain: a prospective cohort study. *BJOG.* 2006;113(7):792–796.
17. Johannesson U, de Boussard CN, Brodda Jansen G, Bohm-Starke N. Evidence of diffuse noxious inhibitory controls (DNIC) elicited by cold noxious stimulation in patients with provoked vestibulodynia. *Pain.* 2007;130(1–2):31–39.
18. Weijenborg PTM, Greeven A, Dekker FW, Peters AAW, ter Kuile MM. Clinical course of chronic

pelvic pain in women. *Pain*. 2007;132(Suppl 1): S117–S123.

19. International Pelvic Pain Society: History and physical examination form. *International Pelvic Pain Society, April* 2008. Available at: http://pelvicpain. org/docs/resources/forms/history-and-physical-form-english.aspx. Accessed October 19, 2014.

20. Krieger JN, Lee SWH, Jeon J, Cheah PY, Liong ML, Riley DE. Epidemiology of prostatitis. *Int J Antimicrob Agents*. 2008;31(Suppl 1):85–90.

21. Petrelluzzi KFS, Garcia MC, Petta CA, Grassi-Kassisse DM, Spadari-Bratfisch RC. Salivary cortisol concentrations, stress and quality of life in women with endometriosis and chronic pelvic pain. *Stress*. 2008;11(5):390–397.

22. Schweinhardt P, Kuchinad A, Pukall CF, Bushnell MC. Increased gray matter density in young women with chronic vulvar pain. *Pain*. 2008;140(3):411–419.

23. Baranowski AP. Chronic pelvic pain. *Best Pract Res Clin Gastroenterol*. 2009;23(4):593–610.

24. Ehrstrom S, Kornfeld D, Rylander E, Bohm-Starke N. Chronic stress in women with localized provoked vulvodynia. *J Psychosom Obstet Gynecol*. 2009; 30(1):73–79.

25. Vercellini P, Somigliana E, Viganò P, Abbiati A, Barbara G, Fedele L. Chronic pelvic pain in women: etiology, pathogenesis and diagnostic approach. *Gynecol Endocrinol*. 2009;25(3):149–158.

26. Vincent K. Chronic pelvic pain in women. *Postgrad Med J*. 2009;85(999):24–29.

27. Yunker A, Steege J. Practical guide to laparoscopic pain mapping. *J Minim Invasive Gynecol*. 2010;17(1):8–11.

28. Merskey H, Bogduk N. *Classification of Chronic Pain: Descriptions of Chronic Pain Syndromes and Definitions of Pain Terms*. 2nd ed., revised. Seatle, WA: *IASP Press*; 1994 (revised 2011). Available at: www. iasp-pain.org/PublicationsNews/Content.aspx?Item-Number=1673. Accessed October 19, 2014.

29. Stratton P, Berkley KJ. Chronic pelvic pain and endometriosis: translational evidence of the relationship and implications. *Hum Reprod Update*. 2011;17(3):327–346.

30. Vincent K, Warnaby C, Stagg CJ, Moore J, Kennedy S, Tracey I. Dysmenorrhoea is associated with central changes in otherwise healthy women. *Pain*. 2011;152(9):1966–1975.

31. As-Sanie S, Harris RE, Napadow V, et al. Changes in regional gray matter volume in women with chronic pelvic pain: a voxel-based morphometry study. *Pain*. 2012;153(5):1006–1014.

32. Stacy J, Frawley H, Powell G, Goucke R, Pavy T. Persistent pelvic pain: rising to the challenge. *ANZJOG*. 2012;52(6):502–507.

33. Kaya S, Hermans L, Willems T, Roussel N, Meeus M. Central sensitization in urogynecological chronic pelvic pain: a systematic literature review. *Pain Physician*. 2013;16(4):291–308.

34. Ahangari A. Prevalence of chronic pelvic pain among women: an updated review. *Pain Physician*. 2014;17(2):141–147.

35. Baranowski AP, Lee J, Price C, Hughes J. Pelvic pain: a pathway for care developed for both men and women by the British Pain Society. *Br J Anaesth*. 2014;112(3):452–459.

36. Brawn J, Morotti M, Zondervan KT, Becker CM, Vincent K. Central changes associated with chronic pelvic pain and endometriosis. *Hum Reprod Update*. 2014;20(5):737–747.

37. Hassan S, Muere A, Einstein G. Ovarian hormones and chronic pain: a comprehensive review. *Pain*. 2014;155(12):2448–2460.

38. Steege J, Siedhoff MT. Chronic pelvic pain in women. *Obstet Gynecol*. 2014;124(3):616–629.

39. Vehof J, Zavos HMS, Lachance G, Hammond CJ, Williams FMK. Shared genetic factors underlie chronic pain syndromes. *Pain*. 2014;155(8): 1562–1568.

2

Anatomy of the Abdomen and Pelvis

MONA K. PATEL AND ASSIA T. VALOVSKA

Chronic pelvic pain is a common problem that has been poorly understood for decades. It is defined as pain that occurs below the umbilicus to mid-thigh and lasts for at least six months. The pelvis is home to multiple organ systems, including the reproductive, urogenital, gastrointestinal, and musculoskeletal.[3] In addition to pain arising from dysfunction of these organs, the etiology of the pain can also be neuropathic or myofascial. Earlier theories for the source of this pain had attributed it to visceral organs or somatic structures in the pelvis in combination with a psychological component. The unclear etiology presented a unique challenge for treatment of the pain. Recent clinical investigations have shed more light on the importance of understanding pelvic floor anatomy and physiological function in order to diagnose and appropriately treat pelvic floor dysfunction.[2] The aim of this chapter is to review the pelvic anatomy and its clinical correlations, with special attention to the female.

HISTORY AND PHYSICAL EXAM

The neuroanatomy of the pelvis is quite intricate; hence, it is vital to obtain a detailed history of the pain. Inquiries should be made regarding (but not limited to) distribution of the pain, nervous system involvement, aggravating factors, associated bowel or bladder dysfunction, and sexual function. A broad physical examination can help determine any diffuse involvement of the nervous system and help localize the problem. Sensation and motor functions must both be tested, along with appropriate reflex testing. Patients will frequently be uncomfortable with portions of the physical exam, like sphincter tone testing; therefore, it will be paramount to talk the patients through the testing so they are aware of the steps. The sections below describe the anatomy of the pelvis to help with diagnosis of the origin of pain and appropriate treatment.

Anatomy

Anteriorly, the pelvis contains the bladder and the perivesicular fossa; posteriorly, the rectum and perirectal fossa; and in the middle, the urogenital organs (Figure 2.1).

The Bony Pelvis

The bony pelvis supports all the visceral organs and pelvic muscles. It comprises the ilium, ischium, pubis, sacrum, and coccyx. The ilium, ischium and pubis fuse to form the acetabulum, which articulates with the femoral head. The sacrum meets the ilium posteriorly to form the sacroiliac (SI) joint, which is a synovial joint. The joint is lined by a membrane that produces lubricating fluid and is protected by a capsule. The SI joint permits little movement, and its primary function is weight bearing. Over time, this joint is obliterated, and since it is innervated by lumbar and sacral joints, that obliteration can manifest as back pain or pain along the sciatic distribution. Anteriorly, the pubic bones meet to form the pubis symphysis, which is a fibrocartilage joint. The pelvic rim defines the greater (above) and lesser (below) pelvis.

Muscles of the Pelvis

Muscles of the pelvic floor serve two major purposes: they form the floor upon which the abdominal viscera are supported, and serve the constrictor function for the urethra, vagina, and anal orifice.[1,2,3]

The walls of the pelvis are covered by striated muscles that are invested in fascia. The posterolateral wall is composed of the piriformis muscle, which arises from the anterior and lateral surface of the sacrum and exits via the greater sciatic foramen and attaches to

Topography of the Female Pelvic Viscera: Medial and Paramedial Sagittal Views

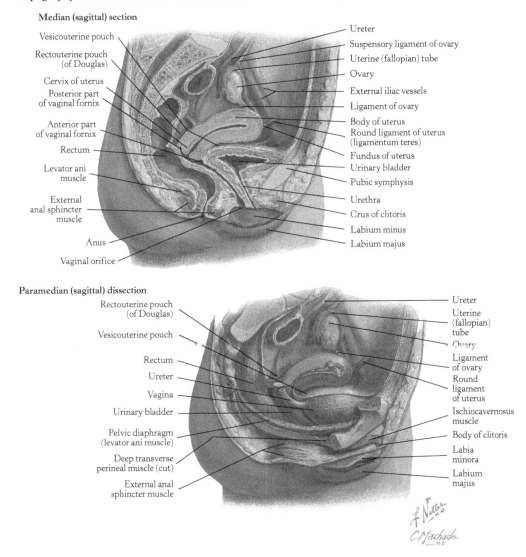

FIGURE 2.1: Topography of the female pelvic viscera: medial and paramedial sagittal views.

the greater trochanter of the femur. It mainly functions as an external/lateral hip rotator. The obturator internus muscle arises from the inferior pubic ramus, ischium and the obturator membrane, as it exits through the lesser sciatic foramen, also to function as an external hip rotator.[3] The obturator externus muscle is flat and triangular in shape and covers the outer surface of the anterior wall of the pelvis. It arises from the medial aspect of the obturator membrane and the inferior ramus of the pubis and ischium and attaches to the lower part of the hip joint into the trochanteric fossa of the femur[1,3] (Figure 2.2). The psoas muscle is a fusiform muscle located at lumbar region of vertebral column and brim of the lesser pelvis; its fibers join with the iliacus muscle, which fills the iliac fossa to form the iliopsoas muscle. It is a strong hip flexor and is innervated by L2–L4.

The pelvic floor is organized between superficial and deep layers. The superficial perineal layer consists of the bulbocavernosus, ischiocavernosus, superficial transverse perineal muscles, and the external anal sphincter. The pudendal nerve innervates these. The deep urogenital diaphragm layer, also innervated by the pudendal

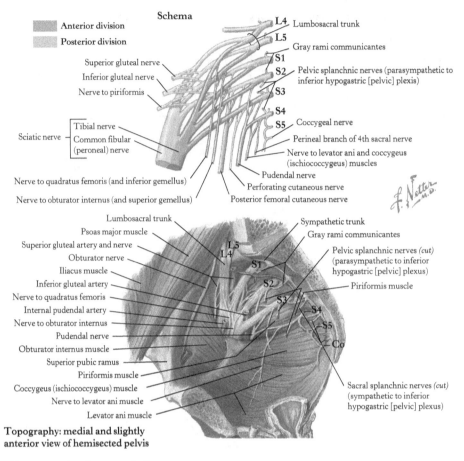

Schema

Anterior division

Posterior division

Superior gluteal nerve
Inferior gluteal nerve
Nerve to piriformis

Sciatic nerve — Tibial nerve
Common fibular (peroneal) nerve

Nerve to quadratus femoris (and inferior gemellus)
Nerve to obturator internus (and superior gemellus)

L4 Lumbosacral trunk
L5
S1   Gray rami communicantes
S2 Pelvic splanchnic nerves (parasympathetic to inferior hypogastric [pelvic] plexis)
S3
S4
S5 Coccygeal nerve
Perineal branch of 4th sacral nerve
Nerve to levator ani and coccygeus (ischiococcygeus) muscles
Pudendal nerve
Perforating cutaneous nerve
Posterior femoral cutaneous nerve

Lumbosacral trunk
Psoas major muscle
Superior gluteal artery and nerve
Obturator nerve
Iliacus muscle
Inferior gluteal artery
Nerve to quadratus femoris
Internal pudendal artery
Nerve to obturator internus
Pudendal nerve
Obturator internus muscle
Superior pubic ramus
Piriformis muscle
Coccygeus (ischiococcygeus) muscle
Nerve to levator ani muscle
Levator ani muscle

Sympathetic trunk
Gray rami communicantes
Pelvic splanchnic nerves (cut) (parasympathetic to inferior hypogastric [pelvic] plexus)
Piriformis muscle

L5
L4
S1
S2
S3
S4
S5
Co

Sacral splanchnic nerves (cut) (sympathetic to inferior hypogastric [pelvic] plexus)

Topography: medial and slightly anterior view of hemisected pelvis

FIGURE 2.2: Sacral and coccygeal plexuses.

nerve, comprises the ureterovaginal sphincter and deep transverse perineal muscle. The pelvic diaphragm forms the floor for the pelvic organs. These muscles connect the pubic symphysis to the coccyx. The pelvic diaphragm separates the pelvic cavity from the perineum (Figure 2.3). The pelvic diaphragm is made up of levator ani and coccygeus muscles. The urogenital diaphragm, also known as the triangular ligament, is a muscular membrane that occupies the area between the pubic symphysis and ischial tuberosities. The urogenital hiatus is U-shaped and houses the urethra, rectum, and vagina.[3] The pelvic diaphragm is primarily supplied by the ventral rami of sacral nerves 2 through 5.

The levator ani muscles serve an important function, as physiologically they are contracted constantly to provide stability to the pelvic floor. The levator ani are made up of the pubococcygeus, puborectalis, and iliococcygeus muscles. The pubococcygeus muscle is divided into the pubovaginalis, puboperinealis, and puboanalis muscles. The anterior attachment is on the inner aspect of the pubic bone and to the lateral walls of the vagina, and to the anus between the internal and external anal sphincters, respectively.[3] All these muscles work together to keep the pelvic floor elevated and the urogenital hiatus narrowed. The puborectalis makes up the medial fibers of the levator ani muscles that attach to the pubic bone and form a U-shaped sling behind the anorectal junction, and functions to draw the junction toward the pubis. The puborectalis is a part of the anal sphincter complex, aiding in fecal continence. The iliococcygeus muscle is the most posterior and thinnest part of the levator ani muscles. Its attachments are the arcus tendineus and the ischial spine. Fibers from both sides come together to form the anococcygeal raphe, also known as the levator plate, which provides support for the rectum, upper vagina, and uterus.

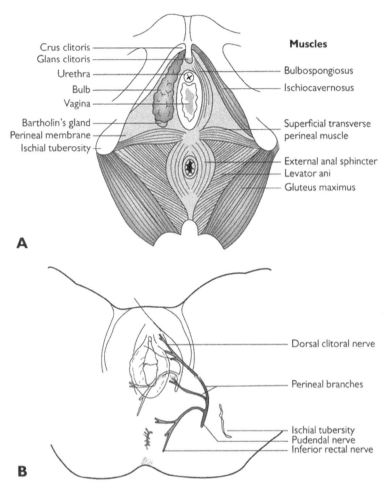

Crus clitoris
Glans clitoris
Urethra
Bulb
Vagina
Bartholin's gland
Perineal membrane
Ischial tuberosity

Muscles

Bulbospongiosus
Ischiocavernosus
Superficial transverse perineal muscle
External anal sphincter
Levator ani
Gluteus maximus

A

Dorsal clitoral nerve

Perineal branches

Ischial tubersity
Pudendal nerve
Inferior rectal nerve

B

FIGURE 2.3: Structures in the anterior (urogenital) and the posterior (anal) perineum, and their relationships.

Reproduced from Harold Ellis, *Clinical Anatomy: Applied Anatomy for Students and Junior Doctors*, figure 99, p. 143. Copyright Wiley, 2010, with permission.

THE NERVOUS SYSTEM

The contents of the pelvis are supplied by the somatic, parasympathetic, and sympathetic components. The lumbar plexus is formed from the ventral rami of spinal nerves T12–L4 on the posterior abdominal wall in the substance of the psoas muscle. Most of the sympathetically derived sensation and functions involve the superior hypogastric plexus and the parasympathetic from the inferior hypogastric plexus.

Somatic Nervous System

Thoracic Innervation

Sensory supply to the abdominal wall is primarily via anterior and lateral cutaneous branches of the rami off T7–T12. These sensory nerves run in a plane between internal oblique and transversus abdominis muscles. The nerve branches advance to the wall of the rectus sheath and supply the skin. Each of these nerves contains a fibrous ring in the rectus sheath that allows the anterior cutaneous nerves to travel freely. However, when the direction of the nerve changes, or with muscle contraction, there can be entrapment of these nerves—namely, anterior abdominis cutaneous nerve entrapment (AACNE). This syndrome is characterized by abdominal pain that can be spontaneous and elicited with palpation. Patients typically have a positive Carnett sign.[4] This sign is produced when the examiner localizes the area of maximal tenderness on the abdominal wall with his/her index finger, followed by asking patient to raise their head and torso with arms crossed over their chest, with finger intact. A positive sign is elicited when the pain is persistent or increased with the maneuver and suggests that the etiology of the pain is more likely to be abdominal wall than visceral in nature.[4] In addition to physical exam signs for diagnosis, ultrasonography (US) can be used to visualize the space between the internal oblique and transversus abdominus muscles for diagnosis and therapeutic purposes. Small amounts of local anesthetic can be injected in the space under the rectus sheath to observe for relief of symptoms. Alleviation of symptoms is diagnostic, and repeat injections with local anesthetic and steroid can be therapeutic.

Lumbar Plexus

The branches of the lumbar plexus are the somatic nerves that help with diagnoses based on the location of pain. The branches include the iliohypogastric (T12, L1), ilioinguinal (L1), genitofemoral (L1, L2), lateral femoral cutaneous (L2, L3, posterior divisions), obturator (L2, L3, L4, anterior divisions), and femoral (L2, L3, L4, anterior) nerves. All these nerves, with the exception of the lateral femoral cutaneous nerve, have both a sensory and a motor component.

The iliohypogastric nerve runs along the lateral abdominal wall between the transversus abdominis and internal oblique muscle, splitting into the lateral branch, which supplies the gluteal region (superolateral), and the anterior branch, which terminates to supply the area of skin just above the pubis. The ilioinguinal nerve supplies the innervation to the skin of the labia majora and mons pubis, along with the skin adjacent to the medial thigh.[1,2,3] As these nerves enter the pelvic canal, they lie anterior to the quadratus lumborum muscles and lateral to the psoas muscle.

The genitofemoral nerve, as the name implies, has two branches. The genital branch passes through the inguinal canal and innervates the labia majora and medial thigh. The femoral branch provides sensation to the anterior thigh. The nerve passes along the medial aspect of the psoas muscle and then posterior to the ureter.[1] As both the ilioinguinal and the genitofemoral nerve innervate the skin adjacent to the medial thigh, irritation to either one of these nerves must be considered when treating patients with neuropathic groin pain. Entrapment of this nerve is commonly seen with inguinal hernia repairs.

The lateral femoral cutaneous nerve ends in two branches (anterior and posterior) that provide sensation to the lateral thigh. This nerve emerges posterior to the psoas muscle, travels laterally to cross the iliacus, and pierces the abdominal wall close to the inguinal ligament to make its way to the lateral thigh. If this nerve gets trapped by staples or sutures, it can result in neuropathic pain over the lateral thigh, a condition termed "meralgia paraesthetica."[2] The obturator nerve runs along with the vein and artery in the obturator canal to terminate in anterior and posterior branches, to supply both sensation and motor innervation to the medial thigh (the major adductors of the thigh). Femoral nerves lie posterior to the psoas major muscle, and then lateral to femoral artery exit the pelvis laterally, to continue to the anterior thigh and split into branches that innervate the hip, knee, anterior thigh, and medial leg. Special attention should be paid to these nerves during abdominal surgery so as to not compress the nerve beneath the psoas muscle or with laterally placed retractors.

Sacral Plexus

The plexus arises lateral to the sacral foramina on the anterior aspect of the piriformis muscle. It is formed by contributions from L4–S4, with each nerve splitting into anterior and posterior divisions. The first branches are the nerve to the quadratus femoris and gemellus inferior (L4, 5 S1 anterior) and the nerve to the obturator internus and gemellus superior (L5, S1, 2 anterior). They travel through the greater sciatic foramen to provide innervation to the respective muscles. The posterior divisions of L4, L5, and S1 come together to form the superior gluteal nerve. The gluteal nerves are anatomically named in relation to the piriformis muscle. The superior gluteal nerve exits through the greater sciatic foramen alongside the gluteal vessels and travels superior to the piriformis to provide innervation to the gluteus medius and minimus, along with the tensor fascia latae. The inferior gluteal nerves also have similar origins (L5, S1, S2 posterior); however, as it transverses through the greater sciatic foramen, it lies inferior to the piriformis muscles and terminates to supply the gluteus maximus.[1,2] Branches of the first and second sacral nerves called the nerve to the piriformis innervate the piriformis muscle itself. Posterior femoral cutaneous nerve (S1, S2 posterior, S2, S3 anterior) provides the cutaneous innervation to the buttock, perineum, and lower extremity after it exits inferiorly through the greater sciatic foramen. Both anterior and posterior branches from L4, L5, and S1–S4 converge into a band to form the largest nerve in the body: the sciatic nerve. This nerve, like the others, also exits via the greater sciatic foramen to the posterior thigh to innervate the major muscles in the posterior thigh, and terminates into the tibial and common peroneal nerve close to the popliteal fossa.[1,2]

The pudendal nerve is composed of anterior contributions from sacral nerves 2–4. It travels between the piriformis and coccygeus muscles to leave the pelvis through the greater sciatic foramen. It then travels laterally to the sacrospinous ligament and reenters the pelvis via the lesser sciatic foramen. The nerve travels in the pudendal or Alcock's canal with the internal pudendal artery and nerve. One of the nerves that arise proximally is the dorsal nerve to the clitoris. This nerve travels in the pudendal canal and along the ischiopubic ramus to terminate and provide cutaneous supply to the clitoris. The second branch, the inferior rectal nerve, also travels in the pudendal canal with the respective vessels to provide innervation to the external anal sphincter (both motor and sensory) and the area adjacent to the sphincter.[1,2,3] The last major branch of the pudendal nerve is the perineal nerve, which is divided into superficial and deep branches. The superficial branch provides cutaneous innervation to the posterior labia and vagina. It also contributes to the mucous membranes of the urethra. The deep branch provides both sensory and motor stimulation to the superficial and deep muscles. The pudendal nerve terminates in the glans clitoris, where it functions purely as a sensory nerve. Cervical, uterosacral, and vulvovaginal areas share afferent fibers entering the dorsal horn of the spinal cord in close proximity. The overlapping nature of vulvar and perineal region innervation makes it challenging to determine the true cause of pelvic pain in many patients.

Coccygeal Plexus

The coccygeal plexus is formed from anterior division of S4, S5, and coccygeal nerves. The muscles innervated by the plexus include the levator ani and coccygeus muscle. The plexus also supplies the sacrococcygeal joint and the skin between the anus and the tip of the coccyx.

Autonomic Nervous System

Sympathetic Nervous System (SNS)

The SNS consists of two neurons that transmit the signal from the spinal cord to the target organ. The shorter, preganglionic neuron descends from the white matter of the spinal cord from levels T1–L2 to synapse with a longer postganglionic neuron at a paravertebral ganglion, which terminates at the target organ. The sympathetic chain runs between the psoas muscle and aorta on the left and between the psoas muscle and inferior vena cava on the right. There are commonly four abdominal sympathetic ganglia. The two trunks converge anterior to the coccyx to form the ganglion impar.

The splanchnic nerves arise from the sympathetic fibers in the thoracic region. Fibers from T5–T9 form the greater splanchnic nerves, which synapse in the celiac plexus and innervate the small intestine and colon. Fibers from T10–T11 form the lesser splanchnic nerves, which supply the small intestine and colon as well but via the superior mesenteric plexus. The least splanchnic nerves arise from T12 and send fibers to form renal and ovarian plexuses.[1,2] The lumbar splanchnic nerves terminate in the inferior mesenteric plexus and supply parts of the colon, and also send branches to the superior rectal plexus to supply the rectum and anal canal along with the internal anal sphincter. As the inferior mesenteric plexus travels caudally, it becomes the superior hypogastric plexus (purely sympathetic in nature), which splits into left and right divisions at the sacral promontory.[1,2] This plexus extends its fibers to the sigmoid colon, uterus, and ureters. Each hypogastric nerve receives contributions from the sacral splanchnic nerves to form the inferior hypogastric or pelvic plexus (combined sympathetic and parasympathetic functions). The plexus terminates in multiple plexuses that supply the bladder (vesical plexus), uterus and vagina (uterovaginal plexus), and the rectum (middle rectal plexus).

Parasympathetic Nervous System (PNS)

The PNS has a craniosacral outflow due to the location of the fibers, which arise from cranial nerves and contributions from the sacral spinal nerves. In contrast to the sympathetic neurons, the presynaptic neuron is long, as it synapses in a ganglion closer to the target organs, resulting in short postsynaptic neurons. The abdominopelvic region is mainly supplied by the vagus nerve. Fibers from the vagus interact with their sympathetic counterpart at the celiac, superior, and inferior mesenteric plexuses; however, they synapse at enteric ganglia (Meissner's plexus and Auerbach's plexus) to act on the small intestine, colon, kidneys, and ureters. The parasympathetic sacral fibers (S2–S4 anterior) supply the digestive tract and the urogenital organs via the pelvic plexus.[1,2]

PAIN PATHWAYS

Somatic nerves are aggravated with noxious stimuli, and the signal is carried to the central nervous system (CNS) via the dorsal root ganglion to produce localized pain. Visceral pain pathways are carried via sympathetic nerves that carry the signals to the spinal cord via the superior and inferior hypogastric plexuses. This is the primary pathway for structures that are intraperitoneal. On the other hand, pelvic splanchnic nerves supply organs that are subperitoneal. These fibers enter the spinal cord via the ventral roots that make them less likely to cause referred pain, as they have less contact with the somatic nerves entering at the same level.

The abdominopelvic anatomy is quite complex and explains in part the difficulty with diagnosing and treating pelvic pain. A good understanding of the structures and the innervation of these structures is therefore critical.

REFERENCES

1. Roberts M. Clinical neuroanatomy of the abdomen and pelvis: implications for surgical treatment of prolapse. *Clin Obstet Gynecol.* 2005;48(3):627–638.
2. Mohammadali M, Sharma A, Mirza N, et al. Neuroanatomy of the female abdominopelvic region: a review with application to pelvic pain syndromes. *Clin Anat.* 2013;26:66–76.
3. Hoffman B, Schorge J, Schaffer J, Halvosron L, Brashaw K, Cunningham F. *Williams Gynecology.* 2nd ed. New York: McGraw Hill Professional; 2012.
4. Kanakarajan S, High K, Naaraja R. Chronic abdominal wall pain and ultrasound- guided abdominal cutaneous nerve infiltration: a case series. *Pain Med.* 2011;12:382–386.

3

Pain Mechanisms in Chronic Pelvic Pain

JUAN DIEGO VILLEGAS-ECHEVERRI, JOSÉ DUVÁN LÓPEZ-JARAMILLO,
ANA LUCÍA HERRERA-BETANCOURT, JORGE DARÍO LÓPEZ-ISANOA,
AND MARÍA DEL PILAR PARDO-BUSTAMANTE

Chronic pelvic pain (CPP) is a severe, disabling condition that affects close to 15–20% of women in childbearing age. Direct costs for the healthcare system amount to nearly US$2.8 billion per year.[1] Moreover, it is estimated that indirect costs associated with disability and absenteeism from work may amount to $15,000,000.000.00.[2,3]

CPP is associated with several physical, psychological and social factors, as well as multiple comorbidities that have a significant negative impact on the quality of life of these patients. In a large number of patients, CPP is associated with depression, chronic fatigue, and sexual dysfunction, and creates disability, physical limitations, and other consequences associated with chronic pain.[3] The causes of CPP are not well known, and the definitive diagnosis of the etiology is difficult, given that pain is rarely associated with a single underlying disorder or contributing factor.

Very frequently, the origin of CPP is associated not only with the presence of gynecological disorders (such as endometriosis, pelvic congestion syndrome, pelvic inflammatory disease, remaining ovary syndrome, or adhesions), but also with non-gynecological diagnoses, including myofascial pain disorders, irritable bowel syndrome, interstitial cystitis/painful bladder syndrome, or fibromyalgia.[3]

Over the past few decades, the understanding of pain processing and perception mechanisms has increased to a large extent, leading to the development of new pharmacological therapies and treatment strategies. However, CPP continues to pose a significant challenge to patients, families, and healthcare practitioners involved in its care. Management of chronic pain requires gaining greater knowledge of its pathophysiology and developing appropriate treatment strategies.[1]

TYPES OF PAIN

There are different neurophysiological mechanisms involved in the production of pain, just as there are multiple sources of pain (Figure 3.1). One way to describe these sources and mechanisms is to divide them into two groups: nociceptive and neuropathic pain. The final treatment decision depends to a large degree on the type of pain and the mechanisms involved.[4]

Nociceptive Pain

Also called "normal" or "physiological," nociceptive pain occurs in response to a noxious stimulus that warns the body regarding actual or impending harm.[4,5] It includes somatic and visceral pain.

Somatic Pain

Somatic pain is the result of injuries involving skin, muscle, ligaments, joints, or bones. It is very localized and circumscribed to the injured area and is usually not accompanied by autonomic reactions such as nausea, vomiting, or diaphoresis.

It usually worsens with physical activity and improves with rest. Receptors respond to stimuli released by the injured cells as a result of different mechanisms, including heat, cold, vibration, chemical insults, and fiber stretching.[5]

Visceral Pain

Visceral pain results from lesions of internal organs.

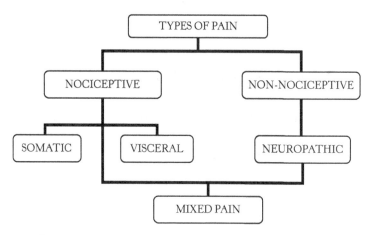

FIGURE 3.1: Types of pain.

Several characteristics describe visceral pain:

- In physiological conditions, noxious stimuli do not evoke painful responses in all organs.
- It is not always associated with a lesion and, consequently, it may be functional in nature.
- It often results in referred somatic pain due to the central convergence of somatic and visceral afferents.
- It tends to be diffuse or poorly localized, probably due to the low concentration of nociceptive afferent fibers inside the viscera. Only 2–10% of the total afferents in the spinal cord originate in visceral nociceptors.

Among others, the multiple generators of visceral pain include capsule distension, visceral muscle fiber distension, ischemia due to vascular abnormalities, bleeding, neoplasms, or mesenteric inflammation or traction.[5]

Neuropathic Pain

Neuropathic pain is also known as "abnormal" or "pathological" pain, and it results from injury and altered transmission of nociceptive information in the peripheral or the central nervous system. It is considered a pathological mechanism per se.[4] It may manifest days, weeks, and even months after the occurrence of the insult.

The main mechanisms leading to neuropathic pain include deafferentation, pathological functional changes that give rise to spontaneous discharges (ectopic foci), direct pathological stimulus due to nerve fiber compression, and activation mediated by the sympathetic nervous system.[6]

Allodynia is pathognomonic, and it is defined as a painful response to stimuli that are usually not painful. The pain is usually described as stinging, tingling, burning, or "needles." It may be continuous or paroxysmal.[7]

PAIN PATHWAYS

Four specific parts of the nervous system transmit painful signals from the periphery to superior centers of the central nervous system (Figure 3.2)[5]:

1. Nociceptors
2. Dorsal horn neurons
3. Ascending tracts
4. Supraspinal projections

Nociceptors

This type of somatosensory receptors, corresponding to *first-order neurons* in the pain pathway, has the ability to distinguish between harmless stimuli and noxious stimuli (free nerve endings). These receptors generate painful signals in response to harmful stimuli.

There are different nociceptors that respond to mechanical, thermal, chemical, or mixed stimuli. Depending on their function, location and characteristics, they are divided into three distinct groups:

1. Skin nociceptors—with three fundamental properties:
   a. High threshold to skin stimulation (they only activate with intense noxious stimuli)
   b. Accurate encoding of the intensity of the stimulus
   c. Absence of spontaneous activity

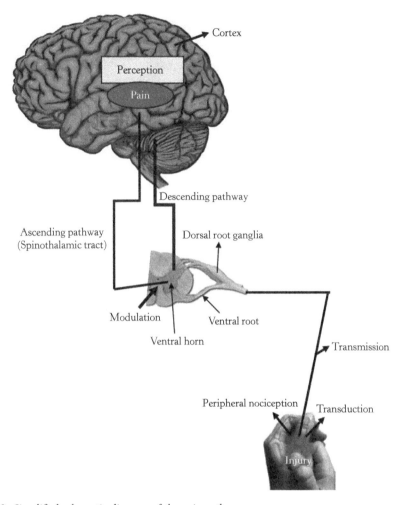

FIGURE 3.2: Simplified schematic diagram of the pain pathway.

Reproduced with permission from: Das V. An introduction to pain pathways and pain "targets." *Progress in Molecular Biology and Translational Science*, Volume 131 (2015). Page 3. Elsevier Inc.

2. Muscle and joint nociceptors
3. Visceral nociceptors

The cell body of the nociceptors is located in the spinal ganglion and penetrates the spinal cord through the posterior horn.

Peripheral fibers, also known as peripheral sensory fibers, conduct painful and somatic signals from the skin, muscle, fascia, vessels, and joint capsules to the dorsal root ganglion. There are three types of fibers, depending on their diameter, myelination, and conduction speed[2,3,8,9]—A (with four subtypes, α, β, and γ, δ), B, and C:

- A δ (myelinated) nerve fibers are smaller in diameter and conduct fast pain at a speed of 5–30 meters per second. Sensation is experienced immediately after the injury and indicates its location.

- B fibers are small in diameter myelinated fibers. They are, in general, the preganglionic fibers of the autonomic nervous system and have a low conduction speed.
- C fibers (non-myelinated) conduct slow pain at a speed below 1.5 meters per second. Given their ability to respond to multiple noxious stimuli, they are known as "polymodal nociceptors."

Second-Order Neurons

There are two types of pain perception second-order neurons:

- Specific nociceptive neurons (SNN)
- Wide dynamic range neurons (WDRN)

They both carry painful signals to the brain through different ascending spinal cord tracts.

SNNs respond exclusively to the activation of nociceptive afferent fibers, and they have limited receptor fields. For this reason, they participate in accurate or fine localization of peripheral noxious stimuli.

WDRNs respond to both harmless as well as harmful stimuli; receive multiple excitatory afferent inputs from sensory, skin, muscle, and visceral receptors, which explains why they lack the ability of accurate localization; and they also become sensitized to repeated stimuli.

Ascending Tracts

Fast Pain

Fast pain travels along the *neospinothalamic tract* through A-δ fibers, ending mainly in the SNNs. The axons of these neurons cross the spinal midline at the anterior white commissure and ascend to the thalamus as the *lateral spinothalamic tract*, also known as the *lateral pain pathway*.

Slow Pain

Slow pain travels along multiple ascending parallel pathways and is transmitted by C fibers ending at the interneurons, which synapse with the WDRNs at the dorsal horn (DH). WDRN axons ascend to the midbrain as the *spinomesencephalic tract*, to the reticular formation as the *spinoreticular tract*, and to the thalamus as the *paleospinothalamic tract*.

Slow painful signals ascend primarily through the *paleospinothalamic tract*, while the other two tracts excite, drive, reflect, and activate descending fibers, also called *intermediate pain pathways*.

The raw input is made conscious at the thalamus, which contains nervous centers responsible for vision, auditory reflexes, balance, and posture, which release pain signals to the brain. The cerebral cortex is responsible for superior thought processes, including emotions and interpretation.

The idea of tracts and fascicles as spinal pathways through which nociceptive input travels in one direction has been abandoned to a certain extent as a result of work suggesting the presence of multiple connections capable of bidirectional transmission (Figure 3.3).[10]

Supraspinal Projections

Pain sensation is composed of two elements: sensory-discriminative and affective. The sensory-discriminative dimension is integrated at the ventral basal complex of the thalamus and the somatosensory cortex (S1 and S2 areas). The nociceptive neurons contained in these areas have characteristics similar to those of the spinal cord, and, based on their properties, they may be classified as multi-receptor WDR neurons, and SN. The affective component of the painful sensation may be localized in the medial thalamic nuclei and areas of the cortex comprising the prefrontal region (PF) and, in particular, the supraorbital region. Traditionally, the thought was that the final integration of the sensory-discriminative and the affective components of pain occurred at a subcortical level, especially in the thalamus and the subthalamic diencephalic nuclei.

Supraspinal Projections: Fast Pain

Most of the fast pain SNN axons converge in the *posterolateral ventral nucleus* (PLV) of the thalamus. Third-order neurons emerge from the PLV and project onto the primary (SI) and secondary (SII) somatosensory cortex. These projections enable the interpretation of the sensory characteristics of pain such as location, intensity, and quality.

Supraspinal Projections: Slow Pain

The tracts that conduct slow pain (spinomesencephalic, spinoreticular, and paleospinothalamic) end in different areas of the brain. The *spinomesencephalic* tract conducts the painful signals to the upper periaqueductual gray colliculus and finally to the hypothalamus and the raphe nucleus. These areas control eye- and head-turning towards the noxious stimulus.[11] The *spinoreticular* tract ends in the brainstem reticular formation. The *paleospinothalamic* tract projects to the thalamic midline and intralaminar nuclei and also to the basal ganglia (BG), the prefrontal cortex (PF), anterior cingulate cortex (ACC), and primary motor cortex (M1). Activity in the spinoreticular and paleospinothalamic tracts results in excitation, avoidance, and affective and autonomic responses to pain.[3]

As shown by PET (positron emission tomography) imaging studies (Figure 3.4), the areas of the brain most frequently involved in the pain process include the:

- Anterior cingulate cortex (limbic system) and locus ceruleus: cognitive and reasoning functions (feed-forward, action,

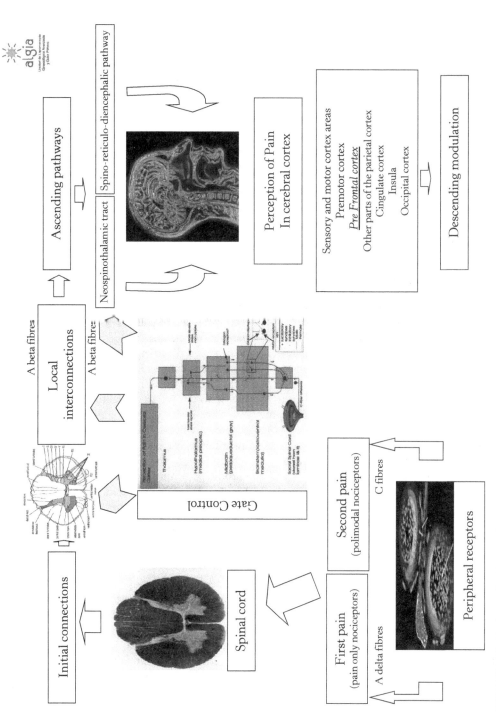

FIGURE 3.3: Pathways for the neural response to pain.

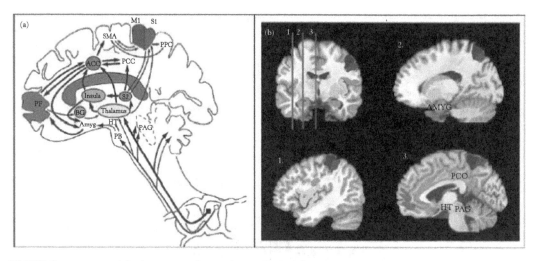

FIGURE 3.4: Areas of the brain most frequently involved in the pain process.

Reproduced with permission from: Apkarian AV, Bushnell MC, Treede RD, Zubieta JK. Human brain mechanisms of pain perception and regulation in health and disease. *European Journal of Pain.* 2005;9(4):463–484.[11]

empathy, and emotion), and integration of emotional stimuli with attention functions
- Insular cortex (limbic system): processing of converging information in order to create emotionally relevant context
- Prefrontal cortex: executive function, working memory (decision to act, memory, and judgement)
- Inferior parietal cortex: related with cognitive variables such as memory and input assessment
- Somatosensory cortex (SI and SII): involved in interpreting the characteristics of pain
- Primary premotor and motor cortex: movement suppression or evocation in relation to current pain
- Thalamus (and amygdala): processing, memory of emotional responses

The role of the basal ganglia (striated, globus pallidus, substantia nigra) in nociception and pain suggests that they may be involved in determining the intensity of pain, discriminating the affective and cognitive dimensions of pain, modulating nociceptive input, and the input of nociceptive information to superior motor areas.

WHY IS ACUTE PAIN DIFFERENT FROM CHRONIC PAIN?

Acute pain and chronic pain are totally different entities in terms of their etiology as well as their course, diagnosis, treatment, and prognosis. Therefore, they need to be considered and managed as such.

While acute pain is a symptom of tissue damage or an associated disease, chronic pain is in itself a disorder. Some individuals suffering from acute pain as a result of their own conditions or of environmental effects may fall into the vicious cycle leading to chronic pain and disability.

Acute pain is caused by a specific disease or injury, it plays a useful biological role, and is self-limiting in the majority of cases. In contrast, chronic pain must be considered as a disease in its own right. Many times, there is no evident triggering factor. When associated with a disease or tissue injury, its resolution takes longer than normal. Chronic pain does not serve any specific biological purpose and has no recognizable ending point.[12]

Therapy for acute pain aims to treat the origin and to interrupt the transmission of nociceptive signaling. On the other hand, chronic pain therapy must be based on a multidisciplinary approach and involves more than a single therapeutic modality. Although the treatment of chronic pain often does not result in a completely pain-free condition, understanding the basis of chronic pain may lead to adequate management and significant relief. Chronic pain patients always expect complete relief of their symptoms with treatment, and many believe that their pain is attributable to an unrecognized disorder. For this reason, it is very important for healthcare providers and patients alike to understand the differences between acute and chronic pain so that management plans and outcomes can be based on realistic expectations.[12,13]

In many chronic pain disorders, there is a weak relationship between abnormal physical findings and the intensity of pain, and with time, it becomes nonexistent. Consequently, chronic pain is an entity with a pathophysiology of its own, its own signs and symptoms, and continues beyond the resolution of any causal disease. In many cases, it is even impossible to identify the original etiological factor that triggered persistent pain.[14]

EMOTIONAL STATES AND PAIN MODULATION

The perception of painful stimuli is profoundly influenced by emotional variables whose neurobiological bases have not been clearly elucidated.[15,16,17]

From the neurobiological perspective, pain perception results from a complex neural process involving closely related emotional, cognitive, and behavioral components. Price[18] has proposed a dual pathway for affective pain processing. Apart from the direct spinothalamic pathway, there is a corticolimbic pathway that goes from the primary and secondary somatosensory cortex to parietal and insular structures; then to the amygdala, the perirhinal cortex, and the hippocampus; and finally converges on the same structures that are activated directly through the direct pathway. This second pathway integrates the sensory characteristics of the pain with information coming from different sensory systems, leading to learning and memory. In this way, a cognitive aspect is added, related in the long term to the affective processing of pain.[18] Emotional modulation may occur very early on in the perception of the stimulus and may be beyond the awareness of the individual.[19]

Fendt and Fanselow propose a more important role for the cognitive impact of the nociceptive stimulus. Predictable pain may elicit fear and hypoalgesia because of the body's need to improve action, whereas unpredictable pain causes anxiety and greater arousal, giving rise to hyperalgesia.[20]

Inherent to some mental disorders is altered perception of pain, either under- or up-regulated, although without any apparent relationship, as is the case in borderline personality disorder, eating disorders, depression, and schizophrenia.[15]

In post-traumatic stress disorder, where there is a lower sensitivity to pain, reduced activity has been reported in several regions of the brain associated with the emotional and cognitive processing of pain, including deactivation of the amygdala and the ventral lateral prefrontal cortex. These findings point to the influence of cognitive and emotional processes on altered pain perception in those patients.

On the other side, major depression could be used as an example. Theoretically, there are at least three reasons to explain increased pain sensitivity in this syndrome. First, the main characteristic of depression is dysphoric mood, and the experimental induction of sadness in healthy subjects leads to an increase in pain perception. Second, the absence of control and the feeling of impotence and despair are important factors in the development and maintenance of depression, and the absence of control of experimental pain in healthy subjects is also related with increased pain intensity. Finally, depressed individuals suffer frequently from clinical pain, and patients with chronic pain show a high prevalence of depressive disorders.[21,22,23,24]

Therefore, we might say that dysfunctional cognitive and emotional processing inherent to mental disorders exercise different influences on pain. Research on the interrelation between altered pain perception and altered emotional processing in mental disorders might be very useful in understanding the interaction between pain and emotion in general.[15]

It has been proposed that emotions involve two motivational systems: the appetitive system, evoked by pleasant stimuli such as eating and sex, and an avoidance system activated by unpleasant stimuli that produce anxiety, withdrawal or aggression, and defensive behavior.[25,26]

Pain and negative emotions may influence each other. There are reports in the sense that the risk of developing musculoskeletal pain may be twice as high in people suffering from depression as it is in healthy controls.[27]

It has been suggested that the underlying mechanism is that the avoidance system elicited by negative emotions selects this pathway and increases the reflexive defensive response and pain perception.[25,28] Stressful situations increase adrenalin levels in the body; together with other neuromodulators, adrenalin acts as an important modulator of pain perception at a spinal and supraspinal level.[29,30,31]

Chronic pain continues to be difficult to treat, and it causes suffering for millions of people. The evidence available at the present time sheds some light on pain transformation and modulation, but much more research is still required in order to complete the process.[32]

The amygdala is located in the medial temporal lobe and consists of interconnected nuclei. Of these, the basal lateral amygdala, which can be described in simple terms as the "entry point," receives input from all the sensory systems and the thalamus.[33] The central amygdala is considered the "exit point," with projections to the hypothalamus, basal nuclei, and brainstem. These connections are involved in the generation of autonomic and endocrine responses to affective stimuli.[34,35] The amygdala is involved in the evaluation of the emotional components and the modulation of autonomic responses (breathing, sweating, increased blood pressure, and heart rate) associated with pain. In threatening situations, it appears to be involved in stress-related analgesia, which is partly modulated by noradrenaline; modulation of these negative emotions is a component of pain therapy. It also participates in the evaluation of positive emotions and the activation of the appetitive system, reducing defensive reflexes. Consequently, it appears to be involved in the enhancement (hyperalgesia) and reduction or inhibition (hypoalgesia, analgesia) of painful signals. For this reason, recent approaches to the treatment of pain include cognitive-behavioral therapy as well as relaxation and the use of music for pain relief.[36,37]

Among the multiple pain neuromodulators, noradrenaline is of greater interest due to its hypoalgesic and analgesic effects and its action on the amygdala, although its exact mechanism is not well understood. Noradrenaline levels in the amygdala increase in response to stressful situations. Almost all adrenergic receptors are located in the central amygdala. There is evidence of noradrenaline release and α_2 receptor activation in the central amygdala in stress-induced analgesia.[38]

Catastrophizing

The term *catastrophizing* was coined in 1979 to describe a maladaptive coping style used by patients with anxiety and depressive disorders. New approaches refer to a negative emotional and cognitive response to pain, including a tendency to amplify and focus on painful symptoms as well as on feelings of defenselessness and pessimism. Catastrophizing has emerged as an important determinant of outcomes related to short and long-term pain, and it is consistently associated with heightened pain levels. This relationship is maintained in a wide range of conditions such as neuropathic pain, lumbar pain, scleroderma, and chronic pelvic pain syndromes, where it has been shown that patients with a high level of catastrophizing have increased musculoskeletal sensitivity and heightened sensitivity to pain; moreover, they are at a higher risk of developing persistent painful and post-operative syndromes.[39]

The exact mechanism for the association between catastrophizing and pain is not completely understood. It is proposed that the emotional and cognitive changes that characterize it may alter endogenous inhibitory descending pain pathways, and that it is also associated with greater activity in the pain processing regions of the brain.

There is an ongoing debate on whether catastrophizing is the cause or rather the consequence of chronic pain. There is evidence in healthy adults as well as in adults with chronic pain that catastrophizing remains stable during weeks and months and it may even remain unchanged after the resolution of acute pain and the insult that provoked it.[40]

In summary, pain is a multifaceted experience that affects many aspects of emotional life. Considering that the amygdala is a key component of the neural circuit where emotions are processed, understanding its role in antinociception might have a clear effect on the development of procedures for improving treatment options in chronic pain.[32]

NERVOUS SYSTEM CHANGES IN CHRONIC PAIN

Chronic pain is associated with multiple changes in the central and peripheral nervous systems, which contribute to the persistence of pain and make it difficult to manage. The exact mechanisms involved in the pathophysiology of pain are not fully understood. However, it is believed that both the central as well as the peripheral nervous systems undergo acute and long-term changes that alter the pathways of pain and end up creating lasting abnormal responses that perpetuate the symptoms.[5]

Cross-Talk

"Cross-talk" is the phenomenon wherein strong electrical signals originating in poorly myelinated (or non-myelinated) nerve fibers produce de novo electrical signals in the adjacent afferent fibers that are not involved in the painful stimuli. The development of cross-talk in pelvic organs requires cross afferent stimulus in the pelvis. The afferent information from the main pelvic organs such as the bladder, colon, rectum, and uterus is transmitted over the hypogastric, splanchnic, and pudendal nerves to cell bodies in the thoracolumbar and lumbosacral dorsal root ganglions. Typically, the prodromic afferent stimulus (from the periphery to the central nervous system) from an affected pelvic organ produces an antidromic stimulus (from the center to the periphery) as well as co-sensitization of another "uninvolved" pelvic organ. These abnormal reflex pathways may occur locally in the periphery through collateral axons (dichotomization of the afferent nerve fibers), in the spinal cord (dorsal root reflexes), and/or in the central nervous system. Consequently, the antidromic pathway may produce functional changes in another pelvic organ with little or no organic pathology.[13,41,42,43]

Peripheral Sensitization

Both central and peripheral sensitization (PS) are the main causes of hypersensitivity to pain following tissue damage. Peripheral sensitization may occur in inflammatory pain, in some forms of neuropathic pain, or after persistent nociceptive stimulation. Tissue damage creates dramatic changes in the chemical milieu of peripheral nociceptor endings, releasing potassium ions, substance P, bradykinin, prostaglandins, and other pro-inflammatory substances. Additionally, some intracellular contents such as adenosine triphosphate (ATP) and hydrogen ions are released from the cells. In peripheral sensitization, inflammatory mediators heighten pain perception in response to stimuli, lowering the threshold. Peripheral sensitization is associated with increased sensitivity to mechanical as well as thermal stimuli regardless of whether they are harmless (allodynia) or noxious (hyperalgesia).[14]

Central Sensitization

"Central sensitization" (CS) refers to an increase in the excitability of the spinal and supraspinal neuronal circuits as a result of injury or activation of the peripheral receptors. Central sensitization is a physiological phenomenon of hyperexcitability leading to neuronal dysregulation and hypersensitivity to pathological as well as harmless stimuli.[14] It appears that in CS there is a combination of a neurotransmitter-mediated disorder together with the individual's altered ability to deal with previous cognitive experiences and their impact on daily life.[44] CS is associated with allodynia, hyperalgesia,[45] expansion of the receptive field (with pain extending beyond the peripheral innervation area), and unusually prolonged pain after the painful stimulus has been eliminated. Generally, patients report throbbing pain, a burning sensation, tingling, or numbness. In CS there is pain dissociation leading to an expansion of hyperalgesia beyond the site of injury, and cross-hypersensitivity between several somatic and visceral structures.[46,47]

Given the implications of sensitization, it is important to bear in mind when deciding the medical management of chronic pain that somatic symptoms must be controlled, and central and peripheral pain elements must also be managed.[48]

Visceral–Somatic and Visceral–Visceral Convergence

There is convergence of the somatic as well as the visceral afferents on the same second-order neuron in the dorsal horn of the spinal cord. Only 2–7% of all afferent nerve fibers in each dorsal root ganglion are visceral, and dorsal horn interneurons are largely influenced by somatic fibers. For this reason, stimuli coming to the dorsal spine from the muscle, for example, are much more potent than those generated in the skin. This is why somatic pain is often reported as visceral pain, especially in the abdominal wall.[43,44,45] Afferent activation of a pelvic structure influences the efferent output to another structure. Therefore, any disease or injury in one pathway may influence the abnormal activation of another pathway. This theory may explain symptom or disorder overlaps in chronic pelvic pain.[13,49]

Spinal Cord Wind-up

Repeated low-frequency stimulation of C fibers produces a gradual increase in the discharge frequency of second-order neurons in the spinal cord until they arrive at a state of almost continuous depolarization. This states results in expansion of receptive fields, permanent biochemical changes, lowering of the threshold, and, finally, sensory processing upregulation.[50]

Neuroplasticity and Central Reorganization

It has been proposed that a barrage of painful stimuli to the dorsal horn may lead to cortical reorganization in patients with chronic pain. It was shown that the cortical areas where pain is represented displace medially, possibly indicating an expansion of that representation area to neighboring areas.

The mechanisms involved in cortical reorganization in patients with chronic pain and no neuropathic damage are still unclear. It has been suggested that in the complex regional pain syndrome (CRPS), constant pain may interfere with sensory perception, not only at a cortical level but also at a subcortical and spinal level, modifying the cortical representation regions of the affected areas. For example, in patients with painful phantom limb syndrome, the increased activity of nociceptive stimuli may induce central sensitization and abnormalities in functional connectivity in the periphery and in the spinal neurons. However, it is not possible to conclude that there is always a relationship between cortical reorganization and chronic pain. Chronic pain may cause cortical reorganization, but, alternatively, maladaptive cortical reorganization may, in itself, trigger or perpetuate chronic pain.[51]

PHARMACOLOGY OF CHRONIC PAIN

Pharmacological treatment is one part of the interdisciplinary approach required in cases of chronic pain. One of the goals of interdisciplinary management is to improve function using various strategies and applying pain scales in order to achieve objective improvement.[52] Many drugs are used in the management of chronic pain, including opioids, nonsteroidal anti-inflammatory agents (NSAIDs), paracetamol (acetaminophen), antidepressants, anticonvulsants, muscle relaxants, topical agents, as well as other drugs that cannot be classified under a specific group, as is the case of ketamine.[5,53,54,55,56]

Opioids

Opioids are the most widely sold medications in the United States. Their sales increased nearly 176% between 1997 and 2006, and they are a first-line treatment in acute management of moderate to severe cancer pain. There is

controversy regarding their efficacy, adverse effects, and associated aberrant behaviors. Their sites of analgesic action are the brain, the cisterna magna, the spinal cord, and the afferent nerve endings. A meta-analysis of 41 randomized controlled studies of the efficacy of opioids in osteoarthritis, diabetic neuropathy, lumbar pain, and rheumatoid arthritis concluded that there is a small functional improvement and some improvement in terms of the severity of pain compared with placebo, with similar pain reduction but less functional improvement when compared with other analgesics.[57]

On the basis of these findings, the International Association for the Study of Pain and the European Federation of Neurological Societies[57] recommended opioids for use as the second or third line of treatment for chronic pain, and as first-line treatment in special circumstances, such as exacerbation of neuropathic pain.[5,54]

An exception to the mechanism of opioids is tramadol (serotonin and noradrenalin reuptake inhibitor and μ-agonist opioid), which reduces pain in osteoarthritis, fibromyalgia, and neuropathic pain. However, there is insufficient evidence for determining the effectiveness of tramadol when compared to other opioids.

Before starting the use of opioids, adverse effects have to be considered, including nausea, constipation, drowsiness, and respiratory depression, among others. Of patients followed for a period of 7–24 months, 14% abandoned the treatment. Other adverse effects include hyperalgesia and hypothalamic-pituitary axis (HPA) disorders.

Aside from adverse physical effects, opioids entail the risk of abuse (45%), leading to overdose, mortality, and drug trafficking by patients and practitioners alike. Consequently, physicians must be aware of their therapeutic and non-therapeutic use (abuse, dependence) when prescribing opioids.

NSAIDs

NSAIDs' mechanism of action is to inhibit the pro-inflammatory cyclo-oxygenase (COX) enzyme that produces prostaglandins and arachidonic acid thromboxanes. COX-1 acts to protect the gastrointestinal tract, and COX-2 is the inducible form and is produced in response to inflammation.[5]

These types of medications have not been shown to be useful in neuropathic pain and have not been included in recent guidelines for fibromyalgia. So far, they have been shown to be useful in osteoarthritis, rheumatoid arthritis, and lumbar pain. One of their adverse reactions is gastropathy. Selective inhibitors of COX-2 have fewer gastrointestinal effects, but they have been associated with an increased cardiovascular risk, something that needs to be considered when it comes to long-term use.[54]

Acetaminophen

Acetaminophen has weaker analgesic effect than NSAIDs, but it is a good option for reducing gastrointestinal complications, and its cost is lower. The main complication is unintended overdosing given its broad distribution, over-the-counter sale, and the tight margin between safe and toxic dosing. The US Food and Drug Administration (FDA) issued a warning in 2010 because of the associated liver toxicity.

Antidepressants

Antidepressants have different effects that contribute to analgesia, including their action on N-methyl-D-aspartate (NMDA) receptors; on adenosine, calcium channels; and serotonin, noradrenaline, and opioid systems. A meta-analysis suggested that they are better than placebo in the treatment of chronic pain, with moderate symptom reduction.[58] Efficacy has also been shown in neuropathic pain, fibromyalgia, lumbar pain, and headache, with stronger evidence in relation to neuropathic pain.[59]

Tricyclic antidepressants (amitriptyline and cyclobenzaprine) block serotonin and noradrenaline reuptake. They have adverse cardiovascular effects (hypertension, postural hypotension, arrhythmias); they have been shown to cause falls in elderly patients; and they have tolerability issues.

Selective serotonin reuptake inhibitors (SSRIs), developed with the aim of reducing the adverse effects of the broad range of tricyclic antidepressants, have shown some beneficial effects.[58] They have no effect on adrenalin, acetylcholine, or sodium channels. Duloxetine is used in fibromyalgia and neuropathic pain.[60]

Anticonvulsants

Anticonvulsants' mechanism of action is the modulation of voltage-dependent sodium and calcium channels, glutamate antagonism, upregulation of the γ-aminobutyric acid (GABA) inhibitory system, or a combination of all of these. The best evidence supports mainly the use of three drugs for the management of neuropathic pain: gabapentin, pregabalin, and carbamazepine or oxcarbazepine. The most common adverse effects include drowsiness, dizziness, fatigue, and weight gain.

Muscle Relaxants

Although the mechanism of muscle relaxants is not clear, it is thought to be associated with their sedative effect. They are recommended as sort-term adjuvant therapy. Studies have not shown significant differences among the various muscle relaxants. Cyclobenzaprine has been studied the most and, in low-quality studies, it has been shown to be better than placebo in fibromyalgia and other disorders in terms of improving pain, muscle spasm, and functional status. Long-term therapy is challenging, given that sedation is the most common adverse effect.

Topical Agents

Topical agents are recommended in cases of localized pain. They have the advantage of avoiding the adverse systemic effects of oral medications, as they are delivered to the specific site, avoiding first-passage metabolism and drug interactions. Capsaicin, derived from chili pepper, is one such agent; it acts by depleting substance P from the primary afferent neuron. When compared with placebo, topical agents are effective in reducing neuropathic and musculoskeletal pain, including osteoarthritis. Other substances shown to be effective are topical diclofenac and lidocaine.[61]

Other Medications

Ketamine was introduced in the 1960s; it has an antagonistic effect on the NMDA receptor and has been studied in the treatment of several chronic pain syndromes. Many studies have shown acute analgesic effects, and recent studies have shown long-term effectiveness in improving chronic pain through modulation of the blockade of increased NMDA receptor activity. However, despite positive results, more studies are needed to examine its safety and toxicity with all routes of administration.[62]

There is ongoing theoretical and experimental work in the development of pain management drugs, including the following groups: transient receptor potential ankyrin channel 1 (TRPA), cannabinoid receptors (CB2), GABA A receptor subtypes, and imidazoline receptors.[55,63]

Pharmacogenetics

Natural and synthetic opioid compounds, alone or in combination with other medications, are broadly used as analgesics in patients with acute and chronic pain.[64,65,66,67,68,69] Pharmacological research has characterized three high-affinity neuronal cell membrane receptors whose activation is responsible for the desirable (antinociceptive) and undesirable (respiratory depression, nausea, vomiting, dependence) effects of opioids. Recent molecular biology and pharmacogenetic studies have shed some light on prior pharmacological observations and have served as a basis for new analgesic therapies with better therapeutic outcomes. Most of the knowledge about the genetic regulation of pain has come from studies in animal models, specifically mice.

Several hereditary syndromes of total or partial insensitivity to pain have been identified, including insensitivity to pain associated with sodium channel disorders where the gene involved is the alpha subunit of the voltage-dependent sodium channel known as Na(v). Other variants of pain sensitivity in the population include the μ opioid receptor, catecholamine-O-methyl-transferase gene, guanosine triphosphate cyclohydrolase gene, and melanocortin receptor-1 gene, among others.

In pain management, numerous polymorphisms affect drug pharmacokinetics, contributing in part to the inter-individual variability of drug efficacy and safety. The most important enzymes that metabolize pain medications are those of the cytochrome P450 group, UDP-glucuronyl transferases (UGTs) and sulfotransferases (SULTs). The best studied transport polymorphisms are ATP transporter ligands.

EFFECTS OF ESTROGEN ON CPP

A meta-analysis of experimentally induced pain reported a 30% reduction in somatic sensory pain thresholds during the premenstrual and menstrual phases, coinciding with low estrogen (E) levels during the cycle.[70] This observation is related to the documented finding of an increase in irritable bowel syndrome symptoms during the same phases of the menstrual cycle, with no changes in gut motility observed.[71] Clinically, this correlates with worsening of painful syndromes in reproductive age (e.g., endometriosis) and improvement at menopause and during medically induced hypoestrogenic states.[72]

Estrogen has a direct influence on primary afferent neuron function. Moreover, it plays multiple roles in the cell membrane, cytoplasm, and nucleus, modulating cellular activity by opening ion channels, G protein signaling, and activating transduction signals as trophic factors. Visceral afferent nerve fibers are sensitive to ATP, and indirect evidence suggests that visceral afferents are sensitive to estrogen: (a) visceral pain is affected by hormonal levels in female cycles; (b) there are gender differences in the prevalence of functional disorders involving viscera; and (c) visceral afferents fit within the populations of dorsal root ganglion neurons sensitive to E.[73,74]

It is worth mentioning that estrogen receptors (α and β) are distributed in different regions of the central and peripheral nervous systems and mediate nociception: neurons of the spinal cord dorsal horn and dorsal root ganglion. These findings suggest that E may modulate sensory input at a primary afferent level. Estrogen modulates nociceptive responses in pelvic pain syndromes, but it is not yet clear if it has pronociceptive or anti-nociceptive activity.

Some researchers propose that estrogen modulation of the nociceptive response depends on the type and duration of pain and the participation of other anti-nociceptive mechanisms. Several authors have suggested that gender differences in terms of pain sensitivity and prevalence of chronic pain disorder may be due more to a poor endogenous functioning of pain inhibition responses than to increased nociceptive activity.[73]

Estrogen modulates nociceptive responses in functional pain syndromes. It modulates the response of dorsal root ganglion neurons to ATP, suggesting that visceral afferent nociceptors are also modulated by estrogen. This could explain the clinical and gender differences in visceral hypersensitivity and points to a potential therapeutic target for nociception mediation.[73,75]

REFERENCES

1. Renn CL, Dorsey SG. The physiology and processing of pain: a review. *AACN Clin Iss.* 2005;16(3):277–290; quiz 413–415.
2. As-Sanie S, Harris RE, Harte SE, Tu FF, Neshewat G, Clauw DJ. Increased pressure pain sensitivity in women with chronic pelvic pain. *Obstet Gynecol.* 2013;122(5):1047–1055.
3. Yunker A, Sathe NA, Reynolds WS, Likis FE, Andrews J. Systematic review of therapies for

noncyclic chronic pelvic pain in women. *Obstet Gynecol Surv.* 2012;67(7):417–425.

4. Howard FM. Endometriosis and mechanisms of pelvic pain. *J Minim Invasive Gynecol.* 2009;16(5):540–550.

5. Fornasari D. Pain mechanisms in patients with chronic pain. *Clin Drug Invest.* 2012;32(Suppl 1): 45–152.

6. Koltzenburg M, Scadding J. Neuropathic pain. *Curr Opin Neurol.* 2001;14(5):641–647.

7. Attal N. Neuropathic pain: mechanisms, therapeutic approach, and interpretation of clinical trials. *Continuum.* 2012;18(1):161–175.

8. Schaible HG, Richter F. Pathophysiology of pain. *Langenbeck's Archives of Surgery / Deutsche Gesellschaft fur Chirurgie.* 2004;389(4):237–243.

9. Stucky CL, Gold MS, Zhang X. Mechanisms of pain. *Proc Natl Acad Sci U S A.* 2001;98(21): 11845–11846.

10. Villanueva L, Nathan PW. Multiple pain pathways. In: Devor M, Rowbotham MC, Wiesenfeld-Hallin Z, eds. *Progress in Pain Research and Management.* Vol. 16. Seattle, WA: IASP Press; 2000:371–386.

11. Apkarian AV, Bushnell MC, Treede RD, Zubieta JK. Human brain mechanisms of pain perception and regulation in health and disease. *Eur J Pain.* 2005;9(4):463–484.

12. Grichnik KP, Ferrante FM. The difference between acute and chronic pain. *Mount Sinai J Med NY.* 1991;58(3):217–220.

13. Lamvu G, Steege JF. The anatomy and neurophysiology of pelvic pain. *J Minim Invasive Gynecol.* 2006;13(6):516–522.

14. Siddall PJ, Cousins MJ. Persistent pain as a disease entity: implications for clinical management. *Anesth Analg.* 2004;99(2):510–520, table of contents.

15. Klossika I, Flor H, Kamping S, Bleichhardt G, Trautmann N, Treede RD, et al. Emotional modulation of pain: a clinical perspective. *Pain.* 2006;124(3):264–268.

16. Meagher MW, Arnau RC, Rhudy JL. Pain and emotion: effects of affective picture modulation. *Psychosom Med.* 2001;63(1):79–90.

17. Villemure C, Bushnell MC. Cognitive modulation of pain: how do attention and emotion influence pain processing? *Pain.* 2002;95:195–199.

18. Price DD. Psychological and neural mechanisms of the affective dimension of pain. *Science.* 2000;288:1769–1772.

19. Lang PJ. The emotion probe. Studies of motivation and attention. *Am Psychologist.* 1995;50(5): 372–385.

20. Fendt M, Fanselow MS. The neuroanatomical and neurochemical basis of conditioned fear. *Neurosci Biobehav Rev.* 1999;23(5):743–760.

21. Rainville P, Bao QV, Chretien P. Pain-related emotions modulate experimental pain perception and autonomic responses. *Pain.* 2005;118:306–318.

22. Peterson C, Maier SR, Seligman MEP. *Learned Helplessness: A Theory for the Age of Personal Control.* New York: Oxford University Press; 1993.

23. Williams DC, Golding J, Phillips K, Towell A. Perceived control, locus of control and preparatory information: effects on the perception of an acute pain stimulus. *Pers Indiv Differ.* 2004; 36:1681–1691.

24. Bair MJ, Robinson RL, Katon W, Kroenke K. Depression and pain comorbidity: a literature review. *Arch Intern Med.* 2003;163(20):2433–2445.

25. Lang PJ, Bradley MM, Cuthbert BN, Patrick CJ. Emotion and psychopathology: a startle probe analysis. *Prog Exper Personality Psychopathol Res.* 1993;16:163–199.

26. Wiech K, Tracey I. The influence of negative emotions on pain: behavioral effects and neural mechanisms. *Neuroimage.* 2009;47:987–994.

27. Magni G, Moreschi C, Rigatti-Luchini S, Merskey H. Prospective study on the relationship between depressive symptoms and chronic musculoskeletal pain. *Pain.* 1994;56:289–297.

28. Rhudy JL, Meagher MW. Fear and anxiety: divergent effects on human pain thresholds. *Pain.* 2000;84:65–75.

29. McCarty R. Age-related alterations in sympathetic-adrenal medullary responses to stress. *Gerontology.* 1986;32:172–183.

30. Yoshimura M, Furue H. Mechanisms for the antinociceptive actions of the descending noradrenergic and serotonergic systems in the spinal cord. *J Pharmacologic Sci.* 2006;101(2):107–117.

31. Pertovaara A. The noradrenergic pain regulation system: a potential target for pain therapy. *Eur J Pharmacol.* 2013;716(1–3):2–7.

32. Strobel C, Hunt S, Sullivan R, Sun J, Sah P. Emotional regulation of pain: the role of noradrenaline in the amygdala. *Sci China Life Sci.* 2014;57(4):384–390.

33. Pape HC, Pare D. Plastic synaptic networks of the amygdala for the acquisition, expression, and extinction of conditioned fear. *Physiol Rev.* 2010;90(2):419–463.

34. Sah P, Faber ES, Lopez De Armentia M, Power J. The amygdaloid complex: anatomy and physiology. *Physiol Rev.* 2003;83:803–834.

35. Morilak DA, Cecchi M, Khoshbouei H. Interactions of norepinephrine and galanin in the central amygdala and lateral bed nucleus of the stria terminalis modulate the behavioral response to acute stress. *Life Sci.* 2003;73(6):715–726.

36. Nilsson U. The anxiety- and pain-reducing effects of music interventions: a systematic review. *AORNJ.* 2008;87(4):780–807.

37. Bushnell MC, Ceko M, Low LA. Cognitive and emotional control of pain and its disruption in chronic pain. *Nature Rev Neurosci.* 2013;14(7):502–511.

38. Ortiz JP, Close LN, Heinricher MM, Selden NR. Alpha (2)-noradrenergic antagonist administration into the central nucleus of the amygdala blocks stress-induced hypoalgesia in awake behaving rats. *Neuroscience.* 2008;157:223–228.

39. Seminowicz DA, Davis KD. Cortical responses to pain in healthy individuals depends on pain catastrophizing. *Pain.* 2006;120:297–306.

40. Alappattu MJ, Bishop MD. Psychological factors in chronic pelvic pain in women: relevance and application of the fear-avoidance model of pain. *Physical Ther.* 2011;91(10):1542–1550.

41. Ren K, Dubner R. Neuron-glia crosstalk gets serious: role in pain hypersensitivity. *Curr Opin Anaesth.* 2008;21(5):570–579.

42. Furuta A, Suzuki Y, Hayashi N, Egawa S, Yoshimura N. Transient receptor potential A1 receptor-mediated neural cross-talk and afferent sensitization induced by oxidative stress: implication for the pathogenesis of interstitial cystitis/bladder pain syndrome. *Int J Urol Japan.* 2012;19(5):429–436.

43. Ustinova EE, Fraser MO, Pezzone MA. Crosstalk and sensitization of bladder afferent nerves. *Neurourol Urodynam.* 2010;29(1):77–81.

44. Sarzi-Puttini P, Atzeni F, Mease PJ. Chronic widespread pain: from peripheral to central evolution. *Best Pract Res Clin Rheumatol.* 2011;25(2):133–139.

45. Bennett RM. Emerging concepts in the neurobiology of chronic pain: evidence of abnormal sensory processing in fibromyalgia. *Mayo Clin Proc.* 1999;74(4):385–398.

46. Gustin SM, Peck CC, Cheney LB, Macey PM, Murray GM, Henderson LA. Pain and plasticity: is chronic pain always associated with somatosensory cortex activity and reorganization? *J Neurosci.* 2012;32(43):14874–14884.

47. Garland EL. Pain processing in the human nervous system: a selective review of nociceptive and biobehavioral pathways. *Primary Care.* 2012;39(3):561–571.

48. Phillips K, Clauw DJ. Central pain mechanisms in chronic pain states—maybe it is all in their head. *Best Pract Res Clin Rheumatol.* 2011;25(2):141–154.

49. Chung MK, Chung RP, Gordon D. Interstitial cystitis and endometriosis in patients with chronic pelvic pain: the "Evil Twins" syndrome. *JSLS.* 2005;9(1):25–29.

50. Herrero JF, Laird JM, Lopez-Garcia JA. Wind-up of spinal cord neurones and pain sensation: much ado about something? *Prog Neurobiol.* 2000;61(2):169–203.

51. Flor H. Cortical reorganisation and chronic pain: implications for rehabilitation. *J Rehabil Med.* 2003(41 Suppl):66–72.

52. Willimann P. [Pharmacological treatment of chronic pain]. *Therapeutische Umschau Revue therapeutique.* 2011;68(9):512–516.

53. Sarzi-Puttini P, Vellucci R, Zuccaro SM, Cherubino P, Labianca R, Fornasari D. The appropriate treatment of chronic pain. *Clin Drug Invest.* 2012;32(Suppl 1):21–33.

54. Ashburn MA, Staats PS. Management of chronic pain. *Lancet.* 1999;353(9167):1865–1869.

55. Li JX, Zhang Y. Emerging drug targets for pain treatment. *Eur J Pharmacol.* 2012;681(1–3):1–5.

56. Furlan AD, Sandoval JA, Mailis-Gagnon A, Tunks E. Opioids for chronic noncancer pain: a meta-analysis of effectiveness and side effects. *CMAJ.* 2006;174(11):1589–1594.

57. Attal N, Cruccu G, Baron R, Haanpaa M, Hansson P, Jensen TS, et al. EFNS guidelines on the pharmacological treatment of neuropathic pain: 2010 revision. *Eur J Neurol.* 2010;17(9):1113-e88.

58. Kroenke K, Krebs EE, Bair MJ. Pharmacotherapy of chronic pain: a synthesis of recommendations from systematic reviews. *Gen Hosp Psychiatry.* 2009;31(3):206–219.

59. Verdu B, Decosterd I, Buclin T, Stiefel F, Berney A. Antidepressants for the treatment of chronic pain. *Drugs.* 2008;68:2611–2632.

60. Tan T, Barry P, Reken S, Baker M, Guideline Development G. Pharmacological management of neuropathic pain in non-specialist settings: summary of NICE guidance. *BMJ.* 2010;340:c1079.

61. Stanos SP, Galluzzi KE. Topical therapies in the management of chronic pain. *Postgrad Med.* 2013;125(4 Suppl 1):25–33.

62. Noppers I, Niesters M, Aarts L, Smith T, Sarton E, Dahan A. Ketamine for the treatment of chronic non-cancer pain. *Expert Opin Pharmacother.* 2010;11(14):2417–2429.

63. Turk DC, Wilson HD, Cahana A. Treatment of chronic non-cancer pain. *Lancet.* 2011;377(9784):2226–2235.

64. Gourlay GK. Advances in opioid pharmacology. *Support Care Cancer.* 2005;13(3):153–159.

65. Burlev AV, Shifman EM. [Pharmacogenetical aspects of clinical anaesthesiology]. *Anesteziologiia i reanimatologiia.* 2010(6):83–86.

66. Somogyi AA, Barratt DT, Coller JK. Pharmacogenetics of opioids. *Clin Pharmacol Ther.* 2007;81(3):429–444.

67. Kosarac B, Fox AA, Collard CD. Effect of genetic factors on opioid action. *Curr Opin Anaesth.* 2009;22(4):476–482.

68. Tremblay J, Hamet P. Genetics of pain, opioids, and opioid responsiveness. *Metabolism Clin Exper.* 2010;59(Suppl 1):S5–S8.

69. Svetlik S, Hronova K, Bakhouche H, Matouskova O, Slanar O. Pharmacogenetics of chronic pain and its treatment. *Mediators Inflammation*. 2013;2013: 864319.

70. Riley JL, Robinson ME, Wise EA, Price DD. A meta-analytic review of pain perception across the menstrual cycle. *Pain*. 1999;81:225–235.

71. Heitkemper MM, Cain KC, Jarrett ME, Burr RL, Hertig V, Bond EF. Symptoms across the menstrual cycle in women with irritable bowel syndrome. *Am J Gastroenterol*. 2003;98(2):420–430.

72. Practice Committee of the American Society for Reproductive M. Treatment of pelvic pain associated with endometriosis: a committee opinion. *Fertil Steril*. 2014;101(4):927–935.

73. Chaban V. Estrogen and visceral nociception at the level of primary sensory neurons. *Pain Res Treat*. 2012;2012:1–6.

74. Li Z, Niwa Y, Sakamoto S, Chen X, Nakaya Y. Estrogen modulates a large conductance chloride channel in cultured porcine aortic endothelial cells. *J Cardiovasc Pharmacol*. 2000;35(3): 506–510.

75. Gold MS, Gebhart GF. Nociceptor sensitization in pain pathogenesis. *Nature Med*. 2010;16(11): 1248–1257.

4

Multidisciplinary Approaches to Pelvic Pain Treatment

A Physical Therapist's Perspective

STEPHANIE PRENDERGAST

Pelvic pain is defined as a biopsychosocial syndrome that may include organic, musculoskeletal, peripheral and central neuropathic, and psychosocial impairments. In recent years, a growing group of physicians, psychologists, and pelvic floor physical therapists have become actively involved in the management of pelvic pain syndromes.

The term "pelvic pain" encompasses a long list of symptoms and diagnoses, discussed in more detail in other chapters in this book. Currently, established protocols do not exist for pelvic pain diagnoses such as vulvodynia, interstitial cystitis/painful bladder syndrome, pudendal neuralgia, and nonbacterial chronic prostatitis or chronic pelvic pain syndrome. Symptoms of pelvic pain syndromes can include genital, abdominal, or buttock pain; burning or itching; dysuria; urinary urgency and frequency; constipation; dyspareunia; and anorgasmia and other sexual dysfunction. Patients often do their own online research and then attempt to get a diagnosis through primary care physicians, gynecologists, urologists, and/or gastroenterologists. For this reason, the treatment needs of the patient may lie outside of the diagnosing provider's particular area of expertise. Despite this limitation, the diagnosing provider is well positioned to help a person with pelvic pain formulate an effective treatment plan by implementing an interdisciplinary treatment approach. Because treatment protocols do not exist, a treatment algorithm can be used to illustrate evidence-based treatment options that can be used successfully in varying combinations.

The first part of this chapter will discuss four conservative therapeutic domains. The second part of the chapter will discuss how to use clinical critical reasoning strategies to manage the patient who is not tolerating or not responding to the treatment plan (Figure 4.1).

Regardless of the discipline of the evaluating provider, the first step of the algorithm is to evaluate, treat and rule out organic pathology. In the absence of organic pathology, 85–90% of people with pelvic pain present with musculoskeletal dysfunction. Therefore, one therapeutic treatment domain is physical therapy.[1,2]

Physical therapists treating pelvic pain should have specialized experience in treating high-tone pelvic disorders. Through a history and a physical examination, a physical therapist will examine the patient for physical, psychosocial, and neuropathic impairments. This exam should include:

1. Pelvic girdle and pelvic floor muscle myofascial trigger points, motor control, length and strength
2. Connective tissue restrictions in the trunk, lower extremities, and pelvis
3. Altered neurodynamics of peripheral nerves—tenderness and movement disorders
4. Biomechanical and movement pattern disorders
5. Joint dysfunction
6. Central sensitization
7. Behavioral factors: catastrophizing, fear-avoidance, depression, anxiety, sleep

(Please see chapters 17 and 18 for more detail on physical therapy evaluation and treatment.)

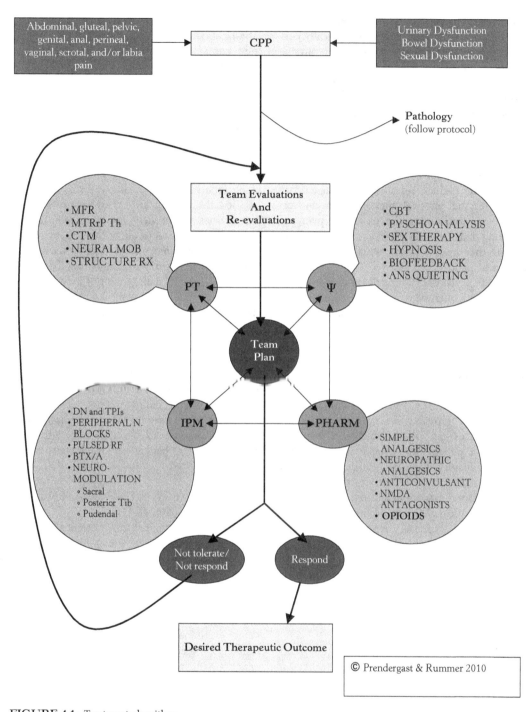

FIGURE 4.1: Treatment algorithm.

Adapted from Prendergast S, Rummer E. Interdisciplinary management of chronic pelvic pain. In: *Chronic Pelvic Pain and Dysfunction*. Chaitow and Jones, eds. New York: Elsevier; 2012:171–185.

Following the evaluation, a physical therapist will develop a comprehensive assessment. An assessment takes into account all past medical information, effective and failed treatments, and the patient's history and etiological factors, and will help link the patient's objective findings to their symptoms. The therapist and patient develop short-term goals, long-term goals, and a treatment plan with an estimated frequency and duration. The treatment plan typically consists of patient education regarding pain physiology, and interdisciplinary treatment approaches, manual therapy techniques, temporary lifestyle modifications, neuromuscular reeducation, and a home exercise program. Generally, patients are treated by a physical therapist once or twice a week for 8–12 weeks. The length of the treatment should be one hour. This often renders the physical therapist one of the medical providers with the highest amount of patient contact. Therefore, the physical therapist can be very useful in coordinating the treatment plan and ensuring that the other providers have the information they need to carry out their role in the treatment plan.

When psychosocial impairments are identified, patients often benefit from services that fall under a second therapeutic treatment domain, categorized as psychosocial behavioral health. Cognitive behavior therapy (CBT), psychoanalysis, sex therapy, hypnosis, biofeedback, and autonomic nervous system quieting (ANSQ) are examples of a few of these treatment strategies.[3] Patient goals and any psychosocial impairments can help the provider determine if and when these services can aid the treatment plan. For example, a patient with dyspareunia who also reports a history of sexual trauma may benefit more from these type of services than a woman who developed dyspareunia as the result of a fall. A person with high levels of anxiety may benefit more from hypnosis than a person without anxiety. Having a comprehensive understanding of the challenges facing the patient and of the particular services can help the team determine which services will be most useful for this particular individual. (See Chapter 16, "Chronic Pelvic Pain and Psychological Disorders," for more detailed information.)

In addition to physical therapy and psychological services, certain patients can benefit from pharmacological intervention to supplement their treatment plan. In an ideal scenario, one pain-management physician helps the team oversee the patient's medication. Simple analgesics, neuropathic agents, anticonvulsants, N-Methyl-D-aspartate (NMDA) agonists, tricyclic antidepressants, and Serontonin Norepinepherine Receptor Inbibitors (SNRI) can be used in varying combinations to treat pain, anxiety, and depression.[4-7] In isolation, these medications rarely provide the desired symptom resolution

for patients. However, managing patient expectations about the intended effects will increase their compliance and can be a useful supplement the treatment plan. Often, the medications are intended to counteract or treat central nervous system disorders and neuropathic pain, and reduce anxiety and depression. It is useful for the provider and the patient to discuss the expected effects of a medication and how they are going to determine if the trial of the medication is successful. Various combinations of pharmacological topical ointments may also be used that can include the above-mentioned medications, hormones, and anesthetic agents. They can also serve to allow the patient to tolerate or become more responsive to treatments in the other therapeutic domains (see Chapter 5, "Pharmacological Management of Pelvic Pain").

Interventional pain management procedures are a fourth therapeutic domain. Dry needling, acupuncture, myofascial trigger point injections, peripheral nerve infiltrations, pulsed radio frequency or ablation, botulinum toxin injections, ketamine infusions, and neuromodulation are a few examples of these types of treatments.[8-11] Like the pharmacology options, these procedures can be very useful when interdisciplinary critical reasoning is used to determine what may provide the most benefit with the lowest risk for the patient.

THE NON-RESPONDING PATIENT

People with polymorphic syndromes such as pelvic pain rarely achieve complete pain resolution with a single treatment in any of the treatment domains. Furthermore, they may not be able to tolerate a particular therapy, or certain therapies may not be available to them. Critical reasoning within the algorithm allows the team to use combinations that are available and reasonable for their particular patient. Commonly, patients will report that individual therapies "are not working." The key is to figure out why, regardless of the treatment. This includes medications, injections, physical therapy, psychology, etc. Commonly, patients with pelvic pain are misinformed or uninformed about why they are doing a particular treatment and what the intended outcome is. For example, patients can be quick to dismiss a medication because their expectation is complete pain resolution. That medication may not resolve their pain but may allow them to tolerate physical therapy, which may be a necessary part of their treatment plan. A patient may not have access to physical therapy and may need pharmaceutical intervention and other strategies to manage their pain. It is important for patients to understand that pain management is useful as they continue to treat the underlying causes.

This strategy can best be described in the form of questions and answers using clinical examples (Cases 4.1 and 4.2, below).

CASE 4.1

A 23-year-old woman with unprovoked vaginal burning and dyspareunia: Her pain gets worse when she sits, and she is unable to wear pants because of her symptoms. She has a history of multiple yeast infections and is a former gymnast.

Treatment Considerations

1. *Is there an active infection? No:* start physical therapy. *Yes:* treat infection and then refer to physical therapy.
2. Physical therapy evaluation reveals myofascial causes of pelvic pain that include external connective tissue dysfunction in the trunk, bony pelvis, and lower extremities, piriformis and obturator internus myofascial trigger points, (+) Tinel's sign at Alcock's canal bilaterally, hypertonic pelvic floor muscles with poor motor control, positive Q-tip test at the vestibule for pain, and vulvar connective tissue restrictions.
3. Physical therapy assessment: It is plausible that this patient had a high-tone pelvic floor because of her gymnastic background. Repetitive yeast infections can then sensitize the vestibular tissue and the pudendal nerve, leading to further muscle hypertonus. The muscles, nerve, and tissue are now impaired enough to generate her described symptoms, even though her infections are resolved. The obturator internus hypertonus and myofascial trigger point can contribute to pudendal nerve irritation, and the pudendal nerve irritation can contribute to pelvic

floor hypertonus and connective tissue dysfunction in the territory of the nerve. Additionally, the vulvar connective tissue restrictions are contributing to the tenderness at the vestibule. The internal and external connective tissue restrictions can be causing her intolerance to pants.

4. Treatment plan: The physical therapist and patient agree to a treatment plan of one visit per week for eight weeks. The plan includes manual therapy to address the above-mentioned issues, and a home exercise program to decrease the high tone, lengthen the pelvic floor, and improve connective tissue integrity. The goals for therapy are to be able to tolerate wearing pants, sitting for two hours without vaginal pain, and to engage in intercourse without pelvic pain symptoms.
5. Problem arises: After three sessions, the patient is frustrated—she reports increased vaginal burning for several days following physical therapy. She is not sure if this treatment is the right treatment. The physical therapist contacts the referring gynecologist to discuss the situation and suggests that the patient speak with her doctor about medication. They modify the physical therapy treatment and stop internal physical therapy, and they continue with the external treatments for a few appointments until it can be better tolerated.
6. The patient returns to physical therapy, her doctor prescribes a tricyclic antidepressant and 2% lidocaine jelly that can be used prior to internal physical therapy to minimize the pain following physical therapy. Even with the lidocaine, the patient still cannot tolerate internal physical therapy.
7. The physical therapist reasons that the burning is not solely coming from the vestibule, or the lidocaine would be more effective. The patient presents with positive Tinel's signs bilaterally on the pudendal nerve branches at Alcock's canal. This patient also presents with bilateral myofascial points in the obturator internus muscles. The physical therapist speaks

with the patient's physician to discuss considering a pudendal nerve block or botox injections to this muscle. They agree that the myofascial trigger points may be aggravating the pudendal nerve and therefore treating the trigger point may be a more useful choice. The physician injects the obturator internus with lidocaine first, which decreases the patient's unprovoked vaginal burning by 50%. This is satisfying to the patient, and botox is then injected. The following week, the patient returns to physical therapy and can tolerate internal therapy. She is also now on a therapeutic dose of the prescribed medication. She continues with physical therapy for 16 more sessions and achieves her goals of pain-free intercourse and the ability to sit and wear pants without vaginal pain.

CASE 4.2

A 25-year-old woman with unprovoked vaginal pain and dyspareunia: She has a history of sexual abuse, anxiety and depression, and a phobia of medical providers.

Treatment Considerations

1. Her gynecologist diagnoses this woman with vulvodynia, and hypertonic pelvic floor muscles were identified. Additionally, the physician recognizes that this patient also has unmanaged anxiety and will suffer emotionally if she needs to attend weekly physical therapy appointments in her current frame of mind.
2. Physical therapy is not an appropriate choice until someone in psychological services treats her anxiety. The patient initially is uninterested in psychological care because she "previously did years of psychoanalysis and it was not helpful." The physician prescribes the patient an SNRI to treat the pain, anxiety, and depression.
3. At the return visit, the patient reports a slight improvement in her pain. The physician discusses physical therapy, but the patient declines, based on the nature of the treatment and her anxiety. Her physician recommends psychological services that are different from psychoanalysis, with the intention of giving her tools to manage her pain and anxiety and also treat her phobia of medical providers. The patient is willing to try hypnosis and cognitive behavioral therapy with this new expectation.
4. Following a successful course of hypnosis and cognitive behavioral therapy, the young woman is ready to start physical therapy. The psychologist calls the physical therapist prior to the first appointment and offers suggestions as to what will be most useful for this particular patient in terms of communication and techniques that may reinforce the psychological improvements. The physical therapist communicates with the patient prior to the appointment that this discussion has occurred and that everyone will work together to coordinate an effective treatment plan.

Cases 4.1 and 4.2 are examples of very different treatment plans for patients with similar symptoms. They present with different underlying etiologies and physical and emotional impairments. Using the algorithm to choose individualized treatments based on a patient's specific assessment can help providers start a reasonable treatment plan. These plans often need to change based on response to treatment, at which time a reevaluation should be used. Because multiple therapeutic combinations exist, interdisciplinary provider and patient communication can help troubleshoot challenges when patients do not respond or cannot tolerate a treatment. Ongoing reevaluations and treatment plan reorganization will lead to more successful outcomes and patient successes.

REFERENCES

1. Tu FF et al. Prevalence of pelvic musculoskeletal disorders in a female chronic pelvic pain clinic. *J Reprod Med.* 2006;51(3):185–189.
2. Butrick CW. Pelvic floor hypertonic disorders: identification and management. *Obstet Gynecol Clin North Am.* 2009;36:707–722.
3. Bergeron S et al. Surgical and behavioral treatments for vestibulodynia: two-and-one-half year

follow-up and predictors of outcome. *Obstet Gynecol.* 2008;111(1):159–166.

4. Richeimer SH et al. Utilization patterns of tricyclic antidepressants in a multidisciplinary pain clinic: a survey. *Clin J Pain.* 1997;13:324–329.

5. Sasaki K et al. Oral gabapentin (neurontin) treatment of refractory genitourinary tract pain. *Tech Urol.* 2001;7:47–49.

6. Hewitt DJ. The use of NMDA-receptor antagonists in the treatment of chronic pain. *Clin J Pain.* 2000;16(Suppl. 2):S73–S79.

7. Visser E, Schug SA. The role of ketamine in pain management. *Biomed Pharmacother.* 2006;60(7): 341–348.

8. Langford C et al. Levator ani trigger point injections: an underutilized treatment for chronic pelvic pain. *Neurourol Urodyn.* 2007;26:59–62.

9. Hough DM et al. Chronic perineal pain caused by pudendal nerve entrapment: anatomy and CT-guided perineural injection technique. *AJR Am J Roentgenol* 2003;181(2):561–567.

10. Dykstra KK, Presthus J. Botulinum toxin type A for the treatment of provoked vestibulodynia. *J Reprod Med.* 2006;51:467–470.

11. Chartier-Kastler E. Sacral neuromodulation for treating the symptoms of overactive bladder syndrome and non-obstructive urinary retention: over 10 years of clinical experience. *BJU Int.* 2008;101(4):417–423.

5

Pharmacological Management of Pelvic Pain

MICHELE L. MATTHEWS AND VESELA KOVACHEVA

The pharmacological approach to the management of pelvic pain involves the use of pharmacotherapeutic agents that can target pathways involved in pain processing, including anticonvulsants, antidepressants, nonsteroidal anti-inflammatory drugs (NSAIDs), local anesthetics, and opioids (Table 5.1). Decision-making with regard to selection of therapies should include factors such as duration of pain, presumed mechanisms of pain, underlying medical conditions, current drug therapy, cost, and convenience. Goals of therapy for the management of pelvic pain should focus on reducing acuity and severity of pain with emphasis on function and quality of life. The effectiveness of these medications along with any adverse effects should be monitored regularly, and the clinician should provide support, reassurance, and encouragement throughout the treatment process.[1] Due to the likelihood that symptoms will wax and wane, modifications to the treatment regimen may be necessary over time.

PHARMACOLOGICAL AGENTS

Acetaminophen

The exact mechanism of action for acetaminophen is unknown, but it is believed to increase the pain threshold by inhibiting prostaglandin (PG) synthesis, much like NSAIDs. However, acetaminophen does not have significant anti-inflammatory effects. It is often used as initial treatment for pelvic pain due to its availability as an over-the-counter medication, although evidence to support its use is lacking, with studies focusing primarily on the treatment of dysmenorrhea. Acetaminophen may be utilized as adjunctive symptomatic treatment, but the risk of hepatotoxicity should be considered and monitored, especially in patients with a history of alcohol use, hepatic dysfunction, concomitant hepatotoxic medications, or underlying conditions that may affect glutathione stores (e.g., anorexia). Additionally, the manufacturers of acetaminophen products have recommended that daily doses not exceed 3 grams per day; however, doses up to 4 grams per day may continue to be recommended under clinician supervision. Acetaminophen is Food and Drug Administration (FDA) pregnancy category B.

Nonsteroidal Anti-Inflammatory Drugs (NSAIDs)

Cyclo-oxygenase (COX) isoenzymes are responsible for various physiological responses. Specifically, COX-1 is responsible for PG synthesis as well as the maintenance of normal renal function, gastric mucosal integrity, and hemostasis, and COX-2 is inducible in many cells in response to certain mediators of inflammation. Nonselective NSAIDs such as naproxen competitively inhibit both COX-1 and COX-2 by blocking arachidonate binding, resulting in analgesic, antipyretic, and anti-inflammatory effects. Celecoxib selectively inhibits the COX-2 isoenzyme. The differences between NSAIDs include not only COX isoenzyme selectivity but also significant inter-patient variability with regard to the efficacy and safety of these medications. This is presumed to be related to differences in the chemical structures.[2] Therefore, treatment failure with one NSAID may not preclude the use of alternative NSAIDs within different chemical classes.

Clinical trials evaluating the efficacy of NSAIDs have focused primarily on pain related to dysmenorrhea and endometriosis.[3,4] However, PGs are implicated in the pathogenesis of various pelvic pain-related diagnoses, including irritable bowel syndrome and interstitial cystitis; therefore, NSAIDs can be beneficial as

TABLE 5.1 PHARMACOLOGICAL THERAPIES FOR CHRONIC PELVIC PAIN

Drug/Therapeutic Class	Initial Adult Dosing	Adverse Effects	Monitoring Parameters
Acetaminophen	500 mg PO every 4 hours	Hepatotoxicity with doses >4 gm/day, concomitant alcohol abuse, or malnutrition	LFTs
Nonselective NSAIDs		GI irritation, GI bleeding, renal toxicity, cardiovascular events	Signs/symptoms of GI bleeding SCr/BUN LFTs
Ibuprofen	400 mg PO every 6 hours; maximum daily dose = 3200 mg		
Naproxen	250 mg PO twice daily; maximum daily dose = 1500 mg		
Indomethacin	25 mg PO 2–3 times per day; maximum daily dose = 200 mg		
Etodolac	200 mg PO every 8 hours; maximum daily dose = 1200 mg		
COX-2 Selective NSAID			
Celecoxib	100 mg PO twice daily or 200 mg PO once daily		
Opioid Analgesics		Sedation, N/V, constipation, cognitive impairment, respiratory depression (regardless of formulation), pruritus, euphoria, dysphoria, hypotension, urinary retention; withdrawal symptoms with abrupt discontinuation; seizures possible at high doses; abnormal pain sensitivity, hormonal changes, and immune modulation with long-term use	Vital signs Oxygen saturation Respiratory rate Level of sedation Bowel movements Urinary output Aberrant drug-related behaviors SCr/BUN LFTs ECG (methadone)
Morphine	IR: 15 mg PO every 4 hours		
Hydromorphone	IR: 2 mg PO every 4 hours		
Oxycodone	IR: 5 mg PO every 4 hours		
Fentanyl	Transdermal: initiate only in opioid-tolerant patients taking ≥ 60 mg of morphine/day or equivalent		
Methadone	2.5 mg PO every 8–12 hours		
Oxymorphone	IR: 5 mg PO every 4 hours		
Hydrocodone	IR combination product containing acetaminophen: 5/325 mg PO every 4–6 hours; maximum of 12 tablets per day		
Buprenorphine	Transdermal: 5 mcg/hour patch applied every 7 days		

(continued)

TABLE 5.1 CONTINUED

Drug/Therapeutic Class	Initial Adult Dosing	Adverse Effects	Monitoring Parameters
Dual Mechanism Analgesics		N/V, sedation, dizziness, dry mouth, headache, respiratory depression, constipation, serotonin syndrome, seizures, blood pressure changes, tolerance, dependence	Vital signs Respiratory rate Oxygen saturation Bowel movements Signs/symptoms of serotonin syndrome
Tramadol	IR: 50 mg PO every 4 hours; maximum daily dose = 400 mg		
Tapentadol	IR: 50 mg PO every 4 hours; maximum daily dose = 600 mg		
Tricyclic antidepressants (TCAs) Amitriptyline Nortriptyline Desipramine	25 mg PO at bedtime	Dry mouth, sedation, mood changes, blurred vision, weight gain, orthostatic hypotension, urinary retention, constipation, arrhythmias	Vital signs ECG Weight Urinary output LFTs Signs/symptoms of bleeding Level of sedation Serum nortriptyline levels (therapeutic range = 50–150 ng/mL)
Serotonin Norepinephrine Reuptake Inhibitors (SNRIs)		Nausea, sedation, mood changes, hypertension, hepatotoxicity	Weight Urinary output LFTs Signs/symptoms of bleeding Level of sedation
Duloxetine	20 mg PO daily		
Milnacipran	12.5 mg PO once on day 1; 12.5 mg PO twice daily on days 2 and 3; 25 mg PO twice daily on days 4–7		
Venlafaxine	IR: 25 mg PO three times daily		
Selective Serotonin Reuptake Inhibitors (SSRIs)		Nausea, xerostomia, mood changes, sedation, sexual dysfunction, bleeding	Weight Urinary output LFTs Signs/symptoms of bleeding Level of sedation ECG (citalopram)
Citalopram	20 mg PO daily		
Sertraline	50 mg PO daily		

(continued)

TABLE 5.1 CONTINUED

Drug/Therapeutic Class	Initial Adult Dosing	Adverse Effects	Monitoring Parameters
Anticonvulsants		Dizziness, somnolence, weight gain, peripheral edema, rash, hepatotoxicity	Weight Chemistry panel Skin exam LFTs SCR/BUN CBC Serum carbamazepine levels (therapeutic range = 2–7 mcg/mL)
Gabapentin	300 mg PO on days 1–3, 300 mg PO twice daily on days 4–6, then 300 mg PO three times a day; may increase as tolerated to 1800-3600 mg/day in three divided doses		
Pregabalin	50–75 mg PO twice daily; may increase as tolerated to 450–600 mg/day in two divided doses		
Carbamazepine	100 mg PO twice daily on day 1, may increase by 100 mg every 12 hours as needed up to a maximum of 1200 mg/day		
Muscle Relaxants		Drowsiness, dizziness, weakness, hypotonia, blood pressure changes, dry mouth	Vital signs Level of sedation LFTs
Baclofen	5 mg PO 2–3 times per day		
Cyclobenzaprine	5 mg PO three times daily		
Tizanidine	2 mg PO every 6–8 hours		
Spasmolytics		Nausea, dizziness, xerostomia, somnolence, blurred vision	SCr/BUN Bowel function
Dicyclomine	20 mg PO four times daily		
Hyoscyamine	0.125–0.25 mg PO or SL every 4 hours or as needed; maximum daily dose = 1.5 mg		

Abbreviations: PO = by mouth/oral; LFTs = liver function tests; GI = gastrointestinal; SCr = serum creatinine; BUN = blood urea nitrogen; IR = immediate-release; N/V = nausea/vomiting; ECG = electrocardiogram; CBC = complete blood count

adjunctive therapy or for the management of acute pain exacerbations. The use of NSAIDs comes with the increased potential for a broad spectrum of adverse gastrointestinal (GI), cardiovascular, renal, and hepatic effects. Risk factors for adverse GI effects include older age, history of prior complicated peptic ulcer disease or upper GI bleed, history of chronic debilitating conditions, use of NSAIDs at high doses, and concurrent use of select medications with bleeding risks (e.g., antiplatelet therapy). NSAIDs and selective COX-2 inhibitors have also been implicated in the development of major cardiovascular events, such as myocardial infarction, stroke, and vascular death; a meta-analysis found that the risks associated with traditional NSAIDs, such as diclofenac and ibuprofen, are similar to those with COX-2 inhibitors, with the exception of naproxen.[5] Therapy considerations include identification of risk factors, selection of NSAIDs based on adverse-effect potential, and initiation of gastroprotective agents (e.g., proton pump inhibitors) for at-risk patients. The FDA pregnancy category for NSAIDs is C for the first two trimesters, but category D in the third trimester.

Antidepressants

Epidemiological studies of chronic pain have shown the strong association between depressive symptoms and the experience of chronic pelvic pain.[6] It has been suggested that the treatment of chronic pain can be improved if depression is considered as part of the patient's clinical presentation[7]; therefore, the use of antidepressants in patients with chronic pelvic pain syndrome may increase the likelihood of a positive outcome and achievement of therapeutic goals.

Tricyclic Antidepressants

Tricyclic antidepressants (TCAs) such as amitriptyline, nortriptyline, and desipramine decrease the reuptake of serotonin and norepinephrine, thereby exerting analgesic effects through the activation of descending inhibitory pain pathways. Amitriptyline possesses strong anticholinergic activity, which may be a favorable effect in select patients such as those with interstitial cystitis, as this can cause a reduction in the urgency and frequency of urination. Additionally, amitriptyline is metabolized to nortriptyline, which accounts for the majority of neurotransmitter activity following administration of amitriptyline. Nortriptyline is more likely to inhibit the reuptake of norepinephrine than serotonin. Desipramine is associated with less anticholinergic activity in comparison to amitriptyline and nortriptyline. The doses for TCAs that are used in the management of chronic pain are often lower than what is needed to exert antidepressant effects, and TCAs are often prescribed to be taken once daily at bedtime due to the risk of sedation.

Studies evaluating the benefit of TCAs have focused on pelvic pain related to various causes including GI, urological, and neurological mechanisms. Amitriptyline has been the most-studied TCA, but with mixed results. In a small study of women with a history of moderate to severe pelvic pain from any cause, amitriptyline was compared to both gabapentin alone and the combination of gabapentin and amitriptyline. Baseline pain scores improved in all three treatment arms over time; however, after 24 months, there were significant differences in pain scores in favor of gabapentin alone or gabapentin plus amitriptyline in comparison to amitriptyline alone.[8] A prospective, randomized study found that four months of treatment with amitriptyline was more effective than placebo in decreasing pelvic pain and urgency in patients with interstitial cystitis.[9] Nortriptyline was studied in a prospective case series of 14 women with chronic pelvic pain with a primary end point of reduction in pain. After two months, 50% of subjects discontinued treatment due to adverse effects; however, six of the seven women who remained in treatment were either pain-free or reported significant pain improvement.[10] With regard to desipramine, a three-month course of treatment was found to be better than placebo in a large, randomized controlled trial in patients with moderate to severe irritable bowel syndrome, especially in those with diarrhea-predominant disease and a history of abuse.[11] A systematic review of studies evaluating the use of antidepressants, including TCAs, for the management of chronic pelvic pain from urological causes suggested that the lack of evidence to support the use of these medications may be due to publication bias.[12] The long-term effects of TCAs for the treatment of pelvic pain are unknown.

Patient education related to proper use of therapy and potential adverse effects is important to ensure their adherence to treatment. Generally, TCAs should be avoided in patients with cardiovascular disease or those that are on medications associated with QT interval prolongation due to the risk of arrhythmias, older adults due to the risk of falls,[13] and patients with a history of seizures. Monitoring parameters for efficacy and safety of TCA therapy should include liver function tests, periodic electrocardiograms, and symptoms of serotonin syndrome. Serum drug levels should be obtained for patients on nortriptyline. TCAs are FDA pregnancy category C.

Selective Serotonin Reuptake Inhibitors/Serotonin Norepinephrine Reuptake Inhibitors

Like TCAs, selective serotonin reuptake inhibitors (SSRIs) and serotonin norepinephrine reuptake inhibitors (SNRIs) increase levels of neurotransmitters within the central nervous system (CNS) to increase inhibitory activity within the descending pain system. The differences between SSRIs and SNRIs are related to their selectivity for neurotransmitters, pharmacokinetics, and cost.

The SSRIs can be effective in patients with depression in the setting of chronic pain; however, the role of these medications in the management of pain has been limited due to lack of evidence. A double-blind, placebo-controlled, randomized crossover trial of sertraline among women with chronic pelvic pain found no difference in pain intensity in comparison to placebo after six weeks.[14] In a small randomized, controlled trial of men with chronic pelvic pain syndrome, the use of sertraline over 13 weeks was not associated with significant improvements in prostatic symptom frequency or severity in comparison to placebo.[15] A prospective case series of 14 patients with chronic pelvic pain who were treated with citalopram showed no significant improvement in pain or disability.[16]

Duloxetine and other SNRIs have been studied and are frequently used in numerous chronic pain syndromes, including peripheral neuropathy and fibromyalgia. For the treatment of interstitial cystitis, approximately 10% of patients rated improvement in overall well-being, but with no significant improvement in pain or urinary urgency.[17] Studies evaluating the role of SNRIs in chronic pelvic pain from other causes are lacking.

Therapy considerations for SSRIs and SNRIs include their adverse-effect profiles, as some of these agents can cause weight gain and sexual dysfunction; risk of drug interactions; pregnancy and lactation; and cost. These drugs should be avoided in patients on other serotonergic medications due to the risk of serotonin syndrome. Expectations of therapy should be discussed, with emphasis on the importance of taking the medication consistently and on the risk of withdrawal with abrupt discontinuation. The use of SNRIs is associated with an increase in noradrenergic activity; therefore, blood pressure and heart rate monitoring should be implemented. Close monitoring of mood is warranted with the use of all antidepressants due to the risk of worsening depression and suicidality. Most commonly used SSRIs are FDA pregnancy category C, with the exception of paroxetine, which is category X due to the risk of congenital cardiovascular malformations during the first trimester.

Anticonvulsants

Anticonvulsants are theorized to interact with voltage-gated calcium channels within the CNS to reduce neuronal hyperactivity. This proposed mechanism has been extrapolated to the management of chronic pain due to the occurrence of wind-up and central sensitization that are commonly associated with neuropathic pain states.

Anticonvulsants are widely used for chronic pain syndromes and have been studied in select pelvic pain models. As previously mentioned, gabapentin was found to be more effective alone or in combination with amitriptyline compared to amitriptyline alone in women with chronic pelvic pain from any cause.[8] In a small case series, gabapentin use was associated with improvement in genitourinary pain that persisted six months after the end of treatment in 47% of patients.[18] A small, prospective case series of 22 women with chronic pelvic pain from any cause found that pregabalin 75 mg twice daily was associated with significant reduction in the mean visual analog scale score, with most benefit in patients with vulvodynia; however, patients were evaluated after only one week of therapy.[19] An open-label trial of lamotrigine showed significant improvement in mood and pain, especially in patients with vulvodynia, after eight weeks of treatment.[20] Based on the limited available evidence, long-term effects of anticonvulsants in the management of chronic pelvic pain are unknown.

Gabapentin and pregabalin can be used safely in patients with hepatic dysfunction due minimal hepatic metabolism; however, dosing must be adjusted in the setting of renal impairment. Gabapentin administration should be separated from antacids due to the risk of drug binding resulting in reduced gabapentin efficacy. Common adverse effects include dizziness, sedation, nausea, weight gain, and peripheral edema. Unlike with other anticonvulsants, such as phenytoin and carbamazepine, monitoring of serum drug levels is not necessary for gabapentin and pregabalin. The primary differences between these two anticonvulsants are related to potency and scheduling as a controlled substance; pregabalin is a Schedule V medication in the United States due to trial data suggestive of abuse potential. It should also be noted that reports of gabapentin abuse are on the rise.[21] Patients should be educated on the importance of adherence to therapy to increase efficacy and minimize risk of withdrawal. Close monitoring of mood and affect is indicated, as these agents may increase the risk of suicidal thoughts. Both gabapentin and pregabalin are FDA pregnancy category C.

Muscle Relaxants

The mechanisms of action for most muscle relaxants are believed to be related to central inhibition of neurons, resulting in muscle relaxation and reduced spasticity. Baclofen, a structural analog of the inhibitory neurotransmitter gamma-aminobutyric acid (GABA), is used extensively for spasticity related to multiple sclerosis and spinal cord injuries. Additionally, baclofen possesses analgesic effects through antagonism of substance P.[22] Tizanidine is structurally related to clonidine and exerts its effects through agonist activity at alpha-2 adrenoreceptors. Cyclobenzaprine has TCA-like activity due to its structural similarities to amitriptyline. Other muscle relaxants such as carisoprodol, metaxalone, and methocarbamol may work more like sedatives, particularly carisoprodol, which is metabolized to a barbiturate (meprobamate).

Evidence to support the use of muscle relaxants for the management of chronic pelvic pain is unavailable; however, if a patient is identified to have a significant muscular component (e.g., iliopsoas spasm or pelvic floor dysfunction), these agents can be very effective. Choice of therapy is often based on patient tolerance, adverse-effect profile, and cost. Adverse effects common to all muscle relaxants include drowsiness, dizziness, and GI effects. CNS depression is additive with other centrally acting medications. The same considerations for the use of TCAs should be applied to cyclobenzaprine. Tizanidine can cause hypotension, and blood pressure should be monitored. Carisoprodol use should be avoided in patients at high risk for medication misuse and abuse. All muscle relaxants are FDA pregnancy category C, with the exception of cyclobenzaprine which is category B.

Spasmolytics

Spasmolytics such as dicyclomine and hyoscyamine induce smooth-muscle relaxation through anticholinergic mechanisms and can be useful for chronic pelvic pain in the setting of irritable bowel syndrome, interstitial cystitis, or in the presence of dysmenorrheal component.[23] Common adverse effects include sedation, constipation, urinary retention, and xerostomia. These agents should be avoided in patients with cardiovascular disease, GI dysmotility, obstructive uropathies, and older adults. Dicyclomine is pregnancy category B, while hyoscyamine is pregnancy category C.

Opioids

Opioids bind to opioid receptors in the CNS to inhibit the transmission of nociceptive input from the periphery to the spinal cord, activate descending inhibitory pathways that modulate transmission in the spinal cord, and alter limbic system activity. Opioids also modify the sensory and affective aspects of pain. Receptors activated by opioids are abundant within the CNS and throughout peripheral tissues. Various types of opioid receptors have been identified, including mu, delta, and kappa receptors, and activation of subtypes of these receptors can lead to analgesia (e.g., mu-1) or adverse effects (e.g., mu-2). Opioids differ based on their chemical structure, receptor activity, and adverse-effect profile.

Commonly used opioids in the management of chronic pain include morphine, oxycodone, oxymorphone, hydromorphone, methadone, tramadol, tapentadol, and fentanyl. Methadone is a pharmacologically long-acting opioid with highly variable pharmacokinetics, resulting in a long half-life and drug accumulation. Tramadol and tapentadol exert weak mu receptor agonist activity as well as inhibition of the reuptake of serotonin and norepinephrine.

Long-term, high-quality studies evaluating opioids for chronic pain are lacking. Nonetheless, the use of opioids for chronic non-cancer pain has increased dramatically, and the incidence of opioid-related adverse effects has risen in a linear fashion relative to increased prescribing, use at high doses, and as a consequence of misuse and abuse.[24] There is fair evidence to support the short-term use of opioids for chronic pain for improvement specifically in pain and quality of life; however, patients included in these studies had failed other therapies and were considered to be at low risk for misuse and abuse.[25]

Frequently, assessment for the appropriateness of opioid therapy is the reason for referral to the pain specialist. A thorough history and physical assessment should be performed, along with a comprehensive benefit-to-harm evaluation. Benefits of opioid therapy include analgesia and improvement in daily function. Risks include overdose, development of physical dependence and tolerance, and possible misuse, abuse, or addiction. Baseline assessment of opioid misuse risk through the use of validated tools such as the Screener and Opioid Assessment in Pain Patients–Revised (SOAPP-R)[26] is highly encouraged, along with urine drug testing and the review of data obtained from a prescription monitoring program. Patients should provide informed consent and sign a treatment agreement prior to the initiation of therapy. Therapy should be assessed on a regular basis and should include evaluation of pain, function, mood, adverse drug effects, and presence of aberrant behavior. Examples of aberrant drug-seeking behavior include multiple "lost" or "stolen" prescriptions, failure to comply with monitoring, current use of alcohol or illicit drugs, multiple prescriptions from different prescribers or pharmacies, or forging, selling, or stealing prescriptions. Ongoing risk management should be performed through the use of periodic urine drug testing and tools such as the Current Opioid Misuse Measure (COMM).[27]

If opioids are considered, choice of therapy should be based on patient-specific factors such as underlying medical conditions, current drug therapy, and pattern of pain (e.g., constant versus intermittent), as well as drug-specific factors including adverse effects, available formulations, and cost. Short-acting opioid formulations may be beneficial for patients with intermittent pain; however, the use of combination opioid formulations (e.g., oxycodone/acetaminophen) should be limited due to the risks associated with the non-opioid component, especially at high doses and for long-term use. The use of extended-release or long-acting opioid formulations results in consistent plasma drug concentrations, and these are recommended for patients with constant chronic pain, although available evidence suggest no significant difference in efficacy or adverse effects in comparison to short-acting formulations.[25] Adverse effects common to all opioids include CNS depression, respiratory depression, constipation, nausea, and pruritus.

Methadone use is associated with cardiac arrhythmias, and baseline and periodic electrocardiograms should be monitored.[28] Long-term opioid use is associated with immunosuppression, endocrine dysfunction, and hyperalgesia.[29,30] Opioids with active metabolites such as morphine should be avoided in patients with renal impairment, and dose adjustments should be implemented in the setting of hepatic dysfunction due to the risk of accumulation. Most opioids are pregnancy category B or C.

Miscellaneous

Adjunctive therapies that target symptoms and/or complications of chronic pelvic pain should be considered.[31] These include medications that may improve sleep, such as sedating antihistamines (e.g., hydroxyzine), or those compounded into vaginal preparations, such as diazepam suppositories for pelvic floor dysfunction.[32] Other examples include the combination use of belladonna and tramadol as a vaginal suppository for neuropathic pain due to Tarlof cysts and pudendal neuralgia. Compounded topical products containing antidepressants, anticonvulsants, NSAIDs, and alpha-2 agonists can be useful for vulvodynia and postherpetic neuralgia, although there is limited available evidence from clinical trials. Intravenous lidocaine may also be considered, although the role of this therapy is limited due to lack of evidence in chronic pelvic pain, adverse effects, and cost.

RATIONAL POLYPHARMACY

The concept of rational polypharmacy in pain management involves the use of one or more drugs to minimize adverse effects, increase adherence, and reduce the need for higher doses of high-risk medications (e.g., opioids) while maintaining or increasing analgesic efficacy. When combining therapies, important considerations include patient factors (e.g., age, organ function), drug mechanisms of action, pharmacokinetics, and adverse effect profiles. A few small studies have demonstrated benefit with the use of rational polypharmacy for the management of chronic pelvic pain.

SUMMARY

The management of chronic pelvic pain can be challenging and complex. A comprehensive pain history and assessment of patient factors can assist with selection of therapy. Beyond pharmacological treatment, a multidisciplinary approach should be implemented to address all aspects of care, including those focusing on the psychological and emotional impact of chronic pelvic pain. Evidence to support most analgesics in the management of chronic pelvic pain is lacking; however, there is robust anecdotal experience to support these therapies.

REFERENCES

1. American College of Obstetricians and Gynecologists (ACOG). Committee on Practice Bulletins—Gynecology. ACOG Practice Bulletin No. 51. Chronic pelvic pain. *Obstet Gynecol.* 2004 Mar;103(3):589–605.

2. Sharma S, Prasad A, Anand KS. Nonsteroidal anti-inflammatory drugs in the management of pain and inflammation: a basis for drug selection. *Am J Ther.* 1999 Jan;6(1):3–11.

3. Marjoribanks J, Proctor M, Farquhar C, Derks RS. Nonsteroidal anti-inflammatory drugs for dysmenorrhoea. *Cochrane Database Syst Rev.* 2010 Jan 20;(1):CD001751. doi: 10.1002/14651858. CD001751.pub2

4. Allen C, Hopewell S, Prentice A, Gregory D. Nonsteroidal anti-inflammatory drugs for pain in women with endometriosis. *Cochrane Database Syst Rev.* 2009 Apr 15;(2):CD004753. doi: 10.1002/ 14651858.CD004753.pub3

5. Bhala N, Emberson J, Merhi A, et al., and the Coxib and traditional NSAID Trialists' (CNT) Collaboration. Vascular and upper gastrointestinal effects of non-steroidal anti-inflammatory drugs: meta-analyses of individual participant data from randomised trials. *Lancet.* 2013;382(9894):769–779.

6. Savidge CJ, Slade P. Psychological aspects of chronic pelvic pain. *J Psychosom Res.* 1997;42(5):433–444.

7. Banks SM, Kerns RD. Explaining high rates of depression in chronic pain: a diathesis-stress framework. *Psychol Bull.* 1996;119:95–110.

8. Sator-Katzenschlager SM, Scharbert G, Kress HG, et al. Chronic pelvic pain treated with gabapentin and amitriptyline: a randomized controlled pilot study. *Wiener klinische Wochenschrift.* 2005;117:761–768.

9. van Ophoven A, Pokupic S, Heinecke A, Hertle L. A prospective, randomized, placebo controlled, double-blind study of amitriptyline for the treatment of interstitial cystitis. *J Urol.* 2004;172:533–536.

10. Walker E, Roy-Byrne P, Katon W, Jemelka R. An open trial of nortriptyline in women with chronic pelvic pain. *Int J Psychiatry Med.* 1991;21:245–252.

11. Drossman D, Toner B, Whitehead W, et al. Cognitive-behavioral therapy versus education and desipramine versus placebo for moderate to severe functional bowel disorders. *Gastroenterology.* 2003;125:19–31.

12. Papandreou C, Skapinakis P, Giannakis D, Sofikitis N, Mavreas V. Antidepressant drugs for chronic urological pelvic pain: an evidence-based review. *Adv Urol.* 2009;2009:797031. doi: 10.1155/2009/ 797031. Epub 2010 Feb 14.

13. American Geriatrics Society, 2012 Beers Criteria Update Expert Panel. American Geriatrics Society updated Beers Criteria for potentially inappropriate medication use in older adults. *J Am Geriatr Soc.* 2012 Apr;60(4):616–631.

14. Engel Jr. CC, Walker EA, Engel AL, Bullis J, Armstrong A. A randomized, double-blind crossover trial of sertraline in women with chronic pelvic pain. *J Psychosom Res.* 1998;44(2):203–207.

15. Lee RA, West RM, Wilson JD. The response to sertraline in men with chronic pelvic pain syndrome. *STIs.* 2005;81(2):147–149.

16. Brown CS, Franks AS, Wan J, Ling FW. Citalopram in the treatment of women with chronic pelvic pain: an open-label trial. *J Reprod Med.* 2008;53(3):191–195.

17. van Ophoven A, Hertle L. The dual serotonin and noradrenaline reuptake inhibitor duloxetine for the treatment of interstitial cystitis: results of an observational study. *J Urol.* 2007;177(2):552–555.

18. Sasaki K, Smith C, Chuang Y, Lee J, Kim J, Chancellor M. Oral gabapentin (neurontin) treatment of refractory genitourinary tract pain. *Tech Urol.* 2001;7:47–49.

19. Sengun HI, Sengun IS. Pregabalin in chronic pelvic pain. *J Neurol Sci [Turkish].* 2013;30(2):265–269.

20. Meltzer-Brody S, Zolnoun D, Steege J, Rinaldi K, Leserman J. Open-label trial of lamotrigine focusing on efficacy in vulvodynia. *J Reprod Med.* 2009;54:171–178.

21. Schifano F. Misuse and abuse of pregabalin and gabapentin: cause for concern? *CNS Drugs.* 2014 Jun;28(6):491–496.

22. Marvizon JC, Grady EF, Stefani E, Bunnett NW, Mayer EA. Substance P release in the dorsal horn assessed by receptor internalization: NMDA receptors counteract a tonic inhibition by GABA(B) receptors. *Eur J Neurosci.* 1999;11:417–426.

23. Trinkley KE, Nahata MC. Treatment of irritable bowel syndrome. *J Clin Pharm Ther.* 2011 Jun;36(3):275–282.

24. Sullivan MD, Howe CQ. Opioid therapy for chronic pain in the United States: promises and perils. *Pain.* 2013 Dec;154(Suppl 1):S94–S100.

25. Manchikanti L et al., American Society of Interventional Pain Physicians. American Society of Interventional Pain Physicians (ASIPP) guidelines

for responsible opioid prescribing in chronic non-cancer pain: Part I—evidence assessment. *Pain Physician*. 2012 Jul;15(3 Suppl): S1–S65.

26. Butler SF, Budman SH, Fernandez KC, Fanciullo GJ, Jamison RN. Cross-validation of a screener to predict opioid misuse in chronic pain patients (SOAPP-R). *J Addict Med*. 2009;3(2):66–73.

27. Butler SF, Budman SH, Fanciullo GJ, Jamison RN. Cross validation of the current opioid misuse measure to monitor chronic pain patients on opioid therapy. *Clin J Pain*. 2010;26(9):770–776.

28. Chou R, Cruciani RA, Fiellin DA, et al. Methadone safety: a clinical practice guideline from the American Pain Society and College on problems of drug dependence, in collaboration with the Heart Rhythm Society. *J Pain*. 2014;15(4):321–337.

29. Brennan MJ. The effect of opioid therapy on endocrine function. *Am J Med*. 2013;126(3 Suppl 1):S12–S18.

30. Pasero C, McCaffery M. Opioid-induced hyperalgesia. *J Perianesth Nurs*. 2012;27(1):46–50.

31. Cheong YC1, Smotra G, Williams AC. Non-surgical interventions for the management of chronic pelvic pain. *Cochrane Database Syst Rev*. 2014 Mar 5;3:CD008797. doi: 10.1002/14651858. CD008797.pub2

32. Rogalski MJ, Kellogg-Spadt S, Hoffmann AR, Fariello JY, Whitmore KE. Retrospective chart review of vaginal diazepam suppository use in high-tone pelvic floor dysfunction. *Int Urogynecol J*. 2010;21:895–899.

6

Dyspareunia and Vulvodynia

*ADEOTI OSHINOWO, ALIN IONESCU, TANYA E. ANIM,
AND GEORGINE LAMVU*

Sexual pain is a common symptom that can have devastating effects on a woman's quality of life and her social and sexual relationships. Research shows that sexual pain is often described by medical providers as *dyspareunia* or *vulvodynia*, and both conditions are associated with significant burden on the healthcare system.[1] Despite the reported high prevalence of these disorders, only one in five women seek help for their pain.[2,3]

The focus of this chapter will be to discuss dyspareunia and vulvodynia as chronic pain syndromes and to provide the reader with a basic understanding of the definition, clinical presentation, and related pathology. This chapter will also review the basic framework for how patients with these conditions should be evaluated and treated.

METHODOLOGY

Relevant research about dyspareunia was identified by searching the biomedical and social sciences databases. Seven research databases were searched for publications from 2005 through to the present (2014), with key articles obtained primarily from PubMed, Ovid, Clinical Key, Cumulative Index to Nursing and Allied Health Literature (CINAHL), and the Cochrane Library. In order to ensure that relevant studies were not missed, the search terms remained broad. These were Medical Subject Headings (MeSH) term/keywords "dyspareunia," and "cervical pain," plus secondary terms in MeSH/keyword/title, "physical examination," "external," "bimanual," "speculum," and truncated language such as "diagnosis" and "pain." Material included was limited to include articles published or available in the English language only. A comprehensive search was made of internet and print resources, including the Agency for Healthcare Research

and Quality (ARHQ), National Guidelines Clearinghouse and the fifth edition of the *Diagnostic and Statistical Manual of Mental Disorders* (DSM-5). Bibliographies of all relevant reviews and primary studies were hand-searched to identify articles not captured by electronic searches.

DEFINITIONS

Dyspareunia is recurrent or persistent genital pain associated with sexual intercourse.[4] The term "dyspareunia" comes from the Greek word "dyspareunos," meaning "bed partners not fitting together."[5] Usually dyspareunia is a symptom of an underlying condition rather than a diagnosis in and of itself. It may be present as a part of a constellation of symptoms from a variety of medical problems that affect the vulva, vagina, and pelvis. Although related, dyspareunia and vulvodynia are two separate entities. Dyspareunia is present either just before, during, or immediately following intercourse. This differentiates it from other pelvic pain syndromes such as vulvodynia in which pain may be present without provocation, or provoked by activities such as intercourse, tampon insertion, when the vulva is touched by clothing, or during movements such as sitting.

Expert authors have used the following terms to describe types of dyspareunia[6]:

- Situational: Pain with intercourse that is limited to specific situations, positions, or a particular partner.
- General Dyspareunia: Pain that is not limited to a specific situation, position, or partner.
- Primary Dyspareunia: Pain with intercourse that has been present since initial intercourse.

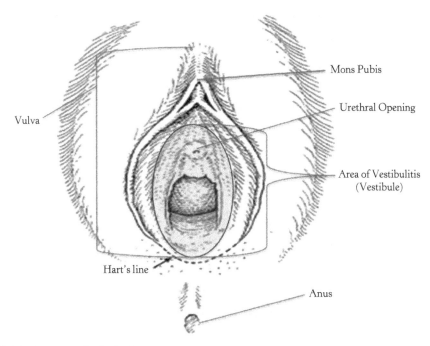

FIGURE 6.1: Anatomy of vulvodynia.

- Secondary Dyspareunia: Pain with intercourse that occurs after a period of pain-free intercourse.

For the purposes of this chapter, we will limit discussion to two types of dyspareunia—superficial and deep.

- Superficial Dyspareunia (SD): Pain limited to the vulvar vestibule or vaginal introitus.[5] This is associated with conditions such as vaginal dermatoses, atrophic vaginitis, and vulvovaginitis.
- Deep Dyspareunia (DD): Pain experienced with deep penetration of the vagina. Typically, this pain has been associated with conditions such as endometriosis, adhesions, fibroids, and cervicitis.[5,7,8]

Unlike dyspareunia, which may have multiple causes; vulvodynia is a chronic lower genital pain syndrome of unknown etiology that manifests as pain and occasional erythema of the vulva without obvious evidence of infectious, dermatological, or neurological cause.[9–11] Patients may present with complaints of vulvar stinging, rawness, burning, and/or irritation.[12,13] The International Society for the Study of Vulvovaginal Disease (ISSVD) recommends that vulvodynia be classified as *generalized* to the entire vulva or *localized* to the vestibule (Figure 6.1).

These two categories can be further subcategorized (Table 6.1) as "provoked vulvodynia" (i.e., with tampon use or sexual activity), "unprovoked vulvodynia" (occurring spontaneously), and "mixed" (both provoked and unprovoked).[14–16] Throughout this chapter, provoked vulvodynia (PVD) will refer to both localized and generalized forms. Pain described as "burning" is highly indicative of PVD.[17]

Continuous pain without any identifiable provoking stimuli is classical for generalized unprovoked vulvodynia, and the pain is often

TABLE 6.1 CLASSIFICATION OF VULVODYNIA AND DYSPAREUNIA

Vulvodynia	Dyspareunia
- Generalized	- Superficial
- Provoked	
- Unprovoked	
- Mixed	
- Localized	
- Provoked	- Deep
- Unprovoked	
- Mixed	

described as severe enough to interfere with wearing clothing, walking, sitting and sleeping.

EPIDEMIOLOGY

The prevalence of vulvodynia is estimated at 3–16% among American women.[16,18] In a recent survey-based study among 2,542 Michigan women, 2,269 of whom completed the survey, it was found that the weighted prevalence of vulvodynia was 8.3%.[16] Interestingly, in this study, African American women were less likely than Caucasian women to screen positive for vulvodynia; although the prevalence among African American women was also substantial (4.2% African American vs. 9.3% Caucasian). Additionally, the researchers found an increased prevalence of vulvodynia among Hispanic women (15.6%) compared to Caucasian women (however, it should be noted that only 2.8% of the population studied identified themselves as Hispanic). The authors postulated that these differences in the prevalence among racial and ethnic groups may reflect a true difference in prevalence, or may reflect differences in symptom reporting or in interpretation of "pain" or "discomfort."[16]

Due to varying definitions of dyspareunia, quantifying the incidence and prevalence of the condition is often difficult, and sources may cite widely ranging figures. The prevalence of dyspareunia in men ranges from 1–5%.[19,20] In the United States, the prevalence of dyspareunia ranges from 12–21% among adult women.[21] One study involving 251 sexually active adolescent females (ages 12–19 years old) also demonstrated a prevalence of 20%.[21] The World Health Organization (WHO) sponsored a meta-analysis of subtypes of chronic pelvic pain. In this meta-analysis it was found that, based on 54 studies with a total of 35,973 participants, the prevalence of dyspareunia was 8–21.1% worldwide. The rates of dyspareunia also differed by country. For instance, the rate of dyspareunia was 1.1% in Sweden, while it was found to be 45% in the US studies.[22]

Kao et al. further delineated many of the issues in acquiring accurate data regarding the prevalence of dyspareunia. Some of the problems they point out are that in many dyspareunia studies they reviewed, only sexually active women were queried regarding dyspareunia. This may lead to selection bias and under-reporting, since women who were not surveyed may have not been sexually active due to the pain they experienced when previously sexually active. The authors also found that many studies did not distinguish subtypes of dyspareunia such as vaginal dryness and soreness,[23] leading to additional selection or response bias.

The impact of dyspareunia on women's lives is poorly studied; however, some information is available about vulvodynia. Not surprisingly, vulvodynia is associated with very poor health-related quality of life, sexual dysfunction, and high rates of psychological distress such as depression and anxiety.[24–31] Vulvodynia patients are also two to three times more likely to have one or more other idiopathic chronic pain conditions such as fibromyalgia, interstitial cystitis (IC), temporomandibular joint disorder (TMJ), or irritable bowel syndrome.[16] The effects of vulvodynia extend past the patient, her family, and her friends. The economic impact to patients and to society associated with vulvodynia has been estimated at $8,862 per patient per 6 *months*; $6,043 (68%) direct healthcare costs, $2,265 (26%) indirect costs, and $553 (6%) direct non-healthcare costs. Based on an annual prevalence of 3–7%,[32] the national economic burden of vulvodynia in the United States ranges from $31 to $72 billion annually.[33]

ETIOLOGY

Vulvodynia is essentially a diagnosis made upon the exclusion of other causes of vulvar pain, for which no obvious etiology can be found.[1] Dyspareunia, on the other hand, is a symptom that may be associated with many other medical conditions (Table 6.2). Dyspareunia may be more common in specific subsets of women. For example, dyspareunia is four times more frequent in women with endometriosis than in controls.[34] Endometriosis affects up to 10% of reproductive-aged women[35] and deep dyspareunia is more commonly associated with endometriosis than is superficial dyspareunia. In fact, superficial dyspareunia is rarely seen in endometriosis, with only a few case reports of vulvar or hymeneal endometriosis noted in literature. Dyspareunia is also especially common in post-menopausal women. In this group of women, the pain is thought to be due to vaginal atrophy, and a substantial proportion of women report improvement in symptoms when they are treated with vaginal topical estrogen therapy. In the smaller percentage of women who do not improve with estrogen therapy, it is important to consider other causes of dyspareunia.[36]

TABLE 6.2 CONDITIONS ASSOCIATED WITH VULVODYNIA

Condition	Definition	Associated Signs and Symptoms
Endometriosis	Occurs when endometrial glandular and/or stromal cells grow outside of the uterine cavity	Infertility/subfertility, dysmenorrhea, abdominal or pelvic pain, ovarian cysts[23,25,26]
Lichen Planus	Inflammatory autoimmune disorder involving keratinized and mucosal surfaces	Itching, burning, postcoital bleeding, dyspareunia, superficial dyspareunia,[27] and pain
Lichen Sclerosis	Chronic, progressive, inflammatory skin condition found most often in the anogenital region	Intense vulvar itching. Skin may appear white, thickened, and excoriated, with edema and resorption of the labia minora, superficial dyspareunia[28,29]
Vaginismus	Involuntary vaginal muscle spasm interfering with sexual intercourse	Superficial (insertional) dyspareunia[30–32]
Vulvovaginal Atrophy (VVA)	Occurs as a result of decreased estrogen and results in thinness of the vaginal mucosa and/or vulvar epithelium, which becomes pale and dry. If the tissues also become inflamed it is termed *atrophic vaginitis*	Dryness, irritation, vaginal bleeding, superficial and deep dyspareunia[4]
Fibroids	Benign uterine tumors that consist of uterine smooth muscle	Superficial dyspareunia, deep dyspareunia[33,34]
Vulvovaginal Candidiasis	Vaginal infection caused by one of the yeast species, most commonly *C. albicans, C. glabrata,* and *C. tropicalis*	Superficial dyspareunia. Vulvovaginal pruritus (50%), vulvovaginal swelling (24%), and dysuria (33%)
Pelvic Inflammatory Disease	Polymicrobial infection of the upper genital tract, typically associated with gonorrhea and/or chlamydia infections	Deep dyspareunia[37,38]
Postpartum State	May be a result of morphological and hormonal changes of the pelvic floor during pregnancy or following delivery, or sequel from vaginal laceration or episiotomy	Deep or superficial dyspareunia[39,40]
Pelvic Floor Surgery	Long-term complications such as pelvic pain and dyspareunia may be as high as 25%	Superficial and deep dyspareunia[41–44]
Sexual Abuse	May include rape or molestation, with or without vaginal penetration	Deep dyspareunia[37]
Pelvic Floor Myalgia	Situation in which the pelvic floor muscles do no not relax or may even contract when relaxation is functionally needed	Superficial and deep dyspareunia[45]
Adnexal Masses	Endometrioma, malignancy, functional ovarian cysts, etc.	Deep dyspareunia
Interstitial Cystitis	Clinical diagnosis with unclear etiology characterized by urinary frequency and urgency, also accompanied by pelvic pain	Urinary urgency and frequency, dysuria, pelvic pain, and deep dyspareunia[46]
Irritable Bowel Syndrome	Chronic disorder characterized by abdominal pain or discomfort associated either with constipation, diarrhea, or alternating symptoms of constipation and diarrhea	Deep dyspareunia

CLINICAL PRESENTATION AND EVALUATION

Patient History

In order to identify sexual pain, the healthcare provider should assume an active role. Presently, about 80% of the time, the patient, rather than the physician, initiates the conversation regarding sexual issues.[37]

Roos et al.[3] proposed a simple screening general "health questionnaire," in which sexual function could be assessed via three questions:

1. Are you sexually active? (yes/no)
2. Is sex painful? (yes/no)
3. Do you have any problems with sex? (yes/no)

Of the 437 women enrolled in this study who had a sexual complaint, 73% complained of dyspareunia, but the complaint was "bothersome" in only 45% of the cases. Thus, upon analysis of the collected data, it became apparent that a fourth question, to address the issue of personal distress, should be introduced in the questionnaire:

4. Are any of your sexual problems bothersome? (yes/no)

Therefore, according to the International Consensus Development Conference on Female Sexual Dysfunction (FSD), a clinical intervention is necessary only if the sexual problem produces sexual distress.

Considering the devastating effects on patients' lives, if sexual pain is identified, then obtaining a thorough and extensive history of the symptoms and associated conditions is crucial. A nonjudgemental approach should be used, maintaining neutrality about sexual practices or preference. The goals of the interview are to[1]:

- Gather relevant information about the patient and their symptoms
- Validate that the patients' symptoms are real
- Exclude other clinical diagnoses that may be contributing to the symptoms
- Educate and reassure

A detailed pain history should be taken to assess the degree of symptoms. The use of pain diaries, quality-of-life questionnaires, and multidimensional pain scales such as the McGill Pain Questionnaire may be more helpful than unidimensional pain scales (such as the Visual Analogue Scale) because they allow patients to provide clinicians with a better description of the quality and intensity of their pain as well as the impact the pain has on their lives.[15,38] Useful questions in evaluating the characteristics of the pain include[17]:

- Onset—lifetime or episode
- Timing—relative to intercourse (before, during or after)
- Location—superficial (entry), or deep
- Intensity
- Duration—continuous, intermittent
- Quality—women with dyspareunia often use terms other than "pain" to describe their discomfort: *itching, burning, stinging, irritation, stabbing* and/or *rawness*.[1]
- Association with other circumstances (specific partner, menstrual cycle, intercourse position)
- Provoked or unprovoked (sexual, nonsexual, or both)
- Precipitating or ameliorating factors
- Previous treatments

Presence of sexual pain should be viewed in the context of sexual difficulty and dysfunction. Among women who have sexual dysfunction, approximately 26% experience pain.[5] Since dyspareunia and sexual dysfunction are closely linked, healthcare providers should inquire specifically about the presence of desire, arousal, adequate lubrication, anorgasmia, vaginismus, and partner-related problems. Identification of psychosexual morbidity is important, as psychosexual counseling may be necessary to complement the medical treatment of pain.[15] A brief reference for the normal sexual cycle is provided in Figure 6.2.[39]

The sexual history is best taken when the patient is clothed and has spent some time interacting with the healthcare provider. Subsequent visits may be required to ensure patient comfort, full disclosure, and complete assessment of the history. Once spousal and sexual abuse has been ruled out, it is generally helpful to invite the partner to be present during the evaluation. Smith et al.[40] showed that partners of patients with PVD may be negatively impacted with regard to some sexual and physical aspects of their relationship; however, Pazmany and colleagues[41] confirmed that partners can also add

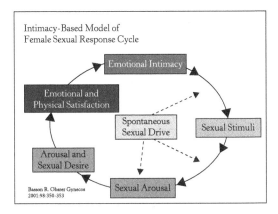

Basson R. Obstet Gynecos
2001;98:350-353

FIGURE 6.2: The stages of the normal sexual cycle.

Reprinted with permission from Basson R. *Obstet Gynecol.* 2001. Aug;98(2):350–353.

insight into the evaluation, thus supporting the involvement of partners in the treatment process.

As in any patient who presents with painful symptoms, the interview of women with dyspareunia should include a full review of the past medical and surgical history. The answers to these questions may help identify additional etiological factors and guide the diagnostic process. For example, entry pain involving the entire vulvar area may suggest vulvitis, vulvar dermatoses, or vulvodynia; while the pain concentrated only at the vaginal opening might be due to vestibulitis, vaginismus, lack of lubrication, or vulvovaginitis. Healthcare providers may choose to characterize the pain by infectious, inflammatory, functional, traumatic, anatomical, or musculoskeletal causes, as listed in Table 6.3.

General Physical Exam

The physical examination should begin with a global assessment of the patient's mood and affect,

before proceeding to a full musculoskeletal and vaginal exam (Figure 6.3). The goals of physical exam are to localize and possibly recreate some of the pain or discomfort, determine the type and location of the pathology, exclude other diagnoses, educate the patient regarding the normal anatomy and sexual function, and reassure her if no pathology is uncovered.[1,6]

Pelvic examinations can be anxiety-producing and painful for a significant number of patients. Before the examination, it is essential to ask the patient regarding her previous experiences with this type of exam.[6,17] A few measures can be taken to facilitate a successful examination[42]:

- Patient should be given as much control as possible over the process.
- Patient should be told what is going to be done before the exam.
- Patient should be made aware of her ability to control the pace of the examination and to terminate the examination at any point.
- Patient should have visual access to the site of examination, if desired.
- Use of a narrow speculum or no speculum.
- Use of a topical anesthetic.

While performing the pelvic examination, the physician should instruct the patient to report if pain is elicited and if the pain experienced during the examination is similar to what she usually feels.

External Musculoskeletal Exam

A systematic pelvic and low back exam should be performed seeking evidence of any pelvic

---

TABLE 6.3 CAUSES OF DYSPAREUNIA AND VULVODYNIA CHARACTERIZED BY COMPONENTS OF THE PATIENT'S HISTORY

History	Conditions
Infectious	Chlamydia, gonorrhea, herpes, syphilis, trichomonas, candida
Inflammatory	Lichen, irritant/contact dermatitis, atrophic vaginitis, IC[a], IBD[b]
Functional	Menstrual history, sexual dysfunction (arousal, anorgasmia)
Traumatic/Surgical	Fissures, mesh erosions, incontinence and prolapse procedures
Anatomical	Imperforated hymen, vaginal septum, uterine fibroids, adnexal masses
Musculoskeletal	Joint or muscle pain, limited mobility, spine or pelvis conditions

[a]Interstitial cystitis
[b]Irritable bowel disorder

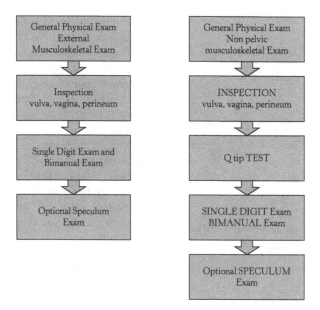

FIGURE 6.3: Components of the dyspareunia and vulvodynia physical examination.

pathology that might be contributing to dyspareunia. Specifically, the musculoskeletal evaluation should involve observation of the patient's gait and posture in the sitting and standing position. Patients with chronic vulvar or vaginal pain often lean to one side in an attempt to avoid the painful side. This often leads to changes in the spine curvature, asymmetry, hypertonicity, and loss of range of motion in the pelvic joints and muscles.[43]

Vulvar Examination

Visual inspection of the external genitalia, perineum, perianal areas of the groin, and the pubic mons is the first step of the vulvar examination. Careful visualization can reveal a number of possible causes for pain, including infection, fissures, inflammation, trauma, and dermatoses.[17] Diffuse or focal erythema and thickening can occur with subclinical human papilloma virus infection, bacterial vaginosis, candidiasis, or dermatitis (i.e., lichen simplex, chronicus or vulvar eczema, or irritants), while thin, dry tissue can suggest atrophy or lichen sclerosis.[6,9,17] Next, a brief neurosensory exam of the vulva and perineum can be done by gently touching the sensory dermatomes T12, L1, S2/S3, S4/S5, and S1 with a cotton swab. This exam is easily done with the cotton and the wooden portion of a cotton-tipped applicator. Clinicians can distinguish between mechanical allodynia and hyperalgesia.[44] Mechanical allodynia is

characterized as pain in response "to a stimulus that does not normally provoke pain,"[44] such as the cotton swab. That is, a patient would report "pain" instead of "cotton ball" when touched with the cotton portion of the applicator. Mechanical allodynia is further differentiated as "static," when it occurs in response to light pressure; or "dynamic" if it occurs in response to light brushing. Conversely, hyperalgesia is characterized as increased sensitivity to a painful or *noxious* stimulus.[44] In this case the patient would report "pain" instead of just a "pin prick" when touched with the wooden portion of the applicator. With this type of sensory examination, the provider can determine if the participant has allodynia, hyperalgesia, hypersensitivity, normal sensation, and a normal anal reflex ("anal wink"). Because pain is a subjective experience, it is recommended that the sensory examination should begin by first educating the patient on the cotton-tip examination such that the baseline is established as "cotton ball" when she is touched with the cotton portion of the applicator, or "pin prick" when she is touched with the wooden portion. Patients should also be instructed that, if they feel a painful sensation, the pain should be quantified using a visual analogue scale (0–10), where 10 is the worst imaginable pain.[44]

Using a similar cotton-tipped applicator technique, the examiner can then proceed to sensory examination of the vulvar vestibule (Figure 6.1).

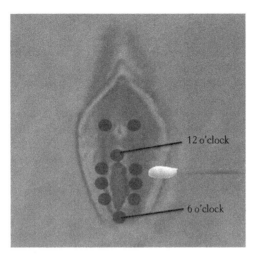

FIGURE 6.4: Cotton-tip sensory evaluation of the vestibule.

Image courtesy of Ronnie J. Fowler II.

Six anatomical sites on the vestibule are determined with reference to the conventional "clock face," with 12 o'clock and 6 o'clock positions corresponding to the anterior and posterior position on the midline, respectively (Figure 6.4).[18]

Women with PVD usually report hyperalgesia and allodynia characterized as exquisite pain located specifically in the vestibule.[1] On the other hand, women with conditions affecting the general anogenital region (infections, dermatoses, neuropathic process) may report a more diffuse pain, including the perineum and labia majora,[17] in addition to having visible inflammatory changes of the skin. In addition, differentiating neuropathic from inflammatory processes can have significant implications for treatment selection and thus is an important part of the examination in women with dyspareunia or vulvodynia.

Single Digit Internal Musculoskeletal and Bi-Manual Examination

The next step in examination should involve a vaginal evaluation with index finger insertion just past the introitus, with as little vestibular contact as possible. This is regarded as the most reliable method for evaluating pelvic muscle tenderness in muscles such as the levator ani, piriformis, and internal obturator.[43,45]

The index finger can be used to palpate the lateral, anterior, and posterior walls of the vagina, the urethra, and pelvic floor muscles; checking for any specific areas of tenderness, any involuntary spasm of the muscles of the introitus, levator sling, and any scars from previous surgery or episiotomy. Having the patient contract the muscles of the pelvic floor while the examiner has the index finger in the vagina helps assess the tone of the pelvic floor and her ability to contract and relax the muscles.[43] Patients with pelvic floor dysfunction will often demonstrate poor contractile function and a tense pelvic floor resting tone.[1,43]

There is evidence that women with PVD can present with pelvic floor muscle dysfunction, characterized by increased pelvic floor muscle tone (i.e., hypertonicity) and activity (i.e., hyperactivity) at rest, poor relaxation capacity following contraction, heightened contractile responses due to pain, and decreased extensibility of the tissues at the vaginal opening. In addition, one study found that women with vaginismus exhibited significantly more hypertonicity and poorer muscle strength in comparison to women with PVD, who in turn had more dysfunction in these areas than non-affected women.[46] Reproducible pain on single-digit palpation of the anterior vaginal wall may provide clues to an inflammatory process involving the vestibule, like vestibulodynia; or involving the bladder, like trigonitis, interstitial cystitis, chronic urethritis, or urethral diverticulum.[6,47]

At the end of the single-digit examination, an abdominal hand can be added to further assess the condition of the uterus, cul-de-sac, and adnexa, and rule out pelvic pathology (masses, adhesions) that may give rise to deep dyspareunia.[1]

Speculum Exam

If tolerated by the patient, a speculum examination should be done, using a small-size, warm, well-lubricated instrument. All efforts should be made to insert the speculum through the hymeneal ring without touching the urethra or vulvar vestibule.[48] Insertion of the speculum should be slow, to allow the pelvic floor muscles to accommodate the speculum. During this portion of the exam, the provider can visualize the internal vaginal tissues for the presence of fissures, vaginal atrophy, and vaginal depth.[17] At this time, cervical cultures, a pap smear, along with vaginal secretions wet-mount should be obtained. Lastly, the cervix can be lightly touched with a cotton-tip applicator to determine if there is any cervical allodynia, a condition that is associated with deep dyspareunia and can result from cervicitis or, more rarely seen, post-excisional therapy for cervical dysplasia.

Diagnostic Tests

A vaginal pH and a sample for Gram stain and cultures should be obtained from the patients with vaginal discharge. Urine cultures, vaginal wet preps, and testing for sexually transmitted infections (STIs: gonorrhea, chlamydia, candida, trichomonas, herpes and syphilis) should be obtained in order to rule out specific infectious causes of dyspareunia.

A normal vaginal pH excludes atrophy and bacterial vaginosis (BV). Large numbers of white blood cells (WBCs) suggest candidiasis, lichen, trichomoniasis, gonorrheal or chlamydial infection, or desquamative vaginitis. Small vulvar biopsies can be helpful in identifying vulvar dermatoses that result in lichenification.

Other tests, like urodynamic testing (incontinence), colposcopy (biopsy of visible lesions, abnormal pap smear, or presence of high-risk human papilloma virus [HPV] strains), cystoscopy (suspected interstitial cystititis), ultrasound or other pelvic imaging (fibroids, ovarian cysts, endometriosis), are indicated on an individual basis.[6,49]

TREATMENT

It is rare that dyspareunia is caused by one factor alone. Organic, musculoskeletal, and psychosocial etiologies, as noted above, can all contribute to dyspareunia. Therefore, most types of long-standing dyspareunia will have overlapping treatments, and an individualized multidisciplinary approach to treatment of dyspareunia is recommended.[1,17] Experts in gynecology, physical therapy, pain management, sexual therapy, and mental health professionals specializing in cognitive and behavioral therapy ideally should work in concert in an effort to treat all possible factors associated with the patient's experience of dyspareunia.

The importance the provider's and the patient's agreement about treatment selection and treatment timeline cannot be overemphasized. Informing the patient from the beginning that treating her pain will be a long process, and that the problem is approached from many different angles, will help align her expectations. Doing so will increase the likelihood of patient compliance with the treatment plan.

Dyspareunia, as with all symptomatology, is a *symptom* whose underlying cause must be treated first. For example, there are both hormonal and non-hormonal treatments for vaginal atrophy and vaginal dryness; topical corticosteroid treatments for dermatoses; pharmacological and surgical treatments for endometriosis; antifungal and antimicrobial therapies for infections causing vulvovaginitis; physical therapy for pelvic floor myalgia; and surgical interventions for uterine fibroids, adnexal pathology, adhesions, and pelvic organ prolapse. Medical and more conservative therapy is almost always preferable to surgery in patients who have a chronic pain diagnosis. It is important to acknowledge that, although the above pathologies are associated with dyspareunia, not all women who have these diagnoses have dyspareunia.

During treatment for dyspareunia, the patient must refrain from intercourse until the pain has resolved (or significantly improved) and until she feels comfortable doing so. Resuming intercourse with pain will only promote more pain and reinforce a cycle of fearful intercourse leading to more pain.[6,50] Treatment for deep dyspareunia caused by organic etiologies will be covered in subsequent chapters (i.e., endometriosis, painful bladder syndrome, pudendal neuralgia, pelvic vascular congestion), and therefore will only be mentioned briefly here.

Validation, Education, and Goal Setting

Often, the patient experiencing dyspareunia or vulvodynia has at some point wondered if it was "all in her head." Validation of the patient's pain, acknowledging that her pain is "real," and giving it a name will help legitimize the patient's pain to herself and her partner.[1] It is important to reeducate the patient and her partner in sexual attitudes and practices, sexual anatomy, physiology, and behavior; thus, giving the patient some knowledge and therefore control of her situation.[6] Education on vulvar care measures is advised: including, but not limited to, avoidance of irritants such as perfumed soaps, detergents, dyes, douches, vaginal sprays, scented tampons; wearing cotton underwear and loose-fitting clothing during the day and none at night; using cotton menstrual pads; gently cleaning the vulva with water and pat-drying (and after cleansing); and using a preservative-free emollient to hold in moisture and provide a barrier to irritation.[38] When the patient resumes intercourse, use of lubrication prior to and during intercourse should be advised.

Medical Therapy

Many pharmacological treatments have been tried to ameliorate dyspareunia and vulvodynia (Table 6.4). Very few of these treatments have been vetted with randomized controlled trials or have sufficient evidence supporting their use for vulvodynia; however, there is a growing consensus amongst vulvar pain specialists about which medical treatments are beneficial.[1,38]

Hormones and Hormone Modulators

Vulvovaginal atrophy (VVA) is a common symptom in the postmenopausal state. Caused by estrogen deficiency, VVA, as mentioned previously, can cause significant dyspareunia. Hormonal medications, such as estrogen containing pills and ointments, progestin-only pills, and newer selective estrogen receptor modulators (SERMs) such as ospemifene and intravaginal Dehydroepiandrosterone (DHEA), can be used to treat dyspareunia caused by VVA. Estrogen therapy restores normal vaginal pH levels, and thickens and revascularizes the epithelium. Superficial cells are increased, and symptoms of atrophy are alleviated.[51] SERMS and intravaginal DHEA modulate estrogenic effects by indirectly stimulating estrogen receptors in the body.

Emollients and Topical Analgesics

Non-hormonal topical emollients can also be used as vaginal moisturizers targeted to increase lubrication during sexual intercourse and provide a barrier, thus specifically treating dyspareunia.[52,53] Topical analgesics, such as lidocaine ointment, have been shown to significantly alleviate pain with intercourse.[54,55] Both emollients and topical analgesics can be compounded with any other topical therapy to provide enhanced effects.

Antidepressants and Anticonvulsants/Neuroleptics

Use of compounded tricyclic antidepressants (TCAs) in a water-based ointment has been shown to provide moderate to excellent

TABLE 6.4 COMMON PHARMACOLOGICAL THERAPIES FOR DYSPAREUNIA AND VULVODYNIA

Drug Class (Route)	Indication	Type
Analgesics (Topical, Injectable)	SD[a], PVD[b]	Lidocaine, Marcaine
Hormones	SD, PVD	Premarin, Estrace, Norethindrone, Mirena
• Estrogens (Topical, Vaginal, Oral)	DD[c]	intrauterine device, DHEA
• Progestins (Oral, Implantable)		
• DHEA (Vaginal)		
SERMs (Oral)	PVS due to VVA[d]	Osphena, Letrozole
Antidepressants (Topical, Oral)	SD, PVD	Amitriptyline, Nortriptyline. Desipramine, Venlafaxine, Fluoxetine, Cymbalta
Anticonvulsants (Topical, Oral)	DD	Gabapentin, Pregabalin
Neuromuscular Blockers (Injectable)	SD, DD, PVD	Botox A
Muscle Relaxants	SD, DD, PVD	Valium, Flexeril, Klonopin
GnRH Agonists (Injectable)	DD due to endometriosis	Leuprolide

[a]Superficial dyspareunia
[b]Provoked dyspareunia
[c]Deep dyspareunia
[d]Vulvovaginal atrophy

improvement of dyspareunia symptoms in patients with vulvodynia.[38,49] Amitriptyline is the best-studied tricyclic; however, the side-effect profile might influence the patient's compliance with treatment.[15] If patients cannot tolerate or are not responding to use of TCAs, anticonvulsants can also be used. Gabapentin is becoming increasingly popular as both an oral and a topical treatment for vulvodynia that is thought to be due to neuropathy. Currently, a randomized control trial is being conducted on the use of extended release gabapentin for the treatment of PVD-related symptoms, including dyspareunia.[56]

Injectables
Pudendal nerve blockade has been used to treat vulvodynia caused by neuralgia.[57] Injection of botulinum toxin A in to the pelvic floor muscles has been shown in some studies to decrease dyspareunia caused by pelvic floor myalgia and contracture.[58,59]

Other Drugs
Deep dyspareunia believed to be caused by endometriosis has been shown to be relieved significantly more when adding gonadotropin-releasing hormone (GnRH) agonist to surgical treatment of endometriosis vs. adding placebo to surgical treatment.[60]

Surgical Therapy
Especially with deep dyspareunia, when there is an underlying organic etiology, surgery can be helpful in mitigating symptoms. Excision of endometriosis,[7,61] hysterectomy, removal of fibroids or adnexal pathology, pelvic organ prolapse procedures, or lysis of adhesions, in those with obvious pathology, could significantly alleviate deep dyspareunia in a patient. However, it is important to note that the surgery in and of itself can be a catalyst for pelvic pain and even dyspareunia in patients. In fact, a study by Vercellini et al. showed that, in patients who had already had one surgery for endometriosis, those who chose progestin-therapy for treatment over repeat surgery had significantly more relief of their pain.[62]

Superficial dyspareunia can be occasionally treated with vulvar surgery: for example, excision of the hymeneal remnant, or perineoplasty to release stenosis for postoperative stricture after colporrhaphy for pelvic organ prolapse. In select patients with vulvovestibulitis causing PVD, a vestibulectomy, in which the vestibule is excised and the vaginal mucosa is advanced to cover the defect, has been shown to alleviate dyspareunia.[63,64]

Physical Therapy
Pelvic floor physical therapy (PFPT) is an important and necessary adjunct to almost all treatment for dyspareunia.[65] A well-trained pelvic floor physical therapist uses techniques like biofeedback with surface electromyography, massage, dilators, and TENS (transcutaneous electrical nerve stimulation) units to help relax the pelvic floor muscles and retrain pain receptors that cause both deep and superficial dyspareunia.[65] PFPT has also been shown to be effective in treating PVD-related dyspareunia as well as sexual and cognitive correlates to PVD.[66] PFPT was also found to be helpful in preventing persistent dyspareunia after vestibulectomy.[67]

Cognitive and Behavioral Therapy
Cognitive behavioral therapy (CBT) has been shown to be effective in conjunction with other therapies, especially as it relates to superficial dyspareunia caused by vaginismus.[68] When patients are able to find a way to curtail their pain-hypervigilance, anxiety, and fear of pain, they are able to decrease their catastrophization of pain, therefore making intercourse less painful.[6,69]

PREVENTION
There is no one preventative measure for dyspareunia or vulvodynia. As noted above, it is important for the patient to be knowledgeable about vulvar care. With regard to the pelvic floor, teaching patients how to properly do pelvic floor exercises will allow them to learn to control their pelvic floor muscles, which may help them with relaxing the pelvic floor. Although Kegel exercises are often recommended in patients with poor pelvic support, Kegels can exacerbate dyspareunia in patients with dyspareunia due to levator ani myalgia.[70]

SUMMARY
The symptom of dyspareunia is multifactorial and requires a multidisciplinary approach to achieve optimal care. Patients with dyspareunia and vulvodynia are a very sensitive population who require attentiveness, attention to detail, and assistance in coordinating care. Ideally, concomitant involvement of a gynecologist who specializes in pelvic pain, a pelvic floor physical therapist, a mental health professional who

specializes in sexual health, and a pain specialist would augment patient care. Making the patient and her partner active participants in her care would also assist in developing a healing environment where she can feel comfortable and optimistic about her care.

ACKNOWLEDGEMENTS

The authors would like to thank the National Vulvodynia Association for providing generous grant support to enable the authors to study vulvodynia; Kaamna Mirchandani (research coordinator and manuscript editor); and Ronnie J. Fowler II (graphic designer and illustrator).

REFERENCES

1. Sadownik LA. Etiology, diagnosis, and clinical management of vulvodynia. *Int J Women Health.* 2014;6:437–449.
2. Moreira EDJr, Brock G, Glasser DB, et al. Help-seeking behaviour for sexual problems: the global study of sexual attitudes and behaviors. *Int J Clin Pract.* 2005;59(1):6–16.
3. Roos AM, Sultan AH, Thakar R. Sexual problems in the gynecology clinic: are we making a mountain out of a molehill? *Int Urogynecol J.* 2012;23(2):145–152.
4. Amato P. Categories of female sexual dysfunction. *Obstet Gynecol Clin N Am.* 2006;33(4):527–534.
5. MacNeill C. Dyspareunia. *Obstet Gynecol Clin N Am.* 2006;33(4):565–577, viii.
6. Howard F. Dyspareunia. In: Howard FM, Perry CP, Carter JE, El-Minawi AM, eds. *Pelvic Pain: Diagnosis and Management.* New York: Lippincott; 2000:112–121.
7. Ferrero S, Abbamonte LH, Giordano M, et al. Deep dyspareunia and sex life after laparoscopic excision of endometriosis. *Hum Reprod.* 2007;22(4):1142–1148.
8. Vercellini P, Somigliana E, Buggio L, et al. "I can't get no satisfaction": deep dyspareunia and sexual functioning in women with rectovaginal endometriosis. *Fertil Steril.* 2012;98(6):1503–1511 e1501.
9. American Menopause Society. *Menopause Practice: A Clinician's Guide.* Mayfield Heights, OH: The North American Menopause Society; 2010.
10. Reed BD. Vulvodynia: diagnosis and management. *Am Fam Physician.* 2006;73(7):1231–1238.
11. Boardman LA, Stockdale CK. Sexual pain. *Clin Obstet Gynecol.* 2009;52(4):682–690.
12. Arnold LD, Bachmann GA, Rosen R, et al. Assessment of vulvodynia symptoms in a sample of US women: a prevalence survey with a nested case control study. *Am J Obstet Gynecol.* 2007;196(2):128.e1-6.
13. Edwards L. New concepts in vulvodynia. *Am J Obstet Gynecol.* 2003;189(3 Suppl):S24–S30.
14. Munday P, Green J, Randall C, et al. Vulval vestibulitis: a common cause of dyspareunia? *BJOG.* 2005;112(4):500–503.
15. Nunns D, Mandal D, Byrne M, et al. Guidelines for the management of vulvodynia. *Br J Dermatol.* 2010;162(6):1180–1185.
16. Reed BD, Harlow SD, Sen A, et al. Prevalence and demographic characteristics of vulvodynia in a population-based sample. *Am J Obstet Gynecol.* 2012;206(2):170.e1-9.
17. Meana M, Binik YM. Dyspareunia: causes and treatments (including provoked vestibulodynia). In Vercellini P, ed. *Chronic Pelvic Pain.* Oxford, UK: Blackwell Publishing Ltd.; 2011:125–136.
18. Moyal-Barracco M, Lynch PJ. ISSVD terminology and classification of vulvodynia: a historical perspective. *J Reprod Med.* 2004;49(10):772–777.
19. Pitts M, Ferris J, Smith A, et al. Prevalence and correlates of three types of pelvic pain in a nationally representative sample of Australian men. *J Sexual Med.* 2008;5(5):1223–1229.
20. Bancroft J. *Human Sexuality and Its Problems* Elsevier Health Sciences; 2009.
21. Landry T, Bergeron S. How young does vulvovaginal pain begin? Prevalence and characteristics of dyspareunia in adolescents. *J Sexual Med.* 2009; 6(4):927–935.
22. Latthe P, Latthe M, Say L, et al. WHO systematic review of prevalence of chronic pelvic pain: a neglected reproductive health morbidity. *BMC Public Health.* 2006;6:177.
23. Kao A, Binik YM, Amsel R, et al. Biopsychosocial predictors of postmenopausal dyspareunia: the role of steroid hormones, vulvovaginal atrophy, cognitive-emotional factors, and dyadic adjustment. *J Sexual Med.* 2012;9(8):2066–2076.
24. Arnold LD, Bachmann GA, Rosen R, et al. Vulvodynia: characteristics and associations with comorbidities and quality of life. *Obstet Gynecol.* 2006;107(3):617–624.
25. Gates EA, Galask RP. Psychological and sexual functioning in women with vulvar vestibulitis. *J Psychosom Obstet Gynaecol.* 2001;22(4):221–228.
26. Meana M, Binik YM, Khalife S, et al. Biopsychosocial profile of women with dyspareunia. *Obstet Gynecol.* 1997;90(4 Pt 1):583–589.
27. Van Lankveld JJ, Weijenborg PT, ter Kuile MM. Psychological profiles of and sexual function in women with vulvar vestibulitis and their partners. *Obstet Gynecol.* 1996;88(1):65–70.
28. Jadresic D, Barton S, Neill S, et al. Psychiatric morbidity in women attending a clinic for vulval problems—is there a higher rate in vulvodynia? *Int J STD AIDS.* 1993;4(4):237–239.

29. Stewart DE, Reicher AE, Gerulath AH, et al. Vulvo-dynia and psychological distress. *Obstet Gynecol.* 1994;84(4):587–590.

30. Nunns D, Mandal D. Psychological and psycho-sexual aspects of vulvar vestibulitis. *Genitourin Med.* 1997;73(6):541–544.

31. Koblenzer CS, Bostrom P. Chronic cutaneous dysesthesia syndrome: a psychotic phenomenon or a depressive symptom? *J Am Acad Dermatol.* 1994;30(2 Pt 2):370–374.

32. Reed BD, Legocki LJ, Plegue MA, et al. Factors associated with vulvodynia incidence. *Obstet Gynecol.* 2014;123(2 Pt 1):225–231.

33. Xie Y, Shi L, Xiong X, et al. Economic burden and quality of life of vulvodynia in the United States. *Curr Med Res Opin.* 2012;28(4):601–608.

34. Jarząbek-Bielecka G, Radomski D, Pawlaczyk M, et al. Dyspareunia as a sexual problem in women with endometriosis. *Archives of Perinatal Medicine*, 2010;16(1):51–53.

35. Ozawa Y, Murakami T, Terada Y, et al. Management of the pain associated with endometriosis: an update of the painful problems. *Tohoku J Exper Med.* 2006;210(3):175–188.

36. Kao A, Binik YM, Kapuscinski A, et al. Dyspareunia in postmenopausal women: a critical review. *Pain Res Management Canada.* 2008;13(3):243–254.

37. Shifren JL, Johannes CB, Monz BU, et al. Help-seeking behavior of women with self-reported distressing sexual problems. *J Women Health.* 2009;18(4):461–468.

38. Haefner HK, Collins ME, Davis GD, et al. The vulvodynia guideline. J Low Genit Tract Dis. 2005;9(1):40–51.

39. Basson R. Female sexual response: the role of drugs in the management of sexual dysfunction. *Obstet Gynecol.* 2001;98(2):350–353.

40. Smith KB, Pukall CF. Sexual function, relation-ship adjustment, and the relational impact of pain in male partners of women with provoked vulvar pain. *J Sexual Med.* 2014;11(5):1283–1293.

41. Pazmany E, Bergeron S, Verhaeghe J, et al. Sexual communication, dyadic adjustment, and psy-chosexual well-being in premenopausal women with self-reported dyspareunia and their part-ners: a controlled study. *J Sexual Med* 2015;12: 516–528.

42. Sutton KS, Pukall CF, Chamberlain S. Pain, psycho-social, sexual, and psychophysical characteristics of women with primary vs. secondary provoked vestibulodynia. *J Sexual Med.* 2009;6(1):205–214.

43. Gyang A, Hartman M, Lamvu G. Musculoskeletal causes of chronic pelvic pain: what a gynecologist should know. *Obstet Gynecol.* 2013;121(3):645–650.

44. Spicher CJ, Mathis F, Degrange B, et al. Static mechanical allodynia (SMA) is a paradoxical painful hypo-aesthesia: observations derived from neuropathic pain patients treated with somato-sensory rehabilitation. *Somatosens Mot Res.* 2008;25(1):77–92.

45. Montenegro ML, Mateus-Vasconcelos EC, Rosa e Silva JC, et al. Importance of pelvic muscle ten-derness evaluation in women with chronic pelvic pain. *Pain Med.* 2010;11(2):224–228.

46. Boyer SC, Goldfinger C, Thibault-Gagnon S, et al. Management of female sexual pain disorders. *Adv Psychosom Med.* 2011;31:83–104.

47. Welk BK, Teichman JM. Dyspareunia response in patients with interstitial cystitis treated with intravesical lidocaine, bicarbonate, and heparin. *Urology.* 2008;71(1):67–70.

48. Sung SC, Jeng CJ, Lin YC. Sexual health care for women with dyspareunia. *J Obstet Gynecol Taiwan.* 2011;50(3):268–274.

49. Pagano R, Wong S. Use of amitriptyline cream in the management of entry dyspareunia due to provoked vestibulodynia. *J Lower Genit Tract Dis.* 2012;16(4):394–397.

50. Howard FM, Perry CP, Carter JE, El-Minawi AM. *Dyspareunia Pelvic Pain Diagnosis and Management.* New York: Lippincott Williams & Wilkins; 2000:529.

51. Panjari M, Davis SR. Vaginal DHEA to treat meno-pause related atrophy: a review of the evidence. *Maturitas.* 2011;70(1):22–25.

52. Kingsberg S, Kellogg S, Krychman M. Treating dys-pareunia caused by vaginal atrophy: a review of treat-ment options using vaginal estrogen therapy. *Int J Women Health.* 2010;1:105–111.

53. Sutton KS, Boyer SC, Goldfinger C, et al. To lube or not to lube: experiences and perceptions of lubri-cant use in women with and without dyspareunia. *J Sexual Med.* 2012;9(1):240–250.

54. Zolnoun DA, Hartmann KE, Steege JF. Overnight 5% lidocaine ointment for treatment of vulvar ves-tibulitis. *Obstet Gynecol.* 2003;102(1):84–87.

55. Bohm-Starke N, Brodda-Jansen G, Linder J, et al. The result of treatment on vestibular and general pain thresholds in women with provoked vestibu-lodynia. *Clin J Pain.* 2007;23(7):598–604.

56. Brown CS, Foster DC, Wan JY, et al. Rationale and design of a multicenter randomized clinical trial of extended release gabapentin in provoked ves-tibulodynia and biological correlates of response. *Contemp Clin Trials.* 2013;36(1):154–165.

57. Rapkin AJ, McDonald JS, Morgan M. Multilevel local anesthetic nerve blockade for the treat-ment of vulvar vestibulitis syndrome. *Am J Obstet Gynecol.* 2008;198(1):41.e1-5.

58. Park AJ, Paraiso MF. Successful use of botulinum toxin type a in the treatment of refractory postop-erative dyspareunia. *Obstet Gynecol.* 2009;114(2 Pt 2):484–487.

59. Nesbitt-Hawes EM, Won H, Jarvis SK, et al. Improvement in pelvic pain with botulinum toxin type A—single vs. repeat injections. *Toxicon*. 2013;63:83–87.

60. Sesti F, Pietropolli A, Capozzolo T, et al. Hormonal suppression treatment or dietary therapy versus placebo in the control of painful symptoms after conservative surgery for endometriosis stage III–IV. A randomized comparative trial. *Fertil Steril*. 2007;88(6):1541–1547.

61. Deguara CS, Pepas L, Davis C. Does minimally invasive surgery for endometriosis improve pelvic symptoms and quality of life? *Curr Opin Obstet Gynecol*. 2012;24(4):241–244.

62. Vercellini P, Frattaruolo MP, Somigliana E, et al. Surgical versus low-dose progestin treatment for endometriosis-associated severe deep dyspareunia, II: effect on sexual functioning, psychological status and health-related quality of life. *Hum Reprod*. 2013;28(5):1221–1230.

63. Tommola P, Unkila-Kallio L, Paavonen J. Surgical treatment of vulvar vestibulitis: a review. *Acta Obstetricia et Gynecologica Scandinavica*. 2010; 89(11):1385–1395.

64. Tommola P, Unkila-Kallio L, Paavonen J. Long-term well-being after surgical or conservative treatment of severe vulvar vestibulitis. *Acta obstetricia et gynecologica Scandinavica*. 2012; 91(9):1086–1093.

65. Rosenbaum TY. Physiotherapy treatment of sexual pain disorders. *J Sex Marit Ther*. 2005;31(4): 329–340.

66. Goldfinger C, Pukall CF, Gentilcore-Saulnier E, et al. A prospective study of pelvic floor physical therapy: pain and psychosexual outcomes in provoked vestibulodynia. *J Sexual Med*. 2009;6(7): 1955–1968.

67. Goetsch MF. Surgery combined with muscle therapy for dyspareunia from vulvar vestibulitis: an observational study. *J Reprod Med*. 2007;52(7): 597–603.

68. Engman M, Wijma K, Wijma B. Long-term coital behaviour in women treated with cognitive behavioral therapy for superficial coital pain and vaginismus. *Cogn Behav Ther*. 2010;39(3): 193–202.

69. Payne KA, Binik YM, Amsel R, et al. When sex hurts, anxiety and fear orient attention towards pain. *Eur J Pain*. 2005;9(4):427–436.

70. DeLancey JO, Sampselle CM, Punch MR. Kegel dyspareunia: levator ani myalgia caused by overexertion. *Obstet Gynecol*. 1993;82(4 Pt 2 Suppl):658–659.

7

Endometriosis

Treatment and Pain Management

ADHAM ZAYED, KARINA GRITSENKO, AND YURY KHELEMSKY

"Endometriosis" is defined as the presence of endometrial tissue outside the uterus. Inflammation of the resulting ectopic tissue results in a spectrum of presenting pain symptoms. It is associated with dysmenorrhea and chronic pelvic pain. The disorder is estrogen-dependent and predominantly affects menstruating women, with a peak of 25–35 years of age. Consequently, its prevalence is probably around 10% of reproductive-age women. The pathogenesis is not clearly understood and is probably multifactorial. The associated morbidity results in increased healthcare costs, and decreased productivity due to work absence, that in the United States are estimated in the billions of dollars.[1] There are many potential treatment options, including both medical and surgical interventions, although, unfortunately, none are definitive. Ongoing research into old and new interventions continues to shape our understanding of this chronic, painful, and debilitating disease.

PATHOPHYSIOLOGY

It is possible that endometriosis is composed of multiple disease processes. There are four main theories of the pathophysiology—with each theory delineating how endometrial tissue becomes ectopic.

The most prevalent theory is that of retrograde menstruation. During menses when the uterine lining is shed, there is retrograde flow of stromal tissues through the fallopian tubes to the ovaries.[2] This can spread to the peritoneum, including the bowel, bladder, vagina, and peritoneal walls.

The Müllerian remnant theory hypothesizes that, during organogenesis, there is spread of endometrial tissue via misdirected Mullerian ducts, resulting in extrauterine stromal implantation, subsequently present at birth, and responsive to hormone changes in puberty.

The endometrial stem cell implantation theory proposes that endometrial precursor cells migrate into the peritoneum, causing endometrial tissue to be developed and differentiated in the peritoneum before subsequent proliferation and shedding.

The last theory is metaplastic change. Extrauterine cells undergo change resulting in an estrogen/progesterone receptor profile similar enough to endometrial tissue that it responds in a similar fashion to these hormonal changes.[3]

The result of all four theories is the presence of extrauterine stromal tissue. The location of this extrauterine tissue does not limit its response to estrogen and progesterone, and thus it responds like native intrauterine cells. Accordingly, there is tissue proliferation during the estrogen-dependent stage of the menstrual cycle. When the tissue is shed corresponding to a drop in progesterone levels, the resulting cells are in their extrauterine location. There can be pain from the active bleeding or from localized inflammation of these ectopic sites.

The presence of endometrial stromal tissue in the peritoneum has been found to stimulate an increased production of inflammatory mediators, including prostaglandins, chemokines, and cytokines. There is a subsequent macrophage-mediated inflammatory response[4] resulting in angiogenesis and lesion growth. Breakdown of red blood cells results in intraperitoneal iron deposition. This results in the production of reactive oxygen species, which causes further localized tissue trauma resulting in progression of depth of implantation of extrauterine endometrial tissue, which further exacerbates the disease. The tissue trauma resulting from these inflammatory processes can lead to nerve sensitization and subsequent pain.

Ectopic tissue can be categorized by its location to help guide management. Superficial peritoneal implants include ectopic tissue on the uterosacral ligament and fallopian tubes. Ectopic tissue can also be in the ovary, known as *endometriomas*, or "chocolate cysts." Deep nodules include endometrial tissue that can be found in the vaginal fornix, bladder, ureters, colon, and pouch of Douglas, or rectal wall. Endometrial tissue has also been described outside the peritoneum and retroperitoneum in the liver, diaphragm, pleura, lung, and umbilicus.

There is a high correlation between endometriosis and infertility. Its causal relationship is not clearly defined in early endometriosis, but is thought to be secondary to the inflammatory cascade causing a hostile environment to egg and/or sperm. In late endometriosis, infertility can occur as a result of anatomical changes (adhesions, cysts, mechanical obstructions) arising secondary to chronic inflammation. Endometriosis has also been associated with hyperalgesia, possibly due to nerve irritation, and a spectrum of social stresses and psychiatric illnesses secondary to complications of chronic pain and the severity of its sequelae.

DIAGNOSIS

Tissue Biopsy

The gold standard for diagnosis is visualization of cell histology under microscope. A biopsy is taken intraoperatively and sent to the pathology laboratory, where it is visualized under the microscope. A positive diagnosis is made when endometrial cells are seen in an extrauterine biopsy. The biopsy is performed via diagnostic laparoscopy, which requires general anesthesia with an endotracheal tube, an operating room, and the time, personnel, sterile equipment and costs associated with it. This is not a practical, cost-worthy, or necessary intervention for most patients. As a result, many diagnoses of endometriosis are presumptive or empirical diagnoses based on a detailed history and physical examination.

History

It is critical to obtain a detailed history due to the varied presentations and comorbid conditions associated with endometriosis. Women most commonly present with dysmenorrhea, but can also present with dyspareunia, dyschezia, dysuria, and intermenstrual pelvic pain. They can also be asymptomatic, with subsequent diagnoses made incidentally. There is some correlation between location of lesions and presenting pain symptoms. This creates a broad differential diagnosis, including gynecological, urological, gastrointestinal, and musculoskeletal pathologies, which must be ruled before a presumptive diagnosis of endometriosis can be made. Endometriosis is present in 87% of women who have been diagnosed with chronic pelvic pain. It is important to obtain a detailed menstrual history and chronologically correlate it with pain symptoms. Although the timing of pain symptoms occurring only during menses is largely suggestive of dysmenorrhea possibly from ectopic lesions, it is not pathognomonic of endometriosis. Endometriosis is often associated with heavy or prolonged menses.

It is also important to obtain a detailed family history. Although the genetic penetrance and expressivity are not yet defined, studies have shown a 51% hereditary component, linked to multiple genetic foci. Social history is also important, as endometriosis has been separately linked in patients with increased alcohol consumption and low exercise levels, respectively. A sexual history can reveal evidence of dyspareunia, and is also important to evaluate any risk of sexually transmitted infections or pregnancy, both intrauterine and ectopic.

Physical Examination

At minimum, the physical should include assessment of vital signs, a detailed abdominal exam, and a detailed gynecological exam, including bimanual palpation, and a rectal exam. Additional components of the physical exam should be performed as suggested by the patient's history to assess for differential diagnoses and comorbid diseases.

Laboratory Studies

There are no laboratory studies that are diagnostic of endometriosis. However, in conjunction with a detailed history and physical exam, some lab results can help narrow the differential diagnosis by ruling out other pathologies. An iron-deficient (microcytic) anemia is largely suggestive of heavy menses in an otherwise healthy menstruating female. There has been some correlation between elevated Ca-125 levels and advanced endometriosis. Labs should be completed as indicated to narrow the list of differential diagnoses.

Imaging

Imaging studies are also not solely diagnostic, although they can be used as aids in diagnosis.

Abdominal ultrasound is not definitive for endometriosis, but it can be used to diagnose endometriomas and other gynecological masses that can cause similar pain symptoms. Directed use of transvaginal ultrasound can be used to visualize endometriosis in the perivaginal or perirectal region. Magnetic resonance imaging is recommended only as a second-line test after a non-diagnostic ultrasound for suspected rectovaginal or bladder lesions.

TREATMENT

There is no absolutely curative treatment for endometriosis. Therefore, treatment is a mix of medical therapies and surgical interventions aimed at both minimizing symptoms and correcting the underlying pathology. The management of endometriosis is largely driven by patient factors. Maintenance of fertility remains the most important factor, as this can restrict the utilization of surgical interventions and medical therapies available. As the gold standard for diagnosis requires a surgical intervention (diagnostic laparoscopy), it is not optimal for many women. Subsequently, a histologically confirmed diagnosis is not required to begin treatment. The treatment regimens discussed herein will focus on the treatment for pain associated with endometriosis, and not with the broader management of infertility associated with endometriosis.

MEDICAL MANAGEMENT

If diagnostic laparoscopy is not chosen, a combined diagnostic-therapeutic medical management regimen can be started. Currently available medical treatments are directed against different parts of the known pathophysiology, ranging from suppression of ovulation to inhibition of the inflammatory cascade. No medical therapy currently available is curative beyond its active treatment course. Furthermore, resolution of symptoms on a treatment regimen is not diagnostic of endometriosis. Pain symptoms are expected to return if a successful medication course is terminated. Subsequently, treatment regimens can be long, repeating courses of patient-driven trial and error, a balance of resolution of symptoms and tolerance of side effects.

GnRH Analogues

Gonadotropin-releasing hormone (GnRH) is normally secreted by the hypothalamus, with receptors located on the anterior pituitary gland. The anterior pituitary secretes follicle-stimulating hormone (FSH) and luteinizing hormone (LH) in response to this stimulation. FSH and LH have subsequent receptors in the ovary, which controls the release of estrogen and progesterone, respectively. Exogenous GnRH analogues bind to GnRH receptors with greater affinity than does endogenous GnRH. There is a subsequent downstream downregulation of receptors resulting in ovarian suppression and a hypoestrogenic environment for the intra- and extrauterine endometrial stroma. This ultimately inhibits the trigger for the subsequent inflammatory cascade. As this treatment results in ovarian suppression, it is not compatible with conception. A recent retrospective systematic review reported a benefit in the suppression of symptoms when compared to placebo or no treatment, although the evidence was of low quality. There was a benefit in reduction of symptoms when compared to danazol, and no observed difference when compared to the levonorgestrel intrauterine device.[5]

Add-Back Therapy

There are known adverse effects to the induced state of hypoestrogenism. In large part, they mimic physiological changes associated with menopause or premature ovarian failure: vasomotor instability, genital atrophy, mood changes, osteopenia, and osteoporosis. Accordingly, add-back therapy can be considered in successful cases of GnRH analogues resolving pain symptoms.[5] It consists of "adding back" some medications to minimize some of the adverse effects of bone resorption caused by GnRH analogues. It can include estrogen, progestins, or progestins plus bisphosphonates. Calcium supplementation is recommended for all patients on add-back therapy to promote bone stability.

Contraceptive Agents

Oral contraceptive agents (estrogen and progesterone, or progesterone only) work the same way for treatment of endometriosis as they do for contraception. In comparing combined estrogen and progesterone pills to progesterone only, the latter may be preferred, as minimizing exogenous estrogen intake theoretically minimizes its downstream proliferation of endometrial tissue. Uninterrupted courses of oral contraceptive agents are theoretically superior to interrupted courses (21 days or otherwise), as there is constant inhibition the trigger of the inflammatory cascade by minimizing endometrial shedding.

Progestin-only agents have also been studied for endometriosis pain. The most promising are norethisterone acetate and dienogest. There are other forms of progestin-only contraceptive agents (subcutaneous implants, intramuscular injections, vaginal insertions) that are used for contraception and have been studied for endometriosis. Although promising, the data are still inconclusive regarding their efficacy specifically for endometriosis pain. A recent systemic retrospective review also showed no difference in efficacy between oral contraceptives and a GnRH analogue.[5]

The levonorgestrel-releasing intrauterine device (IUD) is also an effective device for contraception. Levonorgestrel is a second-generation progestin. After manual placement of the IUD, levonorgestrel is released directly into the uterus at a constant rate to have an effect like other exogenous progestins. The IUD lifespan is up to five years, and it reduces the frequency and regularity of menstruations in most women. Although it is not yet approved by the US Food and Drug Administration (FDA) for endometriosis therapy per se, in theory, any agent that minimizes menstruation is a potentially effective treatment for endometriosis. A recent systematic review showed benefit of this IUD for reduction of pain symptoms versus expectant management.[5]

Danazol

Danazol is an oral androgen, a derivative of 19-nortestosterone. It was the first FDA-approved drug for treatment of endometriosis. The dose ranges from 200–800 mg daily, and it is often recommended not to be continued beyond six months.[6] Danazol has multiple effects in vivo. It decreases the release of gonadotropins from the pituitary, thus blunting the luteinizing hormone surge. It results in a hypoestrogenic environment and endometrial tissue atrophy, both intra- and extrauterine. Additionally, danazol functions to increase circulating levels of testosterone, which results in some undesired side effects, including acne, hirsutism, and change in voice. A recent systematic retrospective review found some benefit in reduction of symptoms for danazol versus placebo, although the evidence was weak.[5] However due to its undesired side-effect profile, it has largely

been replaced by GnRH analogues for treating endometriosis. Like with GnRH analogues, hypoestrogenic side effects can occur, which can be treated by concurrent administration of add-back therapy. Androgenic side effects are found to be dose-dependent, and can sometimes be managed by dose de-escalation.

Non-Steroidal Anti-Inflammatory Drugs (NSAIDs)

NSAIDs (e.g., ibuprofen, naproxen, etc.) have been frequently used for pain control for both endometriosis and dysmenorrhea. These medications inhibit the release of prostaglandins, which have been implicated as inflammatory mediators in endometriosis. However, a recent retrospective failed to show a reduction in symptoms when compared to placebo.[5]

SURGICAL MANAGEMENT

Diagnostic Laparoscopy

If diagnostic laparoscopy for tissue biopsy is desired, surgical removal of lesions can be performed in conjunction. There is some evidence to support decrease of symptoms after diagnostic laparoscopy with removal of lesions versus diagnostic laparoscopy alone. Diagnostic laparoscopy with removal of lesions can be a definitive treatment with complete resolution of symptoms. Lesion removal can be done via excision, coagulation, laser vaporization, or shaving. However, recurrence is common with fertility-sparing surgery where the anatomy is left relatively intact.

Hysterectomy

Severe cases of endometriosis can warrant more extensive surgery. For superficial peritoneal implants, this can be total hysterectomy with bilateral salpingo-oophorectomy, or an ovary-sparing hysterectomy with salpingectomy. If there are no lesions on the ovary, the latter technique may be preferred to prevent the side effects of hypoestrogenism. Even when fertility is sacrificed and this more extensive surgery is performed, endometriosis can still recur, albeit less with bilateral oophorectomy.

Deep Nodule Management

Depending on the location of the lesions, surgical removal of lesions on the colon, bladder, ureters, or vagina can warrant deeper excision of this tissue. For patients with deep lesions, there appear to be improved pain outcomes with more extensive removal, although they are also associated with an increased risk of complications from the more extensive surgery.

Adhesion Management

The chronic inflammatory milieu secondary to ongoing endometriosis exposes the peritoneum to tissue fibrosis and adhesions. Additionally, there is an increased risk of fibrosis and adhesions with every surgical access to the peritoneum, including diagnostic laparoscopy. Management at this point becomes more complicated, as each surgical procedure can increase the risk for future adhesions, which may lead to continued pelvic pain without any guarantee of preventing the recurrence of endometriosis.

Endometrioma Management

It is recommended that endometriomas be surgically managed in symptomatic or asymptomatic patients to prevent their progression to ovarian torsion, ovarian rupture, and infertility. Surgical management is typically incision and drainage or complete excision. Due to an endometrioma's proximity to the ovary, excision carries an increased risk of infertility or ovarian dysfunction. There is some evidence that supports decreased recurrence of endometriomas with excisional surgery.[7] However, there is an increased risk of ovarian dysfunction or infertility in repeated surgeries for recurrent endometriomas. In cases of recurrent endometriomas after surgery, the decision to reoperate must be made on a case-by-case basis.

Post-Surgical Medical Management

Although post-surgical drugs are prescribed frequently, there are no set guidelines for post-surgical medical management, as there has been no benefit for any agent shown in the literature. With potential recurrence after surgical intervention, medical management versus further surgical intervention must be considered on a case-by-case basis.

PROSPECTIVE FUTURE THERAPIES

Randomized controlled trials have been performed to evaluate the efficacy of other potential medical therapies. Overall, the limited results limit their potential recommendation to patients with refractory disease to initial treatment regimens. These newer agents all target the inflammatory cascade, which has been implicated in the pathology of early endometriosis. However, there are still limited medical interventions to manage the intraabdominal fibrosis and adhesions caused by the chronic inflammation in late endometriosis.[3]

Anti-Inflammatory Agents

Similar in mechanism of action to other nonsteroidal anti-inflammatory agents, specific cyclooxygenase-2 (COX-2) inhibitors like rofecoxib have shown promising results regarding symptom control.[8] Pentoxifylline has also been studied in randomized controlled trials, with some promising results.[9]

Antiangiogenics

Antiangiogenics such as rapamycin have been tested in animal models, with promising results. By interfering with cell proliferation, it is hypothesized, they can minimize proliferation of lesions, albeit with the unwanted side effect of limiting in vivo angiogenesis for normal tissue growth. They have not been thoroughly tested in humans to warrant their use at this time, however.

Aromatase Inhibitors

Aromatase stimulates the expression of estrogen in endometrial tissue, causing tissue proliferation. It has a higher expression rate in extrauterine endometrial tissue. Targeted use of aromatase inhibitors is thought to decrease endometrial proliferation. They have been studied in combination with and compared to GnRH agonists.[10]

Immunomodulators

Immunomodulators such as anti-tumor necrosis factor agents have been studied in limited human trials. They are thought to inhibit the immune response causing the inflammatory cascade. Recent studies of intraperitoneal administration and direct injection both have had encouraging results.

Selective Estrogen Response Modulators

These agents have endometrial estrogen receptor antagonism while maintaining estrogen receptor agonism elsewhere in the body. Further studies are required. Statins, valproic acid, and trichostatin A have all been studied but require further testing in larger randomized controlled trials before recommendations can be made on their use in endometriosis.

OTHER SURGICAL INTERVENTIONS

Surgical Interruption of Nerve Pathways

Uterine nerve ablation and presacral nerve ablation have both been performed, with varying results for treatment of chronic pelvic pain associated with endometriosis and dysmenorrhea. Uterine nerve ablation involves ablation of the nerve in the uterosacral ligament near its connection to the uterus. Presacral nerve ablation involves transection of the sacral nerve plexus at the level of the superior hypogastric plexus. The limited studies of uterine nerve ablation show no benefit in treatment of endometriosis pain. There may be a role for presacral nerve ablation, although more studies are needed.[11]

Laparoscopic Helium Plasma Coagulation

Helium plasma coagulation is another method to remove lesions via laparoscopy.[12] A beam of helium is directed at the lesions in a manner to vaporize this ectopic tissue. Its efficacy compared to traditional lesion excision is unclear, and more studies are recommended.

ALTERNATIVE MEDICINES

A recent retrospective review showed weak evidence that auricular acupuncture was beneficial when compared to Chinese herbal medicines, with a different study showing no difference between Chinese herbal medicine and danazol.[5] Since danazol is not the gold standard of treatment, further research is required before conclusive recommendations can be made. Considering the high morbidity and high recurrence rate of the disease, it is premature to categorically rule out alternative therapies, as there is a lack of conclusive evidence regarding many of the allopathic interventions currently being used.

CONCLUSION

Considering the prevalence, morbidity, and healthcare costs associated with endometriosis, trials exploring effectiveness of existing therapies, as well as augmenting the development of novel therapies, are urgently required.

REFERENCES

1. Simoens S, Hummelshoj L, D'Hooghe T. Endometriosis: cost estimates and methodological perspective. *Hum Reprod Update.* 2007;13:395–404.
2. Giudice LC. Clinical practice. Endometriosis. *N Engl J Med.* 2010;362:2389–2398.
3. Vercellini P, Vigano P, Somigliana E, Fedele L. Endometriosis: pathogenesis and treatment. *Nature Rev Endocrinol.* 2014;10:261–275.
4. Bacci M, Capobianco A, Monno A, et al. Macrophages are alternatively activated in patients with endometriosis and required for growth and vascularization of lesions in a mouse model of disease. *Am J Pathol.* 2009;175:547–556.
5. Brown J, Farquhar C. Endometriosis: an overview of Cochrane Reviews. *Cochrane Database Syst Rev.* 2014;3:Cd009590.
6. Johnson NP, Hummelshoj L. Consensus on current management of endometriosis. *Hum Reprod.* 2013;28:1552–1568.
7. Hart RJ, Hickey M, Maouris P, Buckett W. Excisional surgery versus ablative surgery for ovarian endometriomata. *Cochrane Database Syst Rev.* 2008:Cd004992.
8. Cobellis L, Razzi S, De Simone S, et al. The treatment with a COX-2 specific inhibitor is effective in the management of pain related to endometriosis. *Eur J Obstet Gynecol Reprod Biol.* 2004;116:100–102.
9. Kamencic H, Thiel JA. Pentoxifylline after conservative surgery for endometriosis: a randomized, controlled trial. *J Minim Invasive Gynecol.* 2008;15:62–66.
10. Ferrero S, Gillott DJ, Venturini PL, Remorgida V. Use of aromatase inhibitors to treat endometriosis-related pain symptoms: a systematic review. *Reprod Biol Endocrinol.* 2011;9:89.
11. Proctor ML, Latthe PM, Farquhar CM, Khan KS, Johnson NP. Surgical interruption of pelvic nerve pathways for primary and secondary dysmenorrhoea. *Cochrane Database Syst Rev.* 2005:Cd001896.
12. Hill N, McQueen J, Morey R, et al. Over one thousand patients with early stage endometriosis treated with the Helica Thermal Coagulator (HELICA): safety aspects. *Arch Gynecol Obstet.* 2006;274:203–205.

8

Painful Bladder Syndrome
and Interstitial Cystitis in Women

SYBIL G. DESSIE AND EMAN ELKADRY

Painful bladder syndrome (PBS) is a chronic disorder affecting millions of women (Konkle, 2012). This disorder can have significant negative impact on patients' quality of life, and major financial implications as well as decreased productivity (Nickel, 2010; Robinson, 2011). Unfortunately, the syndrome is not well understood and is often diagnosed late in a patient's course, or diagnosed incorrectly. Despite ongoing research, there is limited understanding of the pathogenesis of chronic pelvic and bladder pain syndromes, as well as few effective treatments.

DEFINING PAINFUL
BLADDER SYNDROME

The definition of PBS, also known as interstitial cystitis and bladder pain syndrome (BPS), has evolved over time. The term "interstitial cystitis" implies that there is inflammation within the bladder; however, this is true in only about one-third of patients with PBS. There is a wide array of symptoms with multiple possible clinical presentations. This complexity can lead to misdiagnosis and often to delayed treatment (Johnson, 2006).

PBS is defined by the International Continence Society as "the complaint of suprapubic pain related to bladder filling, accompanied by other symptoms such as increased daytime and nighttime frequency, in the absence of proven urinary infection or other obvious pathology" (Abrams, 2002). The European Society of the Study of Bladder Pain Syndrome/Interstitial Cystitis uses the term "bladder pain syndrome," describing it as a "chronic pelvic pain, pressure, or discomfort perceived to be related to the urinary bladder accompanied by at least one other urinary symptom such as persistent urge to void or urinary frequency" (Van De Merwe, 2008). The Society of Urodynamics and Female Urology uses a similar definition, but symptoms must be present for at least six weeks (Hanno, 2010).

More recently, the American Urological Association released guidelines for the diagnosis and treatment of PBS and concluded that there is insufficient literature to provide an evidence-based diagnosis of PBS in clinical practice. However, on the basis of clinical principles, they recommend diagnosis of PBS by excluding other disorders that may present similarly (Hanno, 2011). The definition and terminology used to describe PBS will probably continue to evolve over time as better understanding of the pathophysiology evolves.

PREVALENCE

It is difficult to estimate the prevalence of PBS, given the variable definitions, population sampling, and survey methods used in the current literature. In addition, PBS is often a disease of exclusion due to its poorly understood etiology (Rover, 2000). Estimation of prevalence in the literature ranges from 10–865 cases per 100,000 people (Simon, 1997; Payne, 2007) in self-report studies. Among studies that surveyed patients about PBS symptoms, 2.7–6.5% of American women have symptoms consistent with PBS. PBS is far more common in women than in men (Parsons, 2007).

ETIOLOGY

The cause of PBS is not well understood. Research on the disease's etiology has traditionally been split between two theories. The first theory focuses on the bladder as the main source of pathology and pain and, accordingly, treatment focuses on the bladder. In this model, a bladder insult disrupts the protective layer of the bladder lining known as the glycosaminoglycan (GAG) layer. The GAG layer protects the bladder epithelium from irritation by urine and bacteria. Potential bladder insults, including a distension injury, bacterial bladder infection, or pelvic floor dysfunction with resulting inflammation, can damage the GAG layer. This allows solutes from the urine (such as potassium) to leak into the bladder lining, leading to tissue inflammation and epithelial injury. Tissue injury might also activate c-fibers (which carry nerve signals to the central nervous system). This can:

- lead to the release of substance P (which stimulates inflammation and aids in the transmission of pain),
- activate mast cells leading to histamine release (which can trigger pain)
- trigger an immune or allergic response

In this line of thought, treatment focuses on preventing or managing the factors that lead to tissue injury and pain as well as treatments to heal the GAG layer (Hurst, 2007; Walters, 2007; Engelhardt, 2011).

The other school of thought centers around generalized pelvic neurogenic inflammation causing the bladder to be secondarily affected along with other end organs. As pain in the bladder becomes chronic, there are changes in how painful stimuli are processed neurologically in the central nervous system. This can lead to a lowered pain threshold and pain from non-painful stimuli (such as bladder filling) (Nazif, 2007; Lilius, 1973).

This theory is consistent with the finding that women with PBS have a higher incidence of other painful conditions, such as irritable bowel syndrome, vulvar pain, and fibromyalgia. There also seems to be a higher incidence of PBS with other inflammatory and autoimmune complaints, as well as chronic fatigue syndrome (Koziol, 1994, Alagiri, 1997).

Regardless of the primary insult and resultant pain pathways, there is evidence that the pathophysiology does involve all the pelvic structures, including the pelvic floor. Previous studies of women with interstitial cystitis (IC) have noted hypertonicity of the pelvic floor muscles (Weiss, 2001). These myofascial abnormalities, found on palpation of muscle and other tissue in the pelvis, are thought to contribute to the pain of PBS and irritative urinary symptoms (Peters,

2007; Lilius, 1973; Weiss, 2001; Oyama, 2004). However, it is unclear which is the primary cause and which is the effect.

An emerging body of research implicates systemic factors in the pathogenesis of urological chronic pelvic pain syndromes, including abnormal hypothalamic-pituitary-adrenal (HPA) axis activity and abnormalities in the sympathetic nervous system (Mayson, 2009). It is possible that PBS represents a process with the bladder as the end organ of various inciting events that lead to local bladder inflammation, peripheral and central neural upregulation, alterations in the HPA axis, and changes in central perception and processing of nociceptive stimuli (Mayson, 2009). Similar pathways may also be responsible for vulvodynia and other non-urological pelvic pain syndromes (Aloisi, 2011).

There is evidence to suggest that genetic risk factors contribute to chronic bladder and pelvic pain syndromes (Dimitrakov, 2009; Talati, 2008). Studies have shown familial clustering (Dimitrikov, 2009), and twin studies have also shown a possible genetic link (Wright, 2010). This suggests that a genomic approach to diagnosis and treatment may be useful.

SYMPTOMS

In clinical practice, women with PBS present with symptoms of bladder pain (especially with filling or emptying), bladder pressure, and dysuria, often with urgency, and frequency (defined as voiding eight or more times per 24 hours). Some women also have dyspareunia, feelings of bloating or vaginal pressure, or constipation. Vulvodynia or other end organ pain symptoms are often present as well. Women may report being treated for recurrent urinary tract infections or recurrent vaginal infections, sometimes without testing or culture.

Symptoms often wax and wane over days to months. Patients can sometimes identify things that trigger or exacerbate their pain, including certain foods or drinks, sexual activity, physical activity, menses, or prolonged sitting. The foods and drinks most likely to make symptoms flare include coffee, tea, alcohol, citrus fruits, artificial sweeteners, and hot peppers (Shorter, 2007). Stress is also often cited as an exacerbating factor (Rothrock, 2001).

Women with PBS also have higher rates of depression, history of sexual abuse and symptoms of PTSD, anxiety, and perceived stress (Whitmore, 2002; Wright, 2010). Patients should be screened for these disorders during their evaluation.

DIAGNOSIS

The diagnosis of PBS is based on the presence of characteristic symptoms and the exclusion of other, similar disorders. A medical history and physical exam are important, both in confirming the diagnosis of PBS and in ruling out other possible diagnoses, such as urinary tract cancer or stones, infection, overactive bladder, urinary retention, or a pelvic mass.

The history should focus on the start of symptoms, possible occurrence of an inciting event, whether symptoms are chronic or intermittent, whether there are factors that exacerbate or alleviate symptoms, and the symptom severity (using a 0–10 Likert-style scale or a visual analog scale).

A 24-hour voiding diary can help to quantify how much and what type of beverages the woman is drinking and give an estimate of her bladder capacity. The diary should include the time and volume of each void and the time and volume for all fluid intake. This information can be used to educate the woman about bladder retraining and fluid titration, behavioral techniques that are useful in reducing her frequency and urgency. If dietary triggers are suspected, a food and drink diary can help to narrow down the list of possible triggers.

Standardized questionnaires are used clinically and in research settings for diagnosing and monitoring PBS. Examples include the Pain, Urgency, Frequency Symptom Scale and the O'Leary-Sant Symptom Index and Problem Index questionnaires (O'Leary, 1997). While these questionnaires might be useful for distinguishing PBS from other urinary complaints or monitoring symptom severity over time, experts agree that questionnaires should not be used alone to diagnose PBS (Kushner, 2006).

The physical examination should include a complete gynecological and urological assessment of pelvic structures, including the health of external and vaginal tissues; assessment for vaginal discharge, pelvic masses, and urethral diverticula; as well as a rectal exam. In addition, a complete musculoskeletal assessment should be performed. Women with PBS often exhibit tenderness of abdominal, hip, low back, and thigh muscles. In addition, palpating the pelvic floor muscles, bladder base, and urethra during the bimanual exam usually elicits pain.

To examine the pelvic floor, place one or two fingers inside the vagina and apply pressure to the posterior and lateral vaginal walls while gently pulling towards the introitus. Normally, the woman should note a feeling of pressure during this examination. In women with PBS, there is often moderate to severe pain with palpation of the pelvic floor. This pain may refer to the bladder, urethra, rectum, or surrounding muscles. Laboratory tests should include a urinalysis and urine culture. Vaginal and cervical cultures are also performed as needed.

Cystoscopy and urine cytology should be performed if indicated, based upon physical findings and risk factors. Although cystoscopy is no longer required for diagnosis, it is important to eliminate other bladder pathology and sources of irritation; cystoscopy can usually be performed in the office. Similarly, urodynamics can be performed if the diagnosis is in doubt and can provide information on other lower urinary tract disease (Hanno, 2011).

In some women, it is not possible to complete an internal pelvic exam due to pain. In this case, it is reasonable to perform a pelvic ultrasound or examination under anesthesia (often with cystoscopy), especially if there is concern about underlying pathology.

There is interest in finding a urinary biomarker that could be useful in the diagnosis of PBS. One such biomarker is antiproliferative factor (APF), which was found to have a high sensitivity and specificity for identifying women with PBS. However, further study is needed to define the benefits, costs, and limits to this approach (Forrest, 2008).

Further diagnostic testing, including cystoscopy with hydrodistension, bladder biopsy, and potassium sensitivity testing, is not required to diagnose PBS (Hanno, 2011). In addition, these tests can be painful and can delay the initiation of treatment. In the past, these tests were recommended to confirm the physical findings thought to be pathognomonic of PBS, such as bladder glomerulations, ulcers, and decreased bladder volume under anesthesia. However, studies reveal that healthy women with no symptoms of painful bladder symptom can also have these findings (Waxman, 1998). In addition, these findings are not consistently present in women with PBS (Denson, 2000).

Nevertheless, many physicians continue to recommend and perform these tests, particularly cystoscopy with hydrodistension. Although some women have relief of symptoms after this procedure, it is short-lived and only occurs in about 50% of women (Ottem, 2005). In addition, the procedure is usually performed under general anesthesia or sedation, increasing the costs and risks.

TREATMENT

Treatment for PBS aims to decrease pain and urinary symptoms. The treatment should include a combination of pelvic floor physical therapy, medications, behavior changes, and psychosocial support. Unfortunately, narcotics are the most commonly prescribed class of medications for this disorder (Anger, 2011). The first-line treatment for patients with PBS is education regarding normal bladder function, their disorder, and treatment options (Hanno, 2011). There is no single "best" treatment or combination of treatments for all women. In many cases, a woman will need to try several therapies to find the one(s) that works best. As the evidence for many of these therapies is lacking, treatment is often guided by physician preference and experience, anecdotal evidence, as well as patient preference.

Behavior Modification

Many women with PBS empty their bladder frequently to avoid the pain associated with bladder filling. Making changes in voiding and drinking behaviors can help relieve symptoms of urinary urgency and frequency.

Bladder retraining involves voiding at regularly scheduled intervals during the day and slowly increasing the voiding interval over a period of weeks. The goal of bladder retraining is to restore a normal voiding interval (3–5 hours) and decrease urgency. Initial voiding intervals are chosen based on a woman's current voiding frequency. Distraction techniques are used to delay urges until the appropriate interval. Intervals are slowly increased as the patient becomes more comfortable. Women who are able to follow this regimen often have an improvement in urgency and frequency (Chalken, 1993).

An important adjunct to bladder retraining is fluid titration. This technique moderates the woman's fluid intake so that she drinks small amounts throughout the day rather than larger amounts at infrequent intervals. Although there are few data, we recommend that women drink four to six ounces per hour throughout the day.

This includes all fluids (e.g., milk on cereal, soup). If nocturia is a problem, we recommend that the woman stop drinking three to four hours before bedtime. Obstacles to adherence include patients' work or activity schedule and the required motivation to follow this program. This type of regimen can be used as a general guideline for patients even if they cannot strictly adhere to the schedule.

Other behavior modifications include the recognition and avoidance of pain triggers. This will also give patients a sense of control over their disease, which can help empower them. Ice or heat applied to painful areas such as the bladder or perineum can sometimes be helpful. There are also some data to suggest that guided-imagery techniques can improve symptoms (Carrico, 2008). Stress is a common trigger for PBS flares. Stress-management techniques can also be used to reduce exacerbations of symptoms (Rothrock, 2001).

Activity restrictions are recommended only if an activity is a trigger of pain or worsening symptoms. Although randomized trials are still lacking, exercise seems to improve chronic pain in patients (Fuentes, 2011, Dubin, 2010).

There is widespread belief that particular foods, beverages, or supplements can trigger or exacerbate symptoms of PBS. Clinical studies are limited to retrospective, subjective reports (Shorter, 2007). Studies suggest that foods high in citric acid can exacerbate bladder pain, while foods with alkalinizing agents might provide some symptom relief (Clemens, 2006; Bologna, 2001). Although the evidence is limited, we recommend that women identify and avoid items that are a trigger to their symptoms. Exacerbating foods can be identified with an elimination diet. This might mean avoiding the item completely, or avoiding it only during a symptom flare. We do not recommend eliminating entire food groups without guidance from a registered dietitian (Friedlander, 2012).

Physical Therapy

Physical therapy (PT) for PBS is an important treatment to modify the dysfunctional pelvic floor musculature that contributes to bladder and pelvic pain (Weiss, 2001, Fitzgerald, 2009). It is considered a second-line treatment by the American Urological Association after behavioral modifications (Hanno, 2011). Pelvic floor physical therapy should be performed by a therapist who is experienced with myofascial and other manual-release techniques. Myofascial physical therapy has been shown to be more efficacious than global massage for the treatment of women with PBS (FitzGerald, 2012). The therapy should aim to release tight, tender pelvic floor muscles, trigger points, scarring, connective tissue restrictions, and to desensitize hypersensitive areas. PT is best used in conjunction with other therapeutic modalities, as many women with severe PBS will need a combination of treatments to achieve the best response. In our practice, PT is the most frequently used treatment for PBS. PT can also be used as the primary treatment modality for women who do not wish to take medications or try more invasive approaches.

Pelvic floor physical therapy is usually done in one-hour sessions once or twice per week for at least 10 weeks. Depending upon the duration and severity of symptoms, one year or more of weekly treatment may be required (Kotarinos, 2001). The therapist works on the abdomen, hips, thighs, groin, lower back, and internal pelvic floor muscles (transvaginally or transrectally). Treatment is done in a private room with the patient in the dorsal lithotomy position. Therapists will often supplement treatment sessions with home exercises and stretches. Patient acceptance is high (Fitzgerald, 2009) despite the perceived intrusive nature of PT and occasional pain flares with therapy. Logistical considerations such as insurance coverage, time commitment, geographic distance, and long wait times to begin therapy can impede treatment.

Medications

Oral medications used to treat PBS include pentosan polysulfate sodium (PPS), benzodiazepines, skeletal muscle relaxants, anticholinergics, chemical neuromodulators, and antidepressants. In our practice, we include medications when symptoms are severe enough to preclude waiting for the benefits of PT or behavioral changes to take effect. We often recommend medications in conjunction with both PT and behavioral changes, depending on symptom severity and patient preference.

Pentosan Polysulfate Sodium (PPS)

Pentosan polysulfate sodium is a heparin-like macromolecule that is believed to repair injured areas of the GAG layer. The standard dose is 100 mg three times per day on an empty stomach, although some providers recommend, 200 mg twice per day. Treatment with PPS is recommended for six months before deciding if the drug is effective. If no improvement is seen at six months, it is reasonable to discontinue. In clinical studies, PPS was more effective than placebo in relieving symptoms of pain, urgency, and frequency. However, the margin of benefit was small (Dimitrakov, 2007). It is the only oral medication approved by the US Food and Drug Administration (FDA) for the treatment of PBS (Rourke, 2014).

PPS can also be given intravesically (Offiah, 2013), sometimes in combination with oral PPS (Davis, 2008). A combination of oral and intravesical PPS appears more effective than oral PPS alone (Davis, 2008). Dosing for intravesical PPS is discussed below (see "Intravesical Therapies").

Antidepressants

Amitriptyline is the most commonly prescribed tricyclic antidepressant for PBS. Clinical studies show that amitriptyline can provide modest pain relief, especially when taken at doses greater than 50 mg per day (Foster, 2010). However, side effects such as drowsiness, dizziness, and other anticholinergic side effects can be limiting at this dose. Starting at the lowest possible dose and increasing slowly will help some women adjust to these side effects.

Serotonin-norepinephrine reuptake inhibitors (SNRIs) were developed to treat depression but were found to relieve pain in some people with chronic pain. Two of the drugs in this category, duloxetine and milnacipran, are approved to treat pain; duloxetine is approved to treat physical pain associated with depression, while milnacipran is approved to treat the pain of fibromyalgia. However, it is not clear if other antidepressants would provide a similar benefit. SNRIs are a reasonable option for women with PBS who have chronic pain, especially women who cannot tolerate other treatment options. Side effects of SNRIs can include nausea and drowsiness. Starting with a low dose and increasing slowly can help minimize side effects.

Antihistamines and H-2 Receptor Antagonists

Medications such as cimetidine or hydroxyzine are widely prescribed for treatment of PBS, often in combination with PPS. This is based on anecdotal evidence that the activation of mast cells (as with seasonal allergies) can exacerbate symptoms of PBS. Clinical trials have failed to support the efficacy of hydroxyzine (Sant, 2003);

therefore we do not recommend it. Several small studies have examined the benefit of cimetidine, an H-2 antagonist (Seshadri, 1994, Thilagarajah, 2001). The studies found that cimetidine reduced symptoms among refractory patients.

Benzodiazepines

Medications such as diazepam, clonazepam, and lorazepam can be useful for pain management among PBS patients. While traditionally used for anxiety, the muscle relaxant properties of benzodiazepines can provide relief of pain related to muscle spasms. Similarly, skeletal muscle relaxants, such as cyclobenzaprine and baclofen, may have a limited role in the treatment of PBS. However, there are inadequate data to support long-term use of either benzodiazepines or skeletal muscle relaxants (Leite, 2009).

Treatment is started at a low dose once or twice per day. It is important to discuss the addictive nature of these medications with patients to ensure that they are willing to follow dosing instructions closely. In addition, patients should be prescribed these medications only when severe symptoms are present, as in a flare, not as a preventive treatment. We reserve the use of these medications for severe cases to ease pain symptoms and to allow better sleep. Increased sleep has shown to help lessen PBS symptoms (Nickel, 2009).

Anticholinergic Medications

Anticholinergic medications are often used to address symptoms of urinary urgency, frequency, and nocturia. Examples of commonly prescribed anticholinergics include oxybutynin, solafenicin, trospium, darafenacin, tolterodine, and fesoterodine. These medications are similar in efficacy, but vary in cost, side effects, and dosing frequency. Side effects can be significant, with the most common including dry mouth, constipation, heartburn, blurred vision, and changes in cognition. There are no data on the effect of this class of medication on PBS/IC.

In women with PBS with urinary urge incontinence or significant urgency or frequency symptoms, anticholinergic medications are a reasonable option to consider. Behavior modifications are recommended in combination with anticholinergic treatment.

Neuromodulators

Neuromodulating medications such as gabapentin and pregabalin are anticonvulsants that are also used to treat neuropathic pain. Their mechanism of action for relieving pain is unclear, and data regarding their use with PBS are limited (Sasaki, 2001; Phatak, 2003; Lee, 2010). However, anecdotal experience supports their use, especially in women with chronic, daily pain.

Gabapentin or pregabalin should be started at a low, once-daily dose (usually at bedtime) and slowly titrated up to three times per day over three to four weeks, as tolerated. Side effects, such as drowsiness, dizziness, and difficulty thinking, can be limiting. Pregabalin can also cause peripheral edema and weight gain. If one drug is not effective, this does not preclude trying the other. Finding an effective neuromodulating medication can help obviate the need for narcotics or other potentially addictive mediations.

Narcotics

In women with chronic pain, narcotic pain medications are recommended on a limited basis due to their addictive nature and short-term benefit. In our practice, we refer patients who require narcotics to a pain-management clinic. This allows the medication to be given by a single provider in a controlled fashion to avoid potential abuse.

Upcoming Medications

New medications are being examined to see if they can help patients with PBS, given the minimal efficacy of current oral treatments. Sildenafil was compared to placebo in 48 women with PBS and found to be significantly better at reducing pain at up to three months of treatment (Chen, 2014). Recent literature examining injections of Adalimumab compared to placebo among women with PBS demonstrated no significant change between the two groups (Bosch, 2014). More research is needed on the efficacy of other medications targeted specifically for patients with PBS.

Intravesical Treatments

Intravesical treatments for PBS are instilled by catheter directly into the bladder. The most commonly used treatment includes alkalinized lidocaine, sometimes in combination with heparin or PPS. Clinical studies of lidocaine-based intravesical treatments reveal that they are effective in reducing pain and urgency, at least temporarily (Nickel, 2009; Parsons, 2005). The patient is instructed to hold the solution in the bladder for as long as possible (at least 30 minutes). In clinical practice, not all women benefit from intravesical treatments. In women who do benefit, pain and urgency can be reduced for hours to days. Patients who benefit can be taught to perform this treatment at home one to three times per week, with a return to the office if there are pain flares.

One combination of a lidocaine-based intravesical treatment includes, 200 mg lidocaine, 40,000 units of heparin, and 8.4% of sodium bicarbonate (to reach a total volume of 15 mL). PPS is sometimes substituted for heparin, and is given at a dose of, 200 mg (two 100 mg capsules) mixed with 30 mL buffered saline (Davis, 2008).

Intravesical heparin is given for its proposed benefit in strengthening the bladder surface mucin barrier. This is thought to decrease the sensitivity of the bladder to irritating substances in the urine. However, large-scale studies supporting the benefit of heparin are lacking. In addition, clinical experience reveals that it can take months to greater than one year of intravesical heparin treatment before improvement is noted (Moldwin, 2007).

Other intravesical treatments have been used to treat PBS, including resiniferatoxin, dimethyl sulfoxide (DMSO), Bacillus Calmette-Guérin (BCG), and oxybutynin. Resiniferatoxin is a capsaicin analogue that has equivocal evidence to support its use and can cause pain during instillation (Dawson, 2009); therefore, we do not recommend its use. Similarly, there are limited data on DMSO, which has not been shown to be more effective than placebo (Dawson, 2009). Oxybutynin instillations have been shown to improve bladder capacity and the number of urgency episodes and may be helpful (Offiah, 2013). BCG is associated with no significant efficacy compared to placebo and can have potentially life-threatening complications; therefore, it should not be used (Hanno, 2011).

Botulinum Toxin A

Botulinum toxin A (BTX-A) acts as a neurotoxin that inhibits the release of acetylcholine at the neuromuscular junction, therefore decreasing muscle contractility at the injection site. BTX-A is injected cystoscopically into the bladder at multiple sites. Currently it is has been approved by the FDA for the treatment of overactive bladder but not for any pain syndrome. It has been suggested that BTX-A has anti-nociceptive effects on the afferent pathways in the bladder (Smith, 2004).

In a majority of studies of BTX-A, there were noted improvements in frequency, pain, voided volume, and quality-of-life indicators. Although there were varied methods, populations, and outcome measures in these studies, there does appear to be a trend towards benefit of treatment over placebo. Reported improvement lasted from 5–12 months in most patients (Anger, 2010). In a prospective trial of women suffering from PBS, multiple injections of BTX-A to the bladder trigone were shown to have improved pain symptoms from baseline with minimal complications (Pinto, 2013). Based on this potential improvement, patients with refractory PBS/IC may benefit from BTX-A injections.

Recent studies have also looked at the use of BTX-A in the pelvic floor and levator muscles rather than into the bladder with good success (Adelewo, 2013). We are currently conducting a randomized controlled trial of BTX-A for pelvic pain, including PBS.

Adverse effects of BTX-A are usually temporary and can include dysuria, hematuria, urinary tract infection, voiding difficulty, and the need for intermittent self-catheterization (ISC). Patients must understand the risk of urinary retention and be willing to perform ISC. There have been reports of rare systemic reactions with BTX-A injections, including respiratory distress and even death, mostly in children with spasticity. Patients should be warned about these risks as well.

PROCEDURES

Percutaneous Posterior Tibial Nerve Stimulation

Percutaneous posterior tibial nerve stimulation (PTNS) is a procedure that involves placing a needle (typically an acupuncture needle) through the skin near the medial malleolus. The needle is connected to an electric stimulator to stimulate the posterior tibial nerve during a 30-minute session that is repeated once weekly for 12 weeks.

PTNS was initially designed to treat overactive bladder and urinary urge incontinence. However, studies have yet to support the benefit of PTNS for women with PBS (Zhao, 2004 and, 2008).

Sacral Neurostimulation

Sacral neurostimulation is an FDA-approved treatment for symptoms of frequency, urgency, and urge incontinence. The treatment involves implanting a pacemaker-like device into the hip, which sends mild electrical impulses to the sacral nerves. The patient can control the device with a handheld programmer. It is thought to work by stimulating afferent nerve pathways at S3 site (Wyndaele, 2000). Potential adverse effects of sacral neurostimulation include pain, skin irritation, infection, device problems, and lead movement. The treatment is reversible, and the device can be removed. The battery must be replaced approximately every five years. The data regarding the efficacy of this treatment modality for PBS are limited but somewhat promising. Larger prospective trials are needed before definitive conclusions can be made regarding the use of sacral neuromodulation for patients with PBS (Marcelissen, 2011).

As with BTX-A, sacral neurostimulation is a reasonable option in women with severe, refractory symptoms. The use of test stimulation prior to permanent implantation allows patients to assess the potential benefit of treatment on a temporary, minimally invasive basis.

Surgical Procedures

Several surgical options exist as a last resort when conservative management fails. These include ablation of Hunner's lesions, transurethral resection of the bladder, ileocystoplasty, and urinary diversion. These treatment options carry high morbidity given their invasive nature, and do not guarantee pain relief. For this reason, all other conservative options should be exhausted prior to proceeding with one of these options (Walters, 2007).

Psychosocial Support

The value of psychosocial support for women with chronic pain should not be underestimated. Women with PBS often see multiple healthcare providers in an attempt to find the source of their symptoms. Because of the dearth of evidence supporting best practices in the treatment of PBS, many physicians are unsure how to identify and manage these women. This combination of factors leaves many women feeling frustrated, misunderstood, and unable to find relief from their pain.

All women being evaluated for PBS should be screened for depression, either with informal questions or a validated questionnaire (such as the Beck's Depression Inventory II). Women should also be questioned about any past history of physical or sexual abuse. As noted, several clinical studies have noted that women with PBS have a higher incidence of depression and

past sexual or physical abuse (Goldstein, 2008; Peters, 2007).

Psychosocial support is available from a number of resources, including local and online support groups and social workers or psychotherapists. If anxiety or depression is suspected, the woman should be referred for further evaluation and treatment.

Complementary and Alternative Medicine (CAM) Treatment

There are a wide variety of complementary and alternative medicine (CAM) treatments advertised to treat PBS. As with some traditional treatments, evidence supporting the benefit of most CAM treatment is lacking. However, CAM appeals to many women with PBS due to its perception as being natural, safe, and under the woman's control.

Examples of CAM used for PBS include the following:

- Herbs and nutraceuticals, such as calcium glycerophosphate, L-arginine, mucopolysaccharides, bioflavonoids (such as quercetin), and Chinese herbs (Whitmore, 2002)
- Proprietary herbal blends include Algonot, Cystoprotek, and Cysta-Q (Moldwin, 2007)
- Guided imagery (Carrico, 2008)
- Acupuncture (Rapkin, 1987)
- Exercise and yoga (Ripoll, 2002; Karper, 2004).

PATIENT RESOURCES

There are a number of resources available for women with PBS. This includes online support and information, local support groups, clinical studies, and books.

Online support is available from the following websites:

- Interstitial Cystitis Network (www.ic-network.com)
- Interstitial Cystitis Association (www.ichelp.com)

Reliable sources of information is available from the following websites:

- National Institute of Diabetes and Digestive and Kidney Diseases (http://

kidney.niddk.nih.gov/kudiseases/pubs/
interstitialcystitis/)
- National Association for Continence (www.nafc.org)

For information about participating in a clinical trial:

- http://clinicaltrials.gov/

Books about PBS:

- *A Headache in the Pelvis: A New Understanding and Treatment for Prostatitis and Chronic Pelvic Pain Syndromes*, David Wise
- *The Interstitial Cystitis Survival Guide: Your Guide to the Latest Treatment Options and Coping Strategies* by Robert M. Moldwin

SUMMARY

Painful bladder syndrome is a debilitating, potentially chronic condition that affects many women, yet remains under diagnosed and undertreated. Research into the etiology and pathophysiology of PBS may help better determine treatment approaches. A high index of suspicion should be maintained when seeing women with persistent frequency, urgency, or pain. Additional testing will exclude underlying pathology. Triggers should be identified and treated or avoided as necessary.

Currently, physical therapy and behavioral modification is the first line of treatment used by our practice, but they often need to be combined with medications. Treatment must be individualized based on the patient's symptoms and response to intervention as well as her comfort level with treatment options. Newer modalities, such as Botox and neuromodulation, may be reserved for refractory patients that fail initial management approaches. Multidisciplinary care is often needed to address all patient symptoms, provide treatment of depression, and develop coping skills.

REFERENCES

Abrams P, Cardozo L, Fall M, et al. Standardization Sub-committee of the International Continence Society. The standardisation of terminology of lower urinary tract function: report from the Standardisation Sub-committee of the International Continence Society. *Neurourol Urodyn*. 2002;21(2): 167–178.

Alagiri M, Chottiner S, Ratner V, Slade D, Hanno PM. Interstitial cystitis: unexplained associations with other chronic disease and pain syndromes. *Urology*. 1997 May;49(5A Suppl):52–57.

Aloisi AM, Buonocore M, Merlo L, et al. Chronic pain therapy and hypothalamic-pituitary-adrenal axis impairment. *Psychoneuroendocrinology*. 2011 Aug;36(7):1032–1039.

Anger JT, Weinberg A, Suttorp MJ, et al. Outcomes of intravesical botulinum toxin for idiopathic overactive bladder symptoms: a systematic review of the literature. *J Urol*. 2010;183:2258.

Anger JT, Zabihi N, Clemens JQ, et al. Treatment choice, duration, and cost in patients with interstitial cystitis and painful bladder syndrome. *Int Urogynecol J*. 2011;22:395–400.

Bologna RA, Gomelsky A, Lukban JC, et al. The efficacy of calcium glycerophosphate in the prevention of food-related flares in interstitial cystitis. *Urology*. 2011;57:119–120.

Bosch PC. A randomized, double-blind, placebo controlled trial of adalimumab for interstitial cystitis/bladder pain syndrome. *J Urol*. 2014;191:77–82.

Carrico DJ, Peters KM, Diokno AC. Guided imagery for women with interstitial cystitis: results of a prospective, randomized controlled pilot study. *J Altern Complement Med*. 2008 Jan–Feb;14(1):53–60.

Chaiken DC, Blaivas JG, Blaivas ST. Behavioral therapy for the treatment of refractory interstitial cystitis. *J Urol*. 1993 Jun;149(6):1445.

Chen H, Wang F, Chen W, et al. Efficacy of daily low-dose sildenafil for treating interstitial cystitis: results of a randomized, double-blind, placebo-controlled trial—treatment of interstitial cystitis/painful bladder syndrome with low dose sildenafil. *Urology*. 2014;84:51–56.

Clemens JQ, Brown SO, Kosloff L, Calhoun EA. Predictors of symptom severity in patients with chronic prostatitis and interstitial cystitis. *J Urol*. 2006;175:963–966.

Davis EL, El Khoudary SL, Talbott EO. Safety and efficacy of the use of intravesical and oral pentosan polysulfate sodium for interstitial cystitis: a randomized double-blind clinical trial. *J Urol*. 2008;179(1):177–185.

Dawson TE, Jamison J. Intravesical treatments for painful bladder syndrome/interstitial cystitis. *Cochrane Database Syst Rev*. 2007 Oct 17;(4):CD006113.

Denson MA, Griebling TL, Cohen MB, Kreder KJ. Comparison of cystoscopic and histological findings in patients with suspected interstitial cystitis. *J Urol*. 2000;164:1908.

Dimitrakov J, Guthrie D. Genetics and phenotyping of urological chronic pelvic pain syndrome. *J Urol*. 2009;181:1550.

Dimitrakov J, Kroenke K, Steers WD. Pharmacologic management of painful bladder syndrome/interstitial cystitis: a systematic review. *Arch Intern Med.* 2007;167(18):1922.

Dmochowski R, Chapple C, Nitti VW, et al. Efficacy and safety of onabotulinum toxin A for idiopathic overactive bladder: a double-blind, placebo controlled, randomized, dose ranging trial. *J Urol.* 2010;184:2416.

Dubin R, King-VanVlack C. The trajectory of chronic pain: can a community-based exercise/education program soften the ride? *Pain Res Manag.* 2010 Nov-Dec;15(6):361–368.

Engelhardt PF, Morakis N, Daha LK, et al. Long-term results of intravescial hyaluronan therapy in bladder pain syndrome/interstitial cystitis. *Int Urogynecol J.* 2011;22:401–405.

FitzGerald MP, Anderson RU, Potts J, et al. Randomized multicenter feasibility trial of myofascial physical therapy for the treatment of urological chronic pelvic pain syndromes. *J Urol.* 2009 Aug;182(2):570–580.

FitzGerald MP, Payne CK, Lukacz ES, et al. Randomized multicenter clinical trial of myofascial physical therapy in women with interstitial cystitis/painful bladder syndrome and pelvic floor tenderness. *J Urology.* 2012;187:2113–2118.

Forrest JB, Moldwin R. Diagnostic options for early identification and management of interstitial cystitis/painful bladder syndrome. *Int J Clin Pract.* 2008 Dec;62(12):1926–1934.

Foster HEJr, Hanno PM, Nickel JC, et al. Interstitial Cystitis Collaborative Research Network. Effect of amitriptyline on symptoms in treatment naïve patients with interstitial cystitis/painful bladder syndrome. *J Urol.* 2010 May;183(5):1853–1858.

Friedlander JI, Shorter B, Moldwin R. Diet and its role in interstitial cystitis/bladder pain syndrome (IC/BPS) and comorbid conditions. *BJUI.* 2012;109:1584–1591.

Fuentes CJP, Armijo-Olivo S, Magee DJ, Gross DP. Effects of exercise therapy on endogenous pain-relieving peptides in musculoskeletal pain: a systematic review. *Clin J Pain.* 2011 May;27(4):365–374.

Goldstein HB, Safaeian P, Garrod K, et al. Depression, abuse and its relationship to interstitial cystitis. *Int Urogynecol J Pelvic Floor Dysfunct.* 2008 Dec;19(12): 1683–1686.

Hanno P, Lin A, Nordling J, et al. Bladder Pain Syndrome Committee of the International Consultation on Incontinence. *Neurourol Urodyn.* 2010;29(1):191–198.

Hanno PM, Burks DA, Clemens JQ, et al. AUA guideline for the diagnosis and treatment of interstitial cystitis/bladder pain syndrome. *J Urol.* 2011;185:2162–2170.

Hurst RE, Moldwin RM, Mulholland SG. Bladder defense molecules, urothelial differentiation, urinary biomarkers, and interstitial cystitis. *Urology.* 2007;69:17.

Hwang P, Auclair B, Beechinor D, et al. Efficacy of pentosan polysulfate in the treatment of interstitial cystitis: a meta-analysis. *Urology.* 1997;50(1):39.

Johnson JE, Johnson KE. Ambiguous chronic illness in women: community health nursing concern. *J Community Health Nurs.* 2006;23:159.

Karper WB. Exercise effects on interstitial cystitis: two case reports. *Urol Nurs.* 2004;24:202

Konkle KS, Berry SH, Elliott MN, et al. Comparison of an interstitial cystitis/bladder pain syndrome clinical cohort with symptomatic community women from the RAND interstitial cystitis epidemiology study. *J Urol.* 2012;187: 508–512.

Koziol JA. Epidemiology of interstitial cystitis. *Urol Clin North Am.* 1994 Feb;21(1):7–20.

Kushner L, Moldwin RM. Efficiency of questionnaires used to screen for interstitial cystitis. *J Urol.* 2006 Aug;176(2):587–592.

Lee WC, Han DY, Jeong HJ. Bladder pain syndrome treated with triple therapy with gabapentin, amitriptyline, and a nonsteroidal anti-inflammatory drug. *Int Neuroufol J.* 2010;14:256–260.

Leite FM, Atallah AN, El Dib R, et al. Cyclobenzaprine for the treatment of myofascial pain in adults. *Cochrane Database Syst Rev.* 2009 Jul 8;(3): CD006830.

Lilius HG, Oravisto KJ, Valtonen EJ. Origin of pain in interstitial cystitis. Effect of ultrasound treatment on the concomitant levator ani spasm syndrome. *Scand J Urol Nephrol.* 1973;7:15.

Maher CF, Carey MP, Dwyer PL, Schluter PL. Percutaneous sacral nerve root neuromodulation for intractable interstitial cystitis. *J Urol.* 2001 Mar;165(3):884–886.

Marcelissen T, Jacobs R, van Kerrebroeck P, de Wachter S. Sacral neuromodulation as a treatment for chronic pelvic pain. *J Urol.* 2011;186: 387–393.

Mayson BE, Teichman JM. The relationship between sexual abuse and interstitial cystitis/painful bladder syndrome. *Curr Urol Rep.* 2009;10:441.

Moldwin RM, Evans RJ, Stanford EJ, Rosenberg MT. Rational approaches to the treatment of patients with interstitial cystitis. *Urology.* 2007 Apr;69(4 Suppl):73–81.

Nazif O, Teichman JM, Gebhart GF. Neural upregulation in interstitial cystitis. *Urology.* 2007;69:24.

Nickel JC, Tripp DA, Pontari M, et al. Psychosocial phenotyping in women with interstitial cystitis/painful bladder syndrome: a case control study. *J Urol.* 2010;183:167–172.

Nickel JC, Moldwin R, Lee S, et al. Intravesical alkalinized lidocaine (PSD597) offers sustained relief from symptoms of interstitial cystitis and painful bladder syndrome. *BJU Int.* 2009 Apr;103(7): 910–918.

Nickel JC, Payne CK, Forrest J, et al. The relationship among symptoms, sleep disturbances and quality of life in patients with interstitial cystitis. *J Urol.* 2009;181(6):2555–2561.

Nickel JC, Barkin J, Forrest J. Randomized, double-blind, dose-ranging study of pentosan polysulfate sodium for interstitial cystitis. *Urology.* 2005 Apr;65(4):654–658.

Offiah I, McMahon SB, O'Reilly BA. Interstitial cystitis/bladder pain syndrome: diagnosis and management. *Int Urogynecol J.* 2013 Aug;24(8): 1243–1256.

O'Leary MP, Sant GR, Fowler FJJr. et al. The interstitial cystitis symptom index and problem index. *Urology.* 1997;49:58.

Ottem DP, Teichman JM. What is the value of cystoscopy with hydrodistension for interstitial cystitis? *Urology.* 2005 Sep;66(3):494–499.

Oyama IA, Rejba A, Lukban JC, et al. Modified Thiele massage as therapeutic intervention for female patients with interstitial cystitis and high-tone pelvic floor dysfunction. *Urology.* 2004;64:862.

Parsons CL. Successful downregulation of bladder sensory nerves with combination of heparin and alkalinized lidocaine in patients with interstitial cystitis. *Urology.* 2005;65:45.

Parsons JK, Kurth K, Sant GR. Epidemiologic issues in interstitial cystitis. *Urology.* 2007;69:5–8.

Payne CK, Joyce GF, Wise M, Clemens JQ. Interstitial cystitis and painful bladder syndrome. *J Urol.* 2007;177(6):2042–2049.

Peters KM, Kalinowski SE, Carrico DJ. Fact or fiction—is abuse prevalent in patients with interstitial cystitis? Results from a community survey and clinic population. *J Urol.* 2007;178:891.

Peters KM, Killinger KA, Ibrahim IA. Childhood symptoms and events in women with interstitial cystitis/painful bladder syndrome. *Urology.* 2009;73:258.

Phatak S, Foster HEJr. The management of interstitial cystitis: an update. *Nat Clin Pract Urol.* 2006 Jan;3(1):45–53.

Pinto R, Lopes T, Silva J, et al. Persistent therapeutic effect of repeated injections of onabotulinum toxin A in refractory bladder pain syndrome/interstitial cystitis. *J Urol.* 2013;289: 548–553.

Rapkin AJ, Kames LD. The pain management approach to chronic pelvic pain. *J Reprod Med.* 1987 May;32(5):323–327.

Ripoll E, Mahowald D. Hatha yoga therapy management of urologic disorders. *World J Urol.* 2002;20:306.

Robinson R. The economic burden of interstitial cystitis and painful bladder syndrome. *J Urol.* 2011:22:395–400.

Rothrock NE, Lutgendorf SK, Kreder KJ, et al. Stress and symptoms in patients with interstitial cystitis: a life stress model. *Urology.* 2001;57:422.

Rourke W, Khan SAA, Ahmen K, et al. Painful bladder syndrome/interstitial cystitis: aetiology, evaluation and management. *Archivio Italiano di Urologia e Andrologia.* 2014;86:126–131.

Rovner E, Propert KJ, Brensinger C, et al. Treatments used in women with interstitial cystitis: the interstitial cystitis data base study experience. The Interstitial Cystitis Data Base Study Group. *Urology.* 2000;20;56:940.

Sant GR, Propert KJ, Hanno PM, et al. A pilot clinical trial of oral pentosan polysulfate and oral hydroxyzine in patients with interstitial cystitis. *J Urol.* 2003 Sep;170(3): 810–815.

Sasaki K, Smith CP, Chuang YC, et al. Oral gabapentin (neurontin) treatment of refractory genitourinary tract pain. *Tech Urol.* 2001 Mar;7(1):47–49.

Seshadri P, Emerson L, Morales A. Cimetidine in the treatment of interstitial cystitis. *Urology.* 1994 Oct;44(4):614–616.

Shorter B, Lesser M, Moldwin RM, Kushner L. Effect of comestibles on symptoms of interstitial cystitis. *J Urol.* 2007 Jul;178(1):145–152.

Simon LJ, Landis JR, Erickson DR, Nyberg LM. The interstitial Cystitis Data Base Study: concepts and preliminary baseline descriptive statistics. *Urology.* 1997;49:64.

Smith CP, Radziszewski P, Borkowski A, et al. Botulinum toxin A has antinociceptive effects in treating interstitial cystitis. *Urology.* 2004;64:871.

Talati A, Ponniah K, Strug LJ. Panic disorder, social anxiety disorder, and a possible medical syndrome previously linked to chromosome 13. *Biol Psychiatry.* 2008;63:594.

Thilagarajah R, Witherow RO, Walker MM. Oral cimetidine gives effective symptom relief in painful bladder disease: a prospective, randomized, double-blind placebo-controlled trial. *BJU Int.* 2001 Feb;87(3):207–212.

van de Merwe JP, Nordling J, Bouchelouche P, et al. Diagnostic criteria, classification, and nomenclature for painful bladder syndrome/interstitial cystitis: an ESSIC proposal. *Eur Urol.* 2008 Jan;53(1):60–67.

Walters MD, Karram MM. *Urogynecology and Reconstructive Pelvic Surgery.* 3rd ed. Mosby Elsevier. 2007;377–386.

Waxman JA, Sulak PJ, Kuehl TJ. Cystoscopic findings consistent with interstitial cystitis in normal women undergoing tubal ligation. *J Urol.* 1998;160:1663.

Weiss JM. Pelvic floor myofascial trigger points: manual therapy for interstitial cystitis and the urgency-frequency syndrome. *J Urol.* 2001;166:2226.

Whitmore KE. Complementary and alternative therapies as treatment approaches for interstitial cystitis. *Rev Urol.* 2002;(4 Suppl 1):S28–S35.

Wright LJ, Noonan C, Ahumada S. Psychological distress in twins with urological symptoms. *Gen Hosp Psychiatry.* 2010;32:262.

Zhao J, Nordling J. Posterior tibial nerve stimulation in patients with intractable interstitial cystitis. *BJU Int.* 2004 Jul;94(1):101–104.

Zhao J, Bai J, Zhou Y, Qi G, Du L. Posterior tibial nerve stimulation twice a week in patients with interstitial cystitis. *Urology.* 2008 Jun;71(6):1080–1084.

9

Functional Abdominal Pain Syndrome

JASON LITT, KARINA GRITSENKO, AND YURY KHELEMSKY

Abdominal pain is one of the most common complaints in both adult and pediatric patients.[1] Chronic abdominal pain has a median prevalence rate of 12% in children aged 2–18 years.[2] Unfortunately, many abdominal pain complaints that are worked up by the physician often yield inconclusive or normal results, leaving the patient and parents frustrated.[1] The Rome III Diagnostic Criteria for Functional Gastrointestinal Disorders is the most widely used tool for diagnosis of any of the multiple functional gastrointestinal disorders (FGID) in adults and children. The term "functional disorder" is used to describe conditions in which the patient is symptomatic, but otherwise has unremarkable physical exam findings, laboratory studies, and imaging studies. Functional abdominal pain (FAP) is a functional gastrointestinal disorder that can occur in adults and children.

While the Rome III criteria describe FAP in adults and children, the majority of current research and evidence on the causes and management of FAP take place in the pediatric population. Moreover, in up to 65% of children with functional gastrointestinal (GI) disorders, the disorder continues into adulthood.[3] Accordingly, this chapter will focus primarily on childhood FAP.

Technically speaking, the Rome III criteria identify functional abdominal pain syndrome (FAPS) in adults and differentiate between childhood functional abdominal pain (CFAP) and childhood functional abdominal pain *syndrome* (CFAPS). As the research for the causes and management for all these diagnoses is largely the same, for simplicity, this chapter will refer to FAP as a blanket diagnosis for any of the functional abdominal pain syndromes. Differences will be pointed out where relevant.

DIAGNOSIS

There is a multitude of conditions that present with the chief complaint of abdominal pain.

Inflammatory bowel disease, celiac disease, food allergies or intolerances, chronic abdominal wall pain, and drug reactions are just a few of many diagnoses that are in the differential diagnosis for abdominal pain. While a thorough history and physical exam are always indicated, many physicians will choose to forgo more invasive tests like colonoscopies and endoscopies in the absence of alarming symptoms like rapid and unintentional weight loss, bloody bowel movements, or nocturnal pain causing sleep disturbance.

Historically, FAP has been thought of as a diagnosis of exclusion; however, it is also possible to have FAP with other abdominal comorbidities. As an example, there is a subset of patients with Crohn's disease who will have abdominal pain even when they are in clinical remission. Thus, they are considered to carry diagnoses of both Crohn's disease and FAP.[4] On the other hand, some patients who have been previously diagnosed with FAP later find out they have other medical conditions, or an abdominal wall pain syndrome such as anterior cutaneous nerve entrapment syndrome that is causing their pain.[5] Clearly, FAP can occur as an isolated disorder or with other comorbidities. As in any condition, care should be taken to perform a thorough history and physical to elucidate if FAP is the most likely cause of abdominal pain.

In both adults and children, once other organic conditions have been ruled out, the diagnosis of FAP is made using the Rome III criteria. To diagnose FAP in adults, all of the following criteria must be present for the last three months, with symptom onset being greater than six months prior to diagnosis:

- Continuous or nearly continuous abdominal pain
- No relationship or only occasional relationship of pain with physiological events (e.g., eating, defecation, or menses)

- Some loss of daily functioning
- Malingering is not present
- Insufficient symptoms to meet criteria for other FGID

To diagnose CFAP, these criteria must all be present at least once per week for at least two months prior to diagnosis:

- Episodic or continuous abdominal pain
- Insufficient criteria for other FGIDs
- No evidence of an inflammatory, anatomical, metabolic, or neoplastic process that explains the symptoms

When CFAP occurs and the abdominal pain is severe enough to interfere with daily functioning 25% of the time, and/or is associated with somatic symptoms such as headache, limb pain, or difficulty sleeping, the condition is referred to as childhood functional abdominal pain syndrome (CFAPS).[6]

CAUSES

The cause of FAP is undoubtedly multifactorial. Studies have examined psychological, biological, and social factors that contribute to the development of FAP. While it is likely that some or all of these factors exert different degrees of influence, the bulk of existing research focuses on the psychological nature of this pain disorder.

Looking at the biopsychosocial factors thought to impact the development of FAP, there is often a degree of stress, either emotional or physical, that is experienced by the child. For example, youths who identify as gay, lesbian, or bisexual have been found to have a higher prevalence of FAP.[7] Also, FGIDs, including FAP, have been shown to be more common in children who undergo abdominal surgeries in infancy. For instance, infants who undergo abdominal surgery for pyloric stenosis are four times as likely to have FAP in childhood.[8] While some have hypothesized that this increased risk of FAP is secondary to bowel manipulation and resulting visceral hypersensitivity, some studies have shown that surgeries without bowel manipulation, like an umbilical hernia repair, also increase the likelihood of FAP. This observation suggests that the physical stress of surgery, and the inflammatory state that ensues, might contribute to FAP. Nevertheless, the correlation seen between surgery and FAP is incompletely understood.[9]

It is has been shown that chronic stress is associated with psychophysiological alterations in the autonomic nervous system and endocrine system. Since children with FAP and other FGIDs experience chronic stress secondary to their pain, it is not surprising that, when looking at studies comparing children with FAP to healthy children, there are notable psychophysiological differences in the response to stressful stimuli. This indicates that there is probably a degree of autonomic dysregulation and hypersensitivity in children with FAP in response to stress. In a systematic literature review of peer-reviewed journal articles about children between the ages of 4 and 18 with abdominal pain, there were many studies that looked at the autonomic nervous system in children with chronic abdominal pain versus healthy children. In many of the studies, there were significant differences noted between healthy children and those with chronic abdominal pain. Some studies looked at the pupillary reflex as a reflection of the parasympathetic nervous system and found that children with chronic abdominal pain had a significant lag time in pupillary reaction, in addition to an unstable pupillary recovery pattern. However, other, similar, studies looking at heart rate variability (HRV) as a reflection of the sympathetic and parasympathetic functions have found mixed results as to the likelihood of autonomic dysregulation in children with FAP. While many of these studies are pilot studies and not without their limitations, it does appear that there is an association between chronic abdominal pain (as in FAP) and autonomic nervous system dysregulation. Determining how autonomic dysregulation contributes to the development or progression of FAP will take further research. Of note, the observed hypersensitivity is visceral, as there is no evidence of somatic hypersensitivity.[10,11]

Obese and overweight children have a higher prevalence of FAP and other functional GI disorders than normal-weight children do. In fact, in one study of 450 children between the ages of 4 and 18, almost half of the obese and overweight children were found to have at least one FGID. The research points to stress from the social stigma of obesity, a heightened inflammatory state, and other unknown biophysiological factors present in heavy children as possible causes.[12]

Interestingly, both parents and patients perceive that diet plays a significant role in FAP symptoms, and the vast majority of patients will make changes to their eating habits based on food associations they perceive as precipitating their pain. In many of these instances, when investigated further, it was found that the food item(s) in question was/were not causing the patient pain.[13]

FAP is not only a condition seen in the United States, but has also been shown to be prevalent with similar rates in other countries.[14] Of note, contrary to what some clinicians believe, an association between antibiotic use and FAP in children has never been demonstrated.[15]

MANAGEMENT

Clearly, while there are many theories about what causes FAP, there is still work that needs to be done to elucidate the underlying causes. Accordingly, there are limited well-researched treatment options, which usually consist of a combination of psychological interventions, medications, and dietary alterations in line with the biopsychosocial model of care.[1,13]

Psychological Interventions

Randomized controlled trials have primarily looked at two psychological therapies in regard to FAP: cognitive behavioral therapy (CBT) and hypnosis.[16]

A consistent healthcare provider–patient relationship is instrumental in the treatment approach to FAP. CBT is an effective intervention that is also the most heavily researched treatment in FAP. While CBT is successful at treating symptoms of FAP, other modes of counseling by a trained professional have been shown to be equally advantageous. In fact, patient education and counseling by an experienced pediatrician was shown to be equally efficacious at reducing symptoms in FAP. After one year of treatment, 60% of patients show significant improvement or recovery after receiving either CBT or regular counseling by a pediatrician.[17]

Additionally, hypnosis has been shown to be helpful in reducing symptoms by as much as half in children with FAP.[16] Due to the apparent success of these treatments, it is clear that a key component to management of FAP is counseling. Whether or not the counseling is with a psychological professional trained in either CBT or hypnosis, or with a pediatrician, there is a notable improvement in patient symptoms. Thus, it is imperative that psychological intervention be started as soon as FAP is suspected, and it should be continued throughout the course of illness for optimal improvement.

In addition to psychological counseling, antidepressants have been utilized for the treatment of FAP. While anxiety and depression occur frequently with FAP, antidepressants, specifically the tricyclic antidepressants (TCAs), are known to have antinociceptive properties below the therapeutic range for depression. For this reason, tricyclic antidepressants, namely amitriptyline, have been used in treating patients with FAP.[18] In a multicenter, double-blind, placebo-controlled, randomized trial looking at children with FGID in which abdominal pain was a major component, after four weeks of placebo or amitriptyline, it was found that there was no significant difference in therapeutic response.[19] Contrary to that, in one retrospective study that looked at 98 pediatric patients with FAP who took a TCA, 78.6% of the patients ($n = 77$) responded to treatment after an average of 11 months.[20] As supported by the latter study, one potential limiting factor of the former study is that TCAs often do not show therapeutic benefit until well after one month of initiating treatment. Nevertheless, the risks and benefits of adding an antidepressant to the therapeutic strategy for treating FAP should be weighed based on the patient's symptoms and degree of debilitation. Prior to initiating therapy with the pro-arrhythmogenic TCAs, a screening electrocardiogram (ECG) should be considered to assess for a prolonged QT interval or other major conduction abnormalities.[21]

Medicinal and Dietary Interventions

While it is not a common occurrence, some patients have symptoms that are exacerbated by eating and will avoid activities that might trigger a pain attack. Avoiding specific foods, vomiting after meals, and skipping meals have all been reported.[13] In severe cases, nutritional deficiencies like scurvy, pellagra, and hypovitaminosis A have developed.[22] Thus, extreme care must be taken to ensure healthy eating habits.

Milk products, gluten, and fructose are common culprits that people with FAP will try to eliminate from their diet to improve their symptoms. While many patients will report an improvement of symptoms after these so-called elimination diets, in multiple studies it has been shown that reported food allergies and intolerances are much higher than their actual prevalence when the patients are tested. Furthermore, even when a food allergy or intolerance exists, removing the culprit food will not always improve the symptoms. On the other hand, in one study it was found that fructose intolerance was present in approximately half of the study population of children with FAP, and when placed on a low-fructose diet, the majority of the patients had improved symptoms. Thus it appears that food allergies and intolerances can occur in conjunction with FAP, and while some patients will report improved symptoms with elimination diets, the foods are typically not the sole cause of the pain.[13,23]

When counseling patients on their eating habits, it is important to keep in mind that mastication and digesting stimulate the bowels; and as previously noted, patients with FAP are likely to have a degree of visceral hypersensitivity, which is thought to play a role in symptomatology. Perhaps, in these cases, it is not the food, but the act of eating that triggers the pain attack through the dysfunctional autonomic nervous system regulation and resulting visceral hypersensitivity.[13]

On the other hand, the addition of certain supplements or foods to the diet has been shown to be beneficial for some patients with FAP. The foods that are considered to be potentially helpful by reducing symptoms in FAP have been referred to as "functional foods." Fiber, peppermint oil, and probiotics in particular have been shown to be promising functional foods for FAP.

While the data are controversial, there is some evidence that low fiber intake is a risk factor for FAP. Fiber softens the stool and relieves constipation and gas buildup that can lead to abdominal pain, but studies on fiber supplementation for treating FAP show variable results. One recent double-blind study of 8–16-year-old patients with FAP found that partially hydrolyzed guar gum reduced clinical symptoms compared with placebo.[13]

Peppermint oil acts as an antispasmodic by relaxing GI smooth muscle, and is already widely used for treating symptoms of irritable bowel syndrome (IBS) after many randomized controlled trials have demonstrated its efficacy. While the evidence for using peppermint oil in children is limited, in one two-week double-blinded randomized controlled trial, 76% of 8–17-year-old patients with IBS reported improvements in pain severity.[24] Many authors feel that these findings are generalizable to children with FAP, as the pain experienced is considered to be of similar etiology. Risks with using peppermint oil are limited, but in excess it

can lead to intestinal nephritis and acute renal failure, in addition to causing bronchospasm in infants and children. Peppermint oil can also reduce esophageal pressure and worsen gastroesophageal reflux disease (GERD).

Like peppermint oil, probiotics are not FDA-regulated, and only 10% of probiotic labels give an accurate composition of their bacterial contents. Despite this, probiotics are becoming widely accepted by physicians and patients as a supplement for many GI conditions. In regard to FAP, there is evidence from two randomized controlled trials that *Lactobacillus rhamnosus* strain GG (LGG) significantly reduced abdominal pain in children aged 5–16 years. One of the studies examined 141 children with IBS or FAP over 16 weeks. The children were randomly assigned to receive either a placebo or LGG for eight weeks and then remain in follow-up for an additional eight weeks. The LGG group had a significant reduction of frequency and severity of pain both after eight weeks and then at 16 weeks, suggesting that the benefits of LGG persist beyond cessation of its administration.[25,26] More studies will need to be done to determine the true efficacy of different strains of bacteria and the effect each has on a variety of GI symptoms.[13]

In treating FAP, the clinician should focus on a multimodal treatment strategy that includes psychological intervention, dietary modification, and medication management in order to mitigate the comorbidities associated with FAP and improve the patient's quality of life.

GOALS OF CARE AND PROGNOSIS

While FAP is a frustrating and debilitating condition, the goals of care need to be focused on maintaining quality of life and optimizing functionality, not just for the patient, but for the family, as well. Children with FAP will often miss more school days and have more physician visits than children with inflammatory bowel disease. The parents of children with FAP have a higher prevalence of anxiety disorders and FGIDs, and increased maternal anxiety is associated with worse outcomes.[11]

Pediatric patients with FAP have a higher likelihood of FGID and miscellaneous chronic pain and distress in adolescence and young adulthood. Age at diagnosis, sex, and abdominal pain severity do not predict FGID later in life, but associated somatic and depressive symptoms are significant predictors.[11,27]

Expectations need to be managed, and the patient, along with his/her family, needs to be educated. FAP is a condition that can last a lifetime, and there is no proven treatment with a 100% success rate. Through effective education, counseling, diagnosis of existing comorbidities, and reassurance, most people with FAP can have adequate symptom management to maintain a reasonable quality of life.

COMORBIDITIES

Comorbid psychiatric disorders are prevalent in people with functional pain disorders and, when present, these are associated with a worse outcome.[16] Childhood FAP is associated with a higher risk of anxiety disorders in adolescence and young adulthood. The risk for anxiety disorders is highest if FAP persists into young adulthood, but it is still higher than the general population without FAP, even if the pain resolves in childhood.[28] Additionally, youths with anxiety or depression are more likely to develop FAP.[29]

CURRENT RESEARCH AND THE FUTURE OF FAP

Small trials have looked at novel treatments with medications, yoga, guided imagery, relaxation, and acupuncture for patients with FAP. One study looked at S-adenosylmethionine (SAM-e), a dietary supplement that has efficacy as an antidepressant and a treatment for chronic pain. The study found that patients reported improvement in pain scores over the two months they took doses of SAM-e between 200 mg/d and 1400 mg/d.[30] Other studies have found yoga exercises are effective at reducing symptom intensity and frequency in children with FAP between the ages of 8 and 18.[31] Guided imagery and relaxation, perhaps by its known impact on the autonomic nervous system, has been shown to decrease pain in FAP.[32]

In summary, FAP is a condition that has a profound impact on many children and adolescent patients and will often afflict many of them through adulthood. These patients have a higher risk of depression, anxiety, and an overall lower quality of life. Of paramount importance in caring for these patients is an understanding that FAP is different for every patient, and as such, the cause is often multifactorial. Accordingly, the treatments should be multimodal, including psychological intervention, dietary modification, and medication. In most instances, patient/ parent education and reassurance is the first step to a strong healthcare provider–patient relationship. While adding medications and addressing dietary or situational triggers is occasionally helpful, early psychological intervention and possible referral to an experienced psychologist or psychiatrist have been shown to be the most beneficial for reliable long-term pain relief.

REFERENCES

1. Walker LS, Sherman AL, Bruehl S, Garber J, Smith CA. Functional abdominal pain patient subtypes in childhood predict functional gastrointestinal disorders with chronic pain and psychiatric comorbidities in adolescence and adulthood. *Pain.* 2012;153:1798–1806.
2. Romano C, Porcaro F. *Current Issues in the Management of Pediatric Functional Abdominal Pain. Reviews on Recent Clinical Trials.* 2014;(9)1:13–20.
3. Carlson MJ, Moore CE, Tsai CM, Shulman RJ, Chumpitazi BP. Child and parent perceived food-induced gastrointestinal symptoms and quality of life in children with functional gastrointestinal disorders. *J Acad Nutr Dietet.* 2014;114:403–413.
4. Zimmerman LA, Srinath AI, Goyal A, et al. The overlap of functional abdominal pain in pediatric Crohn's disease. *Inflamm Bowel Dis.* 2013;19:826–831.
5. van Assen T, de Jager-Kievit JW, Scheltinga MR, Roumen RM. Chronic abdominal wall pain misdiagnosed as functional abdominal pain. *JABFM.* 2013;26:738–744.
6. Ford AC, Bercik P, Morgan DG, Bolino C, Pintos-Sanchez MI, Moayyedi P. Characteristics of functional bowel disorder patients: a cross-sectional survey using the Rome III criteria. *Aliment Pharmacol Ther.* 2014;39:312–321.
7. Roberts AL, Rosario M, Corliss HL, Wypij D, Lightdale JR, Austin SB. Sexual orientation and functional pain in U.S. young adults: the mediating role of childhood abuse. *PLoS One.* 2013;8:e54702.
8. Saps M, Bonilla S. Early life events: infants with pyloric stenosis have a higher risk of developing chronic abdominal pain in childhood. *J Pediatr.* 2011;159:551–554 e1.
9. Rosen JM, Adams PN, Saps M. Umbilical hernia repair increases the rate of functional gastrointestinal disorders in children. *J Pediatr.* 2013;163:1065–1068.
10. Gulewitsch MD, Muller J, Enck P, Weimer K, Schwille-Kiuntke J, Schlarb AA. Frequent abdominal pain in childhood and youth: a systematic review of psychophysiological characteristics. *Gastroenterol Res Pract.* 2014;2014:524383.

11. Levy RL, van Tilburg MA. Functional abdominal pain in childhood: background studies and recent research trends. *Pain Res Manag (Can)*. 2012;17:413–417.

12. Phatak UP, Pashankar DS. Prevalence of functional gastrointestinal disorders in obese and overweight children. *Int J Obes*. 2014;(38)10:1324–1327.

13. van Tilburg MA, Felix CT. Diet and functional abdominal pain in children and adolescents. *J Pediatr Gastroenterol Nutr*. 2013;57:141–148.

14. Saps M, Nichols-Vinueza DX, Rosen JM, Velasco-Benitez CA. Prevalence of functional gastrointestinal disorders in Colombian school children. *J Pediatr*. 2014;164:542–545 e1.

15. Uusijarvi A, Bergstrom A, Simren M, et al. Use of antibiotics in infancy and childhood and risk of recurrent abdominal pain—a Swedish birth cohort study. *Neurogastroenterol Motil (Eur)*. 2014;(26)6:841–850.

16. Palsson OS, Whitehead WE. Psychological treatments in functional gastrointestinal disorders: a primer for the gastroenterologist. *Clin Gastroenterol Hepatol*. 2013;11:208–216; quiz, e22–e23.

17. van der Veek SM, Derkx BH, Benninga MA, Boer F, de Haan E. Cognitive behavior therapy for pediatric functional abdominal pain: a randomized controlled trial. *Pediatrics*. 2013;132:e1163–e1172.

18. Bixquert-Jimenez M, Bixquert-Pla L. [Antidepressant therapy in functional gastrointestinal disorders]. *Gastroenterologia y Hepatologia*. 2005;28:485–492.

19. Saps M, Youssef N, Miranda A, et al. Multicenter, randomized, placebo-controlled trial of amitriptyline in children with functional gastrointestinal disorders. *Gastroenterology*. 2009;137:1261–1269.

20. Teitelbaum JE, Arora R. Long-term efficacy of low-dose tricyclic antidepressants for children with functional gastrointestinal disorders. *J Pediatr Gastroenterol Nutr*. 2011;53:260–264.

21. Patra KP, Sankararaman S, Jackson R, Hussain SZ. Significance of screening electrocardiogram before the initiation of amitriptyline therapy in children with functional abdominal pain. *Clin Pediatr*. 2012;51:848–851.

22. Ho EY, Mathy C. Functional abdominal pain causing scurvy, pellagra, and hypovitaminosis A. F1000Research. 2014;3:35.

23. Escobar MA, Jr., Lustig D, Pflugeisen BM, et al. Fructose intolerance/malabsorption and recurrent abdominal pain in children. *J Pediatr Gastroenterol Nutr*. 2014;58:498–501.

24. Kline RM, Kline JJ, Di Palma J, Barbero GJ. Enteric-coated, pH-dependent peppermint oil capsules for the treatment of irritable bowel syndrome in children. *J Pediatr*. 2001;138:125–128.

25. Francavilla R, Miniello V, Magista AM, et al. A randomized controlled trial of Lactobacillus GG in children with functional abdominal pain. *Pediatrics*. 2010;126:e1445–e1452.

26. Gawronska A, Dziechciarz P, Horvath A, Szajewska H. A randomized double-blind placebo-controlled trial of Lactobacillus GG for abdominal pain disorders in children. *Aliment Pharmacol Ther*. 2007;25:177–184.

27. Horst S, Shelby G, Anderson J, et al. Predicting persistence of functional abdominal pain from childhood into young adulthood. *Clin Gastroenterol Hepatol*. 2014; (12)12:2026–2032.

28. Shelby GD, Shirkey KC, Sherman AL, et al. Functional abdominal pain in childhood and long-term vulnerability to anxiety disorders. *Pediatrics*. 2013;132:475–482.

29. Yacob D, Di Lorenzo C, Bridge JA, et al. Prevalence of pain-predominant functional gastrointestinal disorders and somatic symptoms in patients with anxiety or depressive disorders. *J Pediatr*. 2013;163:767–770.

30. Choi LJ, Huang JS. A pilot study of S-adenosylmethionine in treatment of functional abdominal pain in children. *Alt Ther Health Med*. 2013;19:61–64.

31. Brands MM, Purperhart H, Deckers-Kocken JM. A pilot study of yoga treatment in children with functional abdominal pain and irritable bowel syndrome. *Complement Ther Med*. 2011;19:109–114.

32. Ball TM, Shapiro DE, Monheim CJ, Weydert JA. A pilot study of the use of guided imagery for the treatment of recurrent abdominal pain in children. *Clin Pediatr*. 2003;42:527–532.

10

Pudendal Neuralgia

MICHAEL HIBNER AND MARIO E. CASTELLANOS

Pudendal neuralgia is defined as pain in the dermatomal distribution of the pudendal nerve. Symptoms include pain, tingling, or burning in the clitoris/penis, vagina/scrotum, perineum and/or rectum. Classically, symptoms are aggravated with sitting and relieved by standing.[1] Pudendal neuralgia is often associated with other pelvic pain conditions that affect the bowel, bladder, and sexual function, and it therefore has a broad spectrum of presentations. Thus, it is frequently confused with diseases such as vulvodynia, prostatodynia, vaginismus, levator ani syndrome, and painful bladder syndrome. In this chapter, we will use the term "pudendal neuralgia" strictly as a symptom. This definition is in contrast to "pudendal nerve entrapment," which is defined as compression or impingement of the nerve that may be observed during surgery.

HISTORY

The term "pudendal neuralgia" was first used in 1882 in the book *The Change of Life in Health and Disease. A Clinical Treatise of the Diseases of the Ganglionic Nervous System Incidental to Women at the Decline of Life*, by British obstetrician Dr. Edward John Tilt. He described it as "very distressing sensations of heat, aching and itching at the perineal area." He further reported that this sensation is "worsened by walking and over-exertion and relieved by internal exhibition of assafœtida and valerian combined with the external application of opiates and belladonna." In 1987, French physiatrist Gerard Amarenco noticed a group of patients who presented with burning perineal pain who all had a history of extensive cycling and named it the "cyclist syndrome."[2] In 2008, Prof. Roger Robert established the diagnostic criteria for pudendal neuralgia[3] and described pudendal nerve entrapment as a possible cause. He also established that surgical release of the entrapped pudendal nerve may alleviate symptoms.[4]

EPIDEMIOLOGY

Evaluation of patients with chronic pelvic pain is a common practice in gynecological offices. It may account for up to 15% of all patients and has a vast differential diagnosis that crosses into multiple organ systems.[5] Pelvic pain of neuropathic origin is poorly understood and therefore not commonly recognized by practitioners. Pudendal neuralgia is one of the main causes of neuropathic pelvic pain. The exact prevalence of pudendal neuralgia is unknown. The Pudendal Neuralgia Association (tipna.org) website estimates that 1/100,000 people have pudendal neuralgia, but from our personal observations this condition seems to be much more common. The European website Portal for Rare Diseases and Orphan Drugs (orpha.net) estimates that 1–5/10,000 patients have pudendal neuralgia and that approximately 4% of patients with chronic pelvic pain suffer from this condition. All these numbers are estimates and have not been described in any properly designed study.

ANATOMY OF THE PUDENDAL NERVE AND PELVIC FLOOR

The *pudendal* nerve, derived from the Latin word for "shameful," carries motor, sensory, and sympathetic fibers. It is responsible for sensation of the genitals and rectum and is important for maintaining continence via control of the rectal and urethral sphincters.[6] The pudendal nerve is formed by the ventral rami of the second, third, and fourth sacral spinal nerves that join at the level of the cephalad border of the sacrotuberous ligament. It then runs on the ventral surface of the piriformis muscle dorsal to the ischiococcygeus muscle and exits the pelvis through the greater sciatic foramen. The nerve then wraps around the dorsal surface of the sacrospinous ligament and reenters the pelvis through the lesser sciatic foramen, and for a short distance, it runs in the fat of the ischiorectal fossa (Figure 10.1). The internal pudendal vein and artery branch off the internal iliac vessels, joining the nerve just cephalad to the sacrospinous ligament. From there, the vessels accompany all the branches of the pudendal nerve. The pudendal nerve forms three branches: the dorsal clitoral/penile, perineal, and inferior rectal/anal. Branching of the pudendal nerve is highly variable and may occur anywhere along its course.[7] In some cases, the branches may arise separately from the ventral rami. In general, the inferior rectal nerve is the first branch of the pudendal nerve. Branching may occur anywhere from cephalad to the sacrospinous ligament, to within the pudendal nerve canal (Alcock's canal). In some patients, it even pierces through the sacrospinous ligament. The inferior rectal nerve then continues through the ischiorectal fossa to the rectum. It innervates the external anal sphincter and skin around the anus. The main trunk of the nerve enters Alcock's canal, which is a 3–4 cm passage between the aponeurosis of the obturator internus muscle and the muscle itself. The exit of Alcock's canal is located in the medial surface of the ischial tuberosity. The nerve then follows

the inferior edge of the ischiopubic ramus and divides into its two terminal branches—dorsal clitoral/penile and perineal nerves (Figure 10.2). Perineal nerves course medially and accompany the superficial transverse perineal muscle to innervate the perineum and labia/scrotum. The dorsal clitoral nerve accompanies the ischiocavernosus muscle and runs anteriorly and medially between the superior and inferior layers of the fascia of urogenital diaphragm. It then enters the crura of the clitoris on the dorsomedial side and continues to the glans providing sensation to the clitoris. Vasoactive changes leading to erection are controlled by parasympathetic cavernous nerves of the clitoris and are not related to the pudendal nerve.[8]

In general, entrapment of the pudendal nerve may occur in several locations along its course, especially in areas of fixation, acute flexion, and within narrow canals. The first and most common area of the nerve entrapment is within the interligamentous space—the space between the sacrospinous and sacrotuberous ligaments. Entrapment may occur with the fixation of the nerve to the dorsal surface of the sacrospinous ligament or by the falciform process on the ventral surface of the sacrotuberous ligament.[9] When adhesions are absent, entrapment

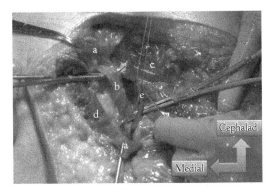

FIGURE 10.1: Pudendal nerve between sacrospinous and sacrotuberous ligaments. Cadaveric dissection of right gluteal region:

a—cut edges of the sacrotuberous ligament

b—sacrospinous ligament

c—piriformis muscle

d—gluteus muscle

e—pudendal nerve

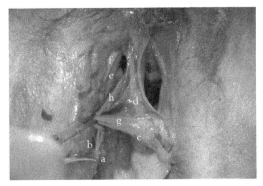

FIGURE 10.2: Pudendal nerve exiting the pudendal nerve (Alcock's) canal. Cadaveric dissection of the right perineal region:

a—ischial tuberosity

b—pudendal nerve exiting pudendal (Alcock's) canal

c—superficial transverse perineal muscle

d—bulbospongiosus muscle

e—ischiocavernosus muscle

f—inferior pubic ramus

g—perineal branch of the pudendal nerve

h—dorsal clitoral branch of the pudendal nerve

may be caused by stretching of the nerve from acute flexion at the sacrospinous ligament or from compression of the nerve within a narrow canal formed by the close proximity of the ligaments. Extreme flexion of the hip or sitting can further narrow the space, causing compression of the nerve.[10] The second potential area of compression is within Alcock's canal. Adhesions may form within the canal, or the canal may be narrowed by spasms of the obturator internus muscle. Other areas of potential compression that are (infrequently) encountered are at the level of the pyriformis muscle and medial to the ischial tuberosity at the ischiopubic ramus. The latter area of compression would affect the perineal and/or dorsal nerve and spare the inferior rectal nerve.

ETIOLOGY

There are four main mechanisms that may give rise to pudendal neuralgia: (1) pelvic floor muscle spasms without true pudendal neuropathy; (2) pelvic floor muscle spasms causing nerve compression; (3) direct injury to the nerve from scar tissue, ligaments, or surgical material; and (4) biochemical injury from disease or infection.[1,11]

Pelvic floor muscle spasms often have a presentation very similar to that of pudendal neuralgia from nerve compression.[12] These muscle spasms may be idiopathic, psychological, related to pelvic floor injury, or caused by some other pain condition in the pelvis. One of the most common diseases in women that cause pelvic floor muscle spasms is endometriosis. Through phenomena called "visceral-somatic convergence," endometriosis implants located on pelvic viscera refer pain to somatic structures via afferent nerves converging at the dorsal horns. These painful muscles lead to vaginal, vulvar, and/or rectal pain that is worse with sitting. In addition, muscle spasms, especially spasms of the obturator internus muscle, may lead to direct compression of the pudendal nerves and its branches as they travel through Alcock's canal and muscle fibers. This compression may lead to pain from physical activity and sitting. Certainly, it is very difficult to distinguish myalgia from neuralgia, since muscle spasms often accompany neuropathic pain.

Pudendal nerve entrapment (PNE) occurs from mechanical injury or compression of the nerve. It is almost always caused by pelvic trauma from events such as surgery, childbirth,

sitting, intercourse, or athletic activity. In our experience, surgery is the most common cause of pudendal nerve entrapment (Box 10.1). Hysterectomy, especially for pelvic organ prolapse, has been implicated as a cause of pudendal nerve entrapment. In these patients, scarring of the pudendal nerve at the interligamentous space is often found during pudendal decompression surgery. Although initially difficult to rationalize, the likely mechanisms of scarring of the nerve may be: (1) secondary to retroperitoneal bleeding during ligation of uterine artery that extends along the course of the pudendal nerve via the pudendal artery; and (2) compression of the nerve at the sacrospinous ligament by long, curved retractors. Pudendal nerve entrapment may also occur after mesh kit placement for repair of vaginal compartment defects (see below "Special Considerations"). In this case, the nerve may be pierced or compressed by the mesh exiting on the posterior side of sacrospinous ligament. In addition, the inferior rectal nerve runs in close proximity to the pathway of the trocar from posterior compartment repair mesh kits and is susceptible to direct injury.[13]

During a vaginal delivery, the pudendal nerve may be stretched or compressed at the level of the ischial spines by the infant's head. Pudendal nerve latency tests have shown that injuries occur after vaginal deliveries.[14] Still, it remains unclear whether traumatic or operative vaginal deliveries predispose patients to developing pudendal nerve entrapment.

Classically, cycling is one of the better-described mechanisms of pudendal nerve entrapment.[2] The narrow seat of the bicycle places pressure on the perineum, leading to repetitive

---

BOX 10.1
CAUSES OF PUDENDAL NEURALGIA

1. Pelvic surgery, especially with use of mesh
2. Pelvic trauma
3. Childbirth
4. Bicycle riding
5. Prolonged sitting
6. Constipation
7. Anal intercourse/use of anal devices
8. Excessive masturbation

micro-trauma. This results in scarring of the nerve medial to the ischial tuberosities and within Alcock's canal. Other causes of pudendal nerve entrapment are instrumentation of the vagina or rectum from use of vibrators or masturbation. It is probably the result of direct nerve injury or stimulation of severe muscles spams causing entrapment. Similarly, athletic activity may lead to hypertrophy of the obturator internus muscle, causing direct compression of the pudendal nerve in the Alcock's canal. If symptoms are noted early enough and activity stops, the patient's symptoms may reverse without any additional treatment.

Another, rare group are patients who developed pudendal neuralgia due to viral infection (herpes zoster, HIV), diabetes, or multiple sclerosis.[15] Treatment of these patients involves treatment of the underlying disease. Nevertheless, their symptoms may persist even after treatment, probably secondary to peripheral and central sensitization.

SYMPTOMS

The hallmark of pudendal neuralgia is burning, neuropathic pain in the distribution of the pudendal nerve that is worse when sitting, and better with lying down. While some patients only have pain when sitting, most patients experience symptoms continuously that is exacerbated by sitting. Pain can be bilateral or unilateral. Patients with pudendal nerve entrapment or direct injuries are more likely to have unilateral pain. If impingement is within the interligamentous space, they may have sharp, stabbing pain deep in the vagina or rectum. Patients may also point to their right or left lower quadrant abdomen or buttocks. This pain is secondary to activation of the nervi nevorum of the pudendal nerve within the interligamentous space.[16]

Pain can involve one, two, or all three branches of the pudendal nerve; therefore, pain may be isolated to the rectum, perineum/vagina, or clitoris, or it may affect a combination of these locations. Pain is usually least in the morning and worse in the evening, indicating myalgia of the pelvic floor muscles. The pain does not wake up the patient at night. There is often improvement of pain with sitting on a toilet seat, as this alleviates pressure from the perineum and sacrospinous ligaments. Allodynia and hyperesthesia are common, leading to discomfort from touch or clothing. Other associated symptoms include allotriesthesia, which is the sensation of a foreign body in the vagina or rectum.

Depending on which branches of the nerve are involved patients can have pain with urination, full bladder, bowel movements, intercourse, or orgasm. Bladder symptoms such as urgency, frequency, and dysuria in the setting of pelvic pain are often mistaken for interstitial cystitis/painful bladder syndrome or overactive bladder.[17] Bowel movements, especially while constipated, may lead to pelvic floor muscle spasms and temporary worsening of symptoms. Some patients report pain with sexual arousal, or have persistent sexual arousal that becomes painful.

Symptoms tend to worsen over time. Comfortable sitting time, or the time it takes to feel uncomfortable with sitting, decreases over time. Also, patients begin to experience pain outside the area of innervation of the pudendal nerve. Legs, lower back, abdomen, and buttocks are common areas of associated pain. Neuralgia may develop of the sciatic, obturator, and/or posterior femoral cutaneous nerves. When patients present with global pain symptoms, it may be difficult to identify pudendal neuralgia as the cause of their symptoms. This difficulty is due to central sensitization.

CENTRAL SENSITIZATION AND COMPLEX REGIONAL PAIN SYNDROME

Central sensitization develops from increased neuron response in the dorsal horn of the spinal cord.[18] This is usually preceded by peripheral sensitization, which is activation of peripheral nerves from inflammation or impingement. Persistent neural activation leads to increased intracellular calcium that in turn and enhances synaptic inputs by increasing the number of synapses on dorsal horn neurons. This mechanism is conducted by N-methyl-D-aspartate (NMDA) receptors. Neuronal excitability follows; thus neurons respond to both noxious and innocuous stimuli, leading to hyperalgesia and allodynia.

Patients with more severe or prolonged pudendal neuralgia often develop symptoms of complex regional pain syndrome (CRPS). Symptoms of CRPS include severe burning, edema, muscle spasm, swelling, changes in skin tenderness and color, joint tenderness, and restricted, painful joint movement. Patients often develop allodynia that extends outside the dermatome of the affected nerve. Type II CRPS begins with nerve injury and causes upregulation in NMDA receptors.

Central sensitization and CRPS can be very difficult to reverse. Ketamine, an anesthetic used in pediatric and veterinary medicine, is used in the treatment of those conditions. Detailed description of use of ketamine in treatment of chronic pelvic neuropathic pain is beyond the scope of this chapter, but several studies have shown its significant benefit in the treatment of chronic pain syndromes.[19]

DIAGNOSIS

History

Pudendal neuralgia is mostly diagnosed based on the patient's history. Establishing the onset and initial setting of pain is very important. The majority of patients develop symptoms after a traumatic event, such as injury to the pelvis.[20] Onset may be immediate or delayed. Common traumatic injuries are pelvic surgery, sport trauma, vaginal delivery, or sexual activity such as vigorous intercourse or the use of vibrators (anal or vaginal). Injury during surgery may occur with hysterectomy, positioning, or mesh placement. It is important to review medical records and operative reports if pain starts after surgery. Pudendal neuralgia may also develop after persistent pelvic infections, prostatitis, and urethritis. This development is likely to be secondary to peripheral sensitization. Nevertheless, some patients report a gradual onset without any identifiable instigating event.

To summarize, patients present with pain located in the area of innervation of pudendal nerve that is unilateral or bilateral. Pain is neuropathic and always worse with sitting. Patients often report that they feel minimal to no pain when they wake up in the morning and worsening pain with daily activities. They also report less pain when sitting on the toilet. Patient often describe feeling a like a ball is lodged in their rectum or vagina, or the sensation of a hot poker. Almost all patients with pudendal neuralgia have pain with intercourse and postcoital dyspareunia. They may also avoid sexual activity or arousal or have symptoms of persistent sexual arousal. The urinary symptoms may range from urgency and frequency to severe dysuria. Quality of life is poor. It affects their work since they cannot sit, and affects their personal relationships with their family.

Examination

Examination for pudendal neuralgia is focused on three things: (1) confirmation of pain in the distribution of the pudendal nerve; (2) evaluation of the pelvic floor muscles; and (3) ruling out other painful conditions that may mimic pudendal neuralgia (see "Differential Diagnosis")[20] (Figure 10.3). A thorough abdominal and pelvic examination should be performed. Attention should be placed on abdominal scars, the presence of any anterior abdominal wall myalgias, and allodynia/hyperalgesia from abdominal and pelvic nerves. During the pelvic examination, careful inspection of the genitals and rectum should be performed for lesions and dermatological changes. Tenderness should be present with palpation of the perineum, vulva, clitoris, and/or anus. Unlike patients with injuries to other nerves, pudendal neuralgia rarely causes sensory deficits, but careful sensory examination can be performed. Because of autonomic dysfunction, there may be identifiable dryness of skin over the affected area. Patients with pudendal neuralgia almost always have spasm of the pelvic floor muscles. Tenderness is often elicited with palpation of the obturator internus muscle and ischiococcygeus muscle. Palpation over the sacrospinous ligament medial to the ischial spine may reproduce symptoms or cause a severe, stabbing, sharp pain, since compression of the pudendal nerve occurs. This response is commonly known as "Tinel's sign." Tinel's sign

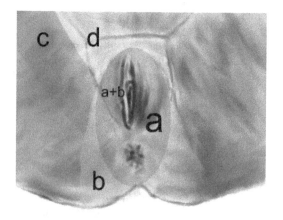

FIGURE 10.3: Innervation of the perineum:
a—pudendal nerve
b—inferior cluneal nerve
c—obturator nerve
d—genitofemoral nerve

may also be present when percussing the dorsal clitoral/penile branch as it emerges from underneath the inferior ramus of the pubic bone.

Electrophysiological Testing

Pudendal Nerve Motor Terminal Latency
Pudendal nerve motor terminal latency is a well-known test to assess for injury to the nerve. The test is a motor nerve conduction study that measures the time it takes for an impulse to travel along the length of the nerve to its target muscle. This time, called the "latency," is measured in milliseconds. In theory, patients with focal compression of the nerve have slow conduction and a prolonged latency. Measurements are obtained with a St. Mark's electrode that is attached to the examiner's gloved index finger. During the test, the tip of the finger that contains a stimulating electrode is placed vaginally or rectally on the sacrospinous ligament. The base of the index finger contains a registering electrode that measures the impulse at the anal sphincter or bulbospongiosus muscle.[21]

Practitioners have questioned the validity of the pudendal nerve motor latency test; therefore, the test remains controversial for the diagnosis of pudendal neuralgia. The test measures motor activity and thus may not be relevant in patients with neuropathic pain without motor deficits. For instance, motor latency is significantly prolonged in many asymptomatic women who delivered vaginally.[22] In our experience, most patients with pudendal neuralgia have normal pudendal nerve latency. Thus, it is possible that prolonged latency does not correlate well with nerve injury. In addition, the latency of the nerve depends on its length, and this length cannot be measured prior to the test. Intra-observer and inter-observer variability in obtaining and interpreting measurements is also high. Therefore, most physicians treating patients for pudendal neuralgia do not rely on this test to diagnose pudendal nerve entrapment.[23]

Electromyography (EMG) is another electrophysiological test to assess pudendal nerve quality. The muscles assessed are the levator muscles of the pelvis, which for the most part are innervated by pudendal nerves. Unfortunately, the validity of that test has never been confirmed, and the fact that other nerves may innervate pelvic floor muscles makes this test less useful.

Quantitative Sensory Testing

Quantitative sensory testing can be used to confirm a neuropathy. Specific tests that have been used are the warmth detection threshold test (WDT), the two-point discrimination test, and the vibration test.[24] These tests rely on asymmetrical presentation where the unaffected side can be compared to the affected side. In the WDT test, a heated probe is applied to the affected area and temperature is increased slowly. The value at which the patient notes a change in temperature is compared with the unaffected side. Similarly, the two-point discrimination test uses two blunt needles that are moved away from each other until the patient can discriminate the sensations. Quantitative sensory testing has been used to diagnose nerve injury in other nerves in the body, but its usefulness in pudendal neuralgia has not been proven in properly designed studies.

Magnetic Resonance Imaging

Magnetic resonance testing can be divided into anatomical scans and functional MRI, also called "MR neurography." Even though the magnetic resonance imaging may turn out to be the best test to assess for compression of the pudendal nerve, the current technology is still not accurate enough to show nerve scarring/compression with high enough certainty and reproducibility.[25]

Pudendal nerve magnetic resonance neurography uses chemical to biochemical properties of the nerve fibers to enhance its signal and distinguish it from the surrounding scar tissue. Signals from nerves are highly organized and run in a parallel direction, while signals from adhesions are very disorganized. Unfortunately, with the small diameters for the pudendal nerve (3–5 mm for the main trunk and 1–2 mm for the branches), this difference in the signal may not be easily seen. There are only a handful of providers who perform MRN of the pudendal nerve. There are no independent studies to confirm these findings or correlation with observations during surgery.

Anatomical scans of the pudendal nerve may prove more useful than the functional scans (Figure 10.4). They can detect compression of the nerve by visualizing scar tissue. The disadvantage is that the resolution of 1.5 and 3 Tesla MRIs are not powerful enough to visualize fine scar tissue less than 1–2 mm. Impingement may be inferred by measuring the pudendal veins. Since the pudendal nerve runs with the pudendal vein and artery, compression of the nerve

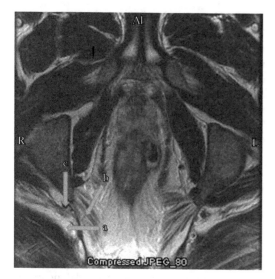

FIGURE 10.4: MRI image of pudendal nerve:
a—sacrotuberous ligament
b—sacrospinous ligament
c—pudendal nerve

would lead to compression of the vein. This can form a varicosity that is visible on the MRI. Similar to functional MRI, the findings of anatomical MRI have never been shown to correlate with surgical observations. Nevertheless, the anatomical MRI may still be important to rule out other conditions such as Tarlov's cyst, pelvic masses, tears in pelvic floor fasciae or tendons, or labrum tears.[26]

Nantes Criteria

Nantes criteria for diagnosing pudendal nerve entrapment were developed by Roger Robert in Nantes, France, and published in 2008.[3] Professor Robert is one of the pioneers of treatment and diagnosis of pudendal neuralgia and is the first person to describe the transgluteal approach to surgical decompression of the pudendal nerve. Nantes criteria were developed to help predict pudendal nerve entrapment and therefore identify patients who are candidates for pudendal neurolysis. This correlation was validated in a randomized study[3] (Box 10.2).

DIFFERENTIAL DIAGNOSIS

The differential diagnosis of genital pain is broad, and common conditions should be ruled out. Pudendal neuralgia shares many similarities with other painful diseases affecting the genital region. Interestingly, those painful diseases are mostly diagnoses of exclusion and therefore may actually represent a subset of pudendal neuralgia in some cases.

1. Pelvic floor tension myalgia (also called levator syndrome or vaginismus) is caused by spastic tender muscles of the pelvic floor that may be idiopathic, psychological, or in response to visceral pain by visceral somatic convergence. Symptoms consists of pain with sitting, physical activity, intercourse, and orgasm.[12] Urinary hesitancy is a hallmark symptom of pelvic floor dysfunction since patients cannot relax the pelvic floor to urinate. Postcoital pain that last for hours to days may also occur. Many patients with pudendal neuralgia share these symptoms since neuralgia may lead to pelvic floor muscle spasms. Thus, pelvic floor tension myalgia must be ruled out in in pudendal neuralgia patients with spastic pelvic floors (see "Treatment" section).

2. Painful bladder syndrome/interstitial cystitis has several symptoms that are identical to some of those in pudendal neuralgia. They include urgency, frequency, dysuria, and pain with full bladder.[17] Pain in patients with painful bladder syndrome/interstitial cystitis is located suprapubically, but it is also often present in the urethra, vagina, labia, perineum, and lower back. Additionally, the etiology of PBS/IC is unknown, and it has been postulated that a neurogenic inflammatory process may play a role in the onset of the disease.[20]

3. Vulvodynia or provoked vestibulodynia are a popular diagnosis of exclusion for patients with vulvar pain without identifiable cause.[27] Vulvar pain in vulvodynia is considered to be neuropathic, and treatments are directed at avoiding stimuli and use of antidepressants. Clearly, neuropathic pain of the vulva could be secondary to pudendal nerve sensitization; therefore, patients with vulvodynia may be suffering from pudendal neuralgia or pudendal nerve entrapment. Additionally, vulvodynia may be secondary to injury

---

BOX 10.2
NANTES CRITERIA

INCLUSION CRITERIA
Pain in the area innervated by the pudendal nerve
Pain does not awaken patients from sleep
Pain with no objective sensory impairment
Pain relieved by diagnostic pudendal block

EXCLUSION CRITERIA
Pain located exclusively in the coccygeal, gluteal, pubic, or hypogastric area (without pain in the area of distribution of pudendal nerve)
Pruritus
Pain exclusively paroxysmal
Abnormality on imaging (MRI, CT) that can account for pain

COMPLEMENTARY CRITERIA
Pain characteristics: burning, shooting, numbing
Allodynia or hyperesthesia
Allotriesthesia (sensation of foreign body)
Pain progressively worse throughout the day
Pain predominantly unilateral
Pain triggered by defecation
Significant tenderness around ischial spine
Abnormal neurophysiology testing Pudendal Nerve Motor Terminal Latency (PNMTL)

ASSOCIATED SIGNS
Buttock pain (around ischial tuberosity)
Referred sciatic pain
Pain referred to the medial side of the thigh
Suprapubic pain
Urinary frequency with full bladder
Pain after orgasm/ejaculation
Dyspareunia or pain after intercourse
Erectile dysfunction
Normal PNMTL

---

of the genitofemoral or posterior femoral cutaneous nerves, as they each have sensory innervation to the area.

TREATMENT

Non-invasive Treatment

Avoidance of Symptoms
Avoidance of painful activities is the single most important treatment of pudendal neuralgia.

Repetitive trauma to the pudendal nerve may increase scarring, while persistent pain increases pelvic floor muscle spasms and may lead to central sensitization. Avoidance of symptoms is extremely effective when pudendal neuralgia is associated with an activities such as cycling, gymnastics, athletics, climbing, and dancing.[28] Patients who stop these activities may improve without further treatment. Nevertheless, this strategy cannot be applied to patients who developed pudendal neuralgia from trauma such as a fall, vaginal delivery, or surgery. In these patients, lifestyle modifications can help manage symptoms. Most patients sit on cushions with a cut-out center to alleviate pressure at the perineum with sitting. Other modifications include using "zero-gravity" chairs and kneeling chairs, standing at work, lying down, and reducing physical activity.

Physical Therapy

Physical therapy is a very important treatment in patients with pudendal neuralgia since muscle spasms are a significant component of their pain. The main role of physical therapy is relaxation of pelvic floor muscles.[1] Therapists address spasm, muscle imbalances, restrictive connective tissues, and other dysfunctions. Therapy is administered as "hands-on" techniques, focusing on posture, range of motion, exercises, stretching, and education. Most of these patients have significant muscle spasm and subsequent muscle shortening throughout the pelvic girdle. Manual techniques that help release the muscle spasms and lengthen the muscle include myofascial release, soft and connective tissue mobilization, and trigger-point release. Other modalities include biofeedback, ultrasonography, and electrical stimulation. Patients who have improvement of muscle spasms may be able to sit longer and perform more physical activities.

Medications

First-line medical therapy for pudendal neuralgia is muscle relaxants.[16] From our experience, oral muscle relaxants do not have much effect on pelvic floor muscles, and the most effective medication is a vaginal suppository with diazepam and baclofen. Diazepam 5,mg is compounded with 4,mg of baclofen into a suppository and inserted vaginally up to twice a day. Belladonna and opium rectal suppositories are also effective, and they have been used for treatment of pelvic pain since the nineteenth century. Belladonna is a mixture of hyoscamine, atropine, and scopolamine and is a potent smooth muscle relaxant. Opium mostly contains morphine and codeine.

Second-line medications are antiepileptic GABA analogues such as gabapentin and pregabaline.[29] They are widely used in treatment of any kind of neuropathic pain and are effective in some patients with pudendal neuralgia. Gabapentin binds to $\alpha 2\delta$ subunit of voltage-dependent calcium channels in the central nervous system. It prevents the formation of new synapses, therefore decreasing neuropathic pain. The usual starting dose for neurontin is 300–900 mg/day in three divided doses, titrated up to a maximum of 3600 mg/day. Lyrica is usually started at 75 mg twice a day. Doses may be increased to a maximum of 600 mg/day in two to three divided doses.

Botulinum Toxin Injections

Botulinum toxin injections into the pelvic floor muscles may benefit patients who have persistent muscle spasms despite adequate pelvic floor physical therapy.[30] Botulinum toxin causes the release of acetylcholine in synapses, thereby inhibiting muscle contraction. Effects from the Botox are seen in about five days, and most patients report improvement of pain in two weeks. Injections are performed transvaginally into the levator ani muscle group and obturator internus muscles bilaterally in patients with global pelvic floor tension myalgia. Alternatively, injections may be focused on areas of spasms. Botox is diluted to 10 units per 1 ml of 0.9% sterile saline and injected in 1 ml increments. This can be done in the office, but sedation is preferred to limit provocation of further muscle spasms from the painful procedure. Some patients improve after one dose, but the majority need repetitive injections every three months when the effects of the toxin wear off. Approximately 60–70% of patients have significant improvement of pain after the botulinum toxin injection.

Interventional Procedures

Pudendal Nerve Blocks

Pudendal nerve blocks are used to help establish the diagnosis of pudendal neuralgia and may provide long-term pain relief. Nerve blocks are injections consisting of a local anesthetic and a steroid and may be performed unguided or with the assistance of imaging technology. Unguided blocks are performed through the vagina, perineum, or buttock by palpating 1 cm medial to the ischial spine. Guided pudendal nerve blocks use ultrasound, fluoroscopy, or computer tomography (CT) to visualize landmarks and confirm injection of solution at the site. All patients with pudendal neuralgia will experience a transient relief of pain regardless of whether a pudendal nerve entrapment is present. In patients in whom no relief is obtained, pudendal neuralgia may be ruled out if a technically successful block can be confirmed. For this reason, CT-guided blocks may be more desirable because one can review images and be certain that the injection was done in the proper location[31] (Figure 10.5).

Some patients also experience long-term relief from the steroid injected. Steroids help reduce inflammation and ectopic nerve activity. One study showed that 92% of patients have some relief after the block, but this number seemed too high in clinical practice.[32] In our experience, it appears that about 30–40% of patients have long-term relief from the block.[20] This observation may be secondary to a large portion of patient in our practice who have a true pudendal nerve entrapment and therefore less likely to respond to steroids.

Pulsed Radiofrequency Ablation

Pulse radiofrequency ablation is a technique in which both thermal and nonthermal energy is delivered to the nerve. This energy is delivered in short 20-millisecond bursts of energy followed by 480 milliseconds of cooling period. Approximately 1600 pulses are applied. The mechanism of pain relief is not known, but it appears that strong electromagnetic fields may cause upregulation of c-Fos protein expression and inhibition of C-fibers.[33] There are several case reports describing good pain relief after this procedure.[34] In a 2013 prospective study, long-term pain relief was seen when patients were followed for 12–18 months.[35]

Surgery

Surgical decompression of the pudendal nerve is reserved for patients with a high suspicion of pudendal nerve entrapment or for patients who have failed to respond to conservative treatments. Since a true pudendal nerve entrapment can only be confirmed with surgery, success of surgery strongly depends on patient selection. Different approaches to access and release the pudendal nerve have been described.

Transgluteal Pudendal Neurolysis

Transgluteal pudendal neurolysis is the most common and successful approach to surgical decompression of the pudendal nerve. This surgical approach allows complete access to the pudendal nerve trunk and visualization of the most common areas of compression (Figure 10.6). It was first described by French neurosurgeon Roger Robert in 1989 and has since been modified by the authors of this chapter to improve visualization, decrease adhesion formation, promote nerve regeneration, help pelvic stability, and improve postsurgical pain.[20,36]

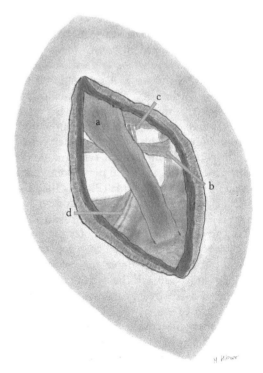

FIGURE 10.6: View during transgluteal pudendal neurolysis (*right*):

a—sacrotuberous ligament

b—sacrospinous ligament

c—pudendal neurovascular bundle in the intraligamentous space

d—pudendal neurovascular bundle in the pudendal nerve (Alcock's) canal

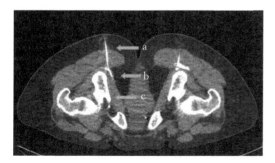

FIGURE 10.5: CT guided pudendal nerve block. Patient prone:

a—needle

b—contrast in the right intraligamentous space

c—right obturator internus muscle

The surgery begins with patients in a prone, jackknife position. The nerve integrity monitoring system is used to help identify the nerve by measuring muscle activity at the external anal sphincter. A transgluteal incision over the sacrotuberous ligament is performed. The ligament is identified and a Z-type incision is made to open up the interligamentous space. This incision helps improve visualization while allowing the surgeon to repair the ligament without using a graft. Although controversial, repair of the ligament is important to maintain pelvic stability.[37] The pudendal nerve is identified using the Nerve Integrity Monitoring System (NIMS) wand and surgical microscope. The nerve is then freed from its surrounding tissue from the level of the piriformis muscle to the distal Alcock's canal. At this point, varicosities of the pudendal vein may be observed, and these veins are typically transected to reduce nerve compression. When the nerve is free, the sacrospinous ligament is transected and the nerve is transposed anteriorly, decreasing the risk of nerve compression and allowing it to run a straighter course. The nerve is then wrapped in any of the commercially available nerve wraps to decrease the risk of re-scarring of the nerve. A pain pump is then placed next to the nerve. This pump allows for continuous two-week block of the nerve and provides excellent postoperative pain control. More importantly, this continuous nerve block may help reverse the central sensitization that many patients with pudendal nerve compression develop. Platelet-rich plasma (PRP) is then used to coat the nerve after surgery.[38] Based on studies, it is believed that Epidermal Growth Factor (EGF) present in the PRP promotes the growth of Schwan cells and therefore the production of myelin, which is responsible for proper nerve function and healing.[18] The sacrotuberous ligament is then repaired and subcutaneous tissue and skin closed.

Measuring objective outcomes of transgluteal pudendal neurolysis or any other treatment for chronic pain is difficult, secondary to broadly varying individual experience of symptoms and its impact on quality of life. Studies from France showed that after surgery, one-third of patients have no pain, one-third have improvement of pain, and one-third have no improvement. Approximately one percent of patients are at risk of getting worse after this procedure. In a sequential randomized control trial, 71.4% of patients in the surgery group had improvement at 12 months, compared to 13.3% of patients in the non-surgery group.[4] Results may depend on the degree of entrapment, nerve integrity, and duration of symptoms.

Transischiorectal Pudendal Neurolysis

Transischiorectal pudendal neurolysis was described by French gynecologist Eric Bautrand in 2003 as an alternative to the transgluteal approach.[39] This procedure is preformed transvaginally in women and through an incision in the perineum in men. One of the advantages of this procedure is that it does not require transection of the sacrotuberous ligament and therefore may decrease the risk of instability of the sacroiliac joint. The biggest drawback to the procedure seems to be the limited visualization of the nerve and poor access to the entire length of the nerve. Also, in male patients, it requires an incision that is painful and difficult to heal. A study from France showed pain resolution in 83% of patients after this procedure; however, this high rate of success was not confirmed by any other practitioner.

Transperineal Pudendal Neurolysis

Transperineal pudendal neurolysis is a procedure developed for patients who have entrapment of terminal branches of the nerve, rather than the main trunk between sacrotuberous and sacrospinous ligaments. It is most suitable for patients with isolated clitoral or perineal pain.[40] In this procedure, the patient is placed in the lithotomy position and an incision is performed lateral to the labia majora in women or the scrotum in men. The nerve is identified at the distal Alcock's canal medial to the ischial tuberosity. The nerve is then freed from scar tissue that usually entraps the nerve to the surface of the ischiopubic ramus. Outcomes of this procedure are not clear.

Endoscopic Transperitoneal Pudendal Neurolysis

The pudendal nerve can be approached through the abdominal cavity either during laparotomy, laparoscopy, or robotic-assisted laparoscopy.[41] After the retroperitoneal space is opened and the internal iliac artery is identified, it can be followed until the internal pudendal artery is found. Sacrospinous ligament is then found anterior to the artery as it leaves the pelvis through the lesser sciatic foramen. This ligament can then be transected, and the pudendal neurovascular bundle is identified posterior to the ligament. This technique allows for access of the interligamentous space and limits visualization to other possible areas of entrapment. In addition, transection of the levator ani muscle may be needed, and this carries potential complications and additional pain. Several surgeons perform transperitoneal pudendal neurolysis. Outcomes are mixed and numbers are too small to assess the outcomes.

Redo Pudendal Neurolysis

Reoperation using a transgluteal approach may be performed for patients who have failed pudendal nerve decompression surgery by other approaches, or for patients who have a recurrence of symptoms after initially successful treatment.[42] Failure of initial surgery may have been secondary to poor visualization of the nerve at the time of surgery, not using preventive measures against adhesions, or reinjury from a fall or trauma. The repeat surgery carries an increased risk of nerve injury from dense fibrosis; therefore, the surgical microscope and NIMS monitor are invaluable. We reported our results from this procedure in nine patients, eight of whom had global improvement and two of whom had complete resolution of pain.

Special Considerations

Post–Vaginal Mesh Pudendal Neuralgia

In 2011 Food and Drug Administration released a warning of potential complications of transvaginal mesh used in the treatment of incontinence and pelvic organ prolapse. Chronic pelvic pain after mesh placement is one of the most serious complications, resulting in decreased productivity and poor quality of life. Many of these patients have pain from pudendal neuralgia from two possible mechanisms. One, the pudendal nerve may be entrapped by the mesh that is anchored to the sacrospinous ligaments, especially if it is attached 1–2 cm from the ischial spine.[13] Second, mesh traveling through or anchored to the obturator internus muscle may cause severe spasms of the pelvic floor, leading to compression and irritation of the pudendal nerve. In these patients, we advocate conservative treatment of pelvic floor, first including physical therapy, Botox injections to pelvic floor, and nerve blocks. If conservative therapy fails, patients will need to have the mesh removed. Published literature shows that the

removal of mesh is beneficial in patients with post–vaginal mesh pain. However, the portion of the mesh that is posterior the sacrospinous ligament cannot be removed through a vaginal or abdominal approach. In patients in whom the pain persists, a transgluteal pudendal neurolysis to remove part of the mesh may be necessary.

Persistent Genital Arousal Disorder

One of the most vexing symptoms in patients with pudendal nerve entrapment is persistent genital arousal disorder (PGAD).[43] Patients have the constant sensation of being on the verge of orgasm and may have to masturbate several times an hour to relieve that tension. Occasionally, patients have spontaneous orgasms, and men can experience ejaculation. This arousal is not related to any feelings of sexual desire. Vibrations, such as riding in a car, may provoke it. PGAD may be caused by pudendal nerve entrapment, but there may be some other causative conditions, such as psychiatric disorders and endocrine disorders. This syndrome may be also potentially be caused by congestion of the veins around the clitoris or penis. Treatment of PGAD is difficult and should be targeted toward the specific etiology causing this condition. In some cases, surgical decompression of the pudendal nerve may be necessary; however, the outcomes in relieving symptoms of PGAD may not be as good at relieving pain.

SUMMARY

Pudendal neuralgia is a debilitating and painful neuropathic condition in the area of innervation of pudendal nerve. Hallmark symptoms include pain with sitting and relief of pain with standing or sitting on a toilet seat. Onset may be gradual or immediately following a traumatic event such as surgery, falls, and vaginal deliveries. The Nantes criteria offer a reproducible way to diagnose pudendal neuralgia. A pudendal nerve block can be performed to confirm the diagnosis. Conservative therapies such as avoidance, lifestyle modifications, and medications are preferred. Surgical decompression is reserved for patients for whom medical management has failed. Despite advances in medicine, pudendal neuralgia is still not well understood, and further research is needed to describe patient phenotypes and to establish diagnosis and treatment. Nevertheless, pudendal neuralgia should be suspected in patients complaining of genital and rectal pain without an identifiable cause to insure prompt referral, patient education, and treatment.

REFERENCES

1. Hibner M, Desai N, Robertson LJ, Nour, M. Pudendal neuralgia. *J Minim Invasive Gynecol.* 2010;17:148–153.

2. Amarenco G, Lanoe Y, Perrigot M, Goudal H. A new canal syndrome: compression of the pudendal nerve in Alcock's canal or perinal paralysis of cyclists. *Presse Med.* 1987;16:399.

3. Labat J-J et al. Diagnostic criteria for pudendal neuralgia by pudendal nerve entrapment (Nantes criteria). *Neurourol Urodyn.* 2008;27:306–310.

4. Robert R, et al. Decompression and transposition of the pudendal nerve in pudendal neuralgia: a randomized controlled trial and long-term evaluation. *Eur Urol.* 2005;47:403–408.

5. Zondervan K, Barlow DH. Epidemiology of chronic pelvic pain. *Best Pract Res Clin Obstet Gynaecol.* 2000;14:403–414.

6. Gray H, Standring S, Ellis H, Berkovitz BKB. *Gray's Anatomy: The Anatomical Basis of Clinical Practice.* New York: Elsevier Churchill Livingstone; 2005: 1364–1371.

7. Mahakkanukrauh P, Surin P, Vaidhayakarn P. Anatomical study of the pudendal nerve adjacent to the sacrospinous ligament. *Clin Anat.* 2005;18: 200–205.

8. Baskin LS, et al. Anatomical studies of the human clitoris. *J Urol.* 1999;162:1015–1020.

9. Labat JJ, Robert R, Bensignor M, Buzelin JM. [Neuralgia of the pudendal nerve. Anatomo-clinical considerations and therapeutical approach]. *J Urol (Paris).* 1990;96:239–244.

10. Brandon K, et al. Excursion of the pudendal nerve and change in the distance between the sacrospinous and sacrotuberous ligament. *Int Pelvic Pain Soc Meet.* 2012.

11. Robert R, et al. Anatomic basis of chronic perineal pain: role of the pudendal nerve. *Surg Radiol Anat.* 1998;20:93–98.

12. Butrick CW. Pelvic floor hypertonic disorders: identification and management. *Obstet Gynecol Clin North Am.* 2009;36:707–722.

13. Castellanos ME, Yi J, Atashroo D, Desai N, Hibner, M. Pudendal neuralgia after posterior vaginal wall repair with mesh kits: an anatomical study and case series. *J Minim Invasive Gynecol.* 2012;19: S72–S73.

14. Lien K-C, Morgan DM, Delancey JOL, Ashton-Miller JA. Pudendal nerve stretch during vaginal birth: a 3D computer simulation. *Am J Obstet Gynecol.* 2005;192:1669–1676.

15. Howard EJ. Postherpetic pudendal neuralgia. *JAMA.* 1985;253:2196.

16. Benson JT, Griffis K. Pudendal neuralgia, a severe pain syndrome. *Am J Obstet Gynecol.* 2005;192:1663–1668.

17. Possover M, Forman, A. Voiding dysfunction associated with pudendal nerve entrapment. *Curr Bladder Dysfunct Rep.* 2012;7:281–285.

18. Campbell JN, Meyer RA. Mechanisms of neuropathic pain. *Neuron.* 2006;52:77–92.

19. Goldberg ME, et al. Multi-day low dose ketamine infusion for the treatment of complex regional pain syndrome. *Pain Physician.* 2005;8:175–179.

20. Hibner M, Castellanos M, Desai N, Balducci J. Pudendal Neuralgia. In: Arulkumaran S, ed. *Global Library of Women's Medicine.* David Bloomer; 2011. doi:10.3843/GLOWM.10468. http://www.glowm.com/section_view/item/691/recordset/18975/value/691

21. Le Tallec de Certaines H, et al. [Comparison between the terminal motor pudendal nerve terminal motor latency, the localization of the perineal neuralgia and the result of infiltrations. Analysis of 53 patients]. *Ann Readapt Med Phys.* 2007;50:65–69.

22. Sultan AH, Kamm MA, Hudson CN. Pudendal nerve damage during labour: prospective study before and after childbirth. *BJOG.* 1994;101:22–28.

23. Tetzschner T, Sørensen M, Rasmussen OO, Lose G, Christiansen J. Reliability of pudendal nerve terminal motor latency. *Int J Colorectal Dis.* 1997;12: 280–284.

24. Walk D, et al. Quantitative sensory testing and mapping: a review of nonautomated quantitative methods for examination of the patient with neuropathic pain. *Clin J Pain.* 2009;25:632–640.

25. Filler AG, et al. Sciatica of nondisc origin and piriformis syndrome: diagnosis by magnetic resonance neurography and interventional magnetic resonance imaging with outcome study of resulting treatment. *J Neurosurg Spine.* 2005;2:99–115.

26. Chen A, Kalinkin O, Castellanos ME, Hibner M. Common MRI findings in patients with symptoms of pudendal neuralgia. *Int Pelvic Pain Soc.* 2012.

27. Shafik A. Pudendal canal syndrome as a cause of vulvodynia and its treatment by pudendal nerve decompression. *Eur J Obstet Gynecol Reprod Biol.* 1998;80:215–220.

28. Antolak SJ. Genitourinary Pain And Inflammation. In: Potts JM, ed. *Current Clinical Urology.* Current Clinical Urology. Totowa, NJ: Humana Press; 2008: 39–56. doi:10.1007/978-1-60327-126-4

29. Backonja M, Glanzman RL. Gabapentin dosing for neuropathic pain: evidence from randomized, placebo-controlled clinical trials. *Clin Ther.* 2003;25: 81–104.

30. Abbott J. The use of botulinum toxin in the pelvic floor for women with chronic pelvic pain—a new answer to old problems? *J Minim Invasive Gynecol.* 2008;16:130–135.

31. Filippiadis DK, et al. CT-guided percutaneous infiltration for the treatment of Alcock's neuralgia. *Pain Physician*. 2011;14:211–215.

32. Fanucci E, et al. Role of interventional radiology in pudendal neuralgia: a description of techniques and review of the literature. *Radiol Med*. 2009;114:425–436.

33. Van Zundert J, et al. Pulsed and continuous radiofrequency current adjacent to the cervical dorsal root ganglion of the rat induces late cellular activity in the dorsal horn. *Anesthesiology*. 2005;102:125–131.

34. Rhame EE, Levey K, Gharibo CG. Successful treatment of refractory pudendal neuralgia with pulsed radiofrequency. *Pain Physician*. 2009;12:633–638.

35. Masala S, et al. CT-guided percutaneous pulse-dose radiofrequency for pudendal neuralgia. *Cardiovasc Intervent Radiol*. 2014;37:476–481.

36. Robert R, Labat JJ, Riant T, Khalfallah M, Hamel O. Neurosurgical treatment of perineal neuralgias. *Adv Tech Stand Neurosurg*. 2007;32:41–59.

37. Vrahas M, Hern TC, Diangelo D, Kellam J, Tile M. Ligamentous contributions to pelvic stability. *Orthopedics*. 1995;18:271–274.

38. Sariguney Y, et al. Effect of platelet-rich plasma on peripheral nerve regeneration. *J Reconstr Microsurg*. 2008;24:159–167.

39. Bautrant E, et al. [Modern algorithm for treating pudendal neuralgia: 212 cases and 104 decompressions]. *J Gynecol Obstet Biol Reprod (Paris)*. 2003;32:705–712.

40. Hruby S, Dellon L, Ebmer J, Höltl W, Aszmann OC. Sensory recovery after decompression of the distal pudendal nerve: anatomical review and quantitative neurosensory data of a prospective clinical study. *Microsurgery*. 2009;29:270–274.

41. Possover M. Laparoscopic management of endopelvic etiologies of pudendal pain in 134 consecutive patients. *J Urol*. 2009;181:1732–1736.

42. Hibner M, Castellanos ME, Drachman D, Balducci J. Repeat operation for treatment of persistent pudendal nerve entrapment after pudendal neurolysis. *J Minim Invasive Gynecol*. 2012;19:325–330.

43. Pink L, Rancourt V, Gordon A. Persistent genital arousal in women with pelvic and genital pain. *J Obstet Gynaecol Can*. 2014;36:324–330.

11

Incapacitating Pelvic Congestion Syndrome

*NEERAJ RASTOGI, NII-KABU KABUTEY, GILLIAN LIEBERMAN,
AND DUCKSOO KIM*

Pain secondary to pelvic venous congestion syndrome (PCS) or pelvic venous incompetence (PVI) is defined as non-cyclical pelvic pain that lasts for at least a six-month duration. The pain is associated with standing, intercourse, and dilated ovarian, periuterine, or vaginal veins. PCS as a clinical entity was first described in 1949 by Taylor, suggesting venous insufficiency as an etiological factor contributing to pelvic pain pathology.[1,2,3] The term "PVI" is preferred to "PCS" or—female varicocele or pelvic vascular congestion (PVC)—because it defines the etio-pathology associated with pelvic congestion and venous engorgement. It usually occurs in premenopausal and multi-parous women.[1,2] Fifteen percent of women experience PCS between the ages of 20 and 50, but not all experience symptoms.[4]

Preliminary diagnostic laboratory tests are obtained to rule out more common pelvic pathologies that can cause pelvic pain. Testing should include a pregnancy test and Pap smear to ensure pregnancy or cervical cancer is not the cause for pain. Pelvic duplex ultrasound (US) and/or computed tomography (CT) scans are usually the first imaging modalities in the evaluation of patients with chronic pelvic pain. Cross-sectional imaging studies are useful to obtain in order to help determine whether there may be an anatomical problem that is causing the problem. Although noninvasive methods such as CT, magnetic resonance imaging (MRI) and pelvic venous duplex ultrasound are increasingly gaining favor as helpful diagnostic tools. Selective ovarian venography[1,2,5] remains the most effective method for both identification of pelvic venous pathology and its ability to provide treatment options. Pelvic varices are treatable by using ovarian suppression, ligation of the pelvic veins, or endovascular embolotherapy with utilization of sclerosant/coils. Procedural interventions, including coil embolization of ovarian the vein,

is usually performed in females with PCS that does not respond to medical treatment.[6,7,8,9,10] In this chapter, we have made an attempt to define *primary* and *secondary* PCS, highlight the role of ovarian venography, and describe the endovascular coil embolization as a safe and effective treatment modality in the management of PCS. Additionally, we review the literature and results of various treatment modalities of unresolved incapacitating pelvic congestion syndrome.

PATHOPHYSIOLOGY

The etiology of pelvic pain can be very difficult to discern. Referred pain from the abdominal viscera and neurogenic and psychogenic factors can all contribute to pelvic pain pathology. Pain within the pelvis can occur with a number of pelvic conditions, such as endometriosis, fibroids, pelvic inflammatory disease, uterine prolapse/malposition, and ovarian cysts.[1,2,3] Therefore, it can be very challenging for physicians who deal with pain involving the pelvis, including primary care doctors, general surgeons, gynecologists, gastroenterologists, pain specialists/anesthesiologists, urological surgeons, and interventional radiologists, to confirm a diagnosis of PCS. Usually, no definitive diagnosis is made in 60% of patients with pelvic pain.[4,11] The presence of varices of the pelvic veins has been shown to be the underlying etiology in most patients with PCS.[1,12,13,14,15] Therefore, primary PCS, which includes congenital or acquired ovarian vein incompetence from non-obstructive causes, is considered a diagnosis of exclusion. Patients with secondary PCS develop ovarian and/or pelvic vein collateral pathways to circumvent the obstruction.

Development of symptomatic varices is caused by a combination of pelvic venous valvular insufficiency and endocrine and mechanical factors. Obstructing anatomical anomalies such as Nutcracker syndrome (NCS), May-Thurner syndrome, uterine malposition, and pelvic tumors may lead to secondary PCS, wherein the ovarian and/or pelvic veins contribute to the development of the collateral pathways to relieve antegrade obstruction. In some cases left retro-aortic renal vein may obstruct the drainage from the left ovarian vein leading to symptomatic pelvic varices. Ovarian veins in premenopausal women are exposed to high concentrations of estradiol and estrone compared to the peripheral circulation.[16] Estrogen overstimulation may be responsible in more than 50% of women diagnosed with PCS. Of note, most patients with PCS do not have amenorrhea or demonstrate hirsutism. Estrogen stimulation leads to venodilatation, which results in the pelvic venous engorgement and thereby weakening of the venous walls, leading to enlargement of the pelvic veins/varicosities. Frequently, ovarian and pelvic varicosities are seen after pregnancy. The capacity of pelvic veins may increase by 60-fold over the non-pregnant state due to increased blood volume during pregnancy, which contributes to venous dilatation and valvular insufficiency. This venous distension may also cause pelvic pain in some woman.

Importantly, contributing factors to PCS include mechanical factors such as damaged or absent venous valves that lead to retrograde flow. Weight gain and anatomical changes in the pelvic structures during pregnancy, external vascular compression such as renal Nutcracker syndrome and iliac vein compression/May-Thurner syndrome may all lead to PCS. "Nutcracker syndrome" is described as the left ovarian vein and the left renal vein's compression by the superior mesenteric artery (Figure 11.1). May-Thurner syndrome can occur due to left common iliac vein compression from the right common iliac artery against the pelvic brim, which may cause iliofemoral deep venous thrombosis with or without the pelvic varices of PCS. Additionally, a few rare cases of combined PCS secondary to both May-Thurner syndrome and NCS have been reported.[10,11,13,14] Mechanical factors result in pooling and delayed clearance of blood in the pelvic and ovarian veins that may be a predisposing factor for venous thrombosis and pelvic pain, secondary to mass effect on the lumbosacral plexus.

CLINICAL PICTURE

Clinical symptoms of pelvic congestion are likely to be the result of the presence of ovarian and pelvic varicosities secondary to PCS. The spectrum is comparable to lower-extremity varicose vein symptomatology, where leg pain and discomfort arises during ambulation resulting from lower extremity venous hypertension, secondary to superficial veins' valvular incompetence, and giving rise to varicose veins.

PCS is associated with constant dull pain in the pelvis, vulvar region, and upper thighs. Heaviness just before the onset of menses, with or without dyspareunia and/or post-coital pain, may also occur. Pelvic examination may demonstrate cervical motion and ovarian point tenderness. Exacerbations of symptoms often occur after prolonged walking/standing or activities that typically increase intra-abdominal pressure. Diurnal variations are frequently reported; the patients are asymptomatic in the morning, and pain typically worsens over time during the day, in the premenstrual period, and/or during pregnancy. The symptoms usually continue to worsen after each subsequent pregnancy; therefore, multiparous women are predisposed to develop PCS due to significant increase in intravascular

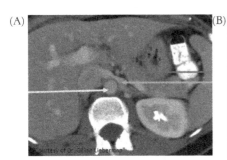 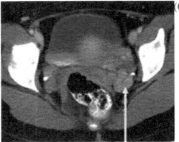 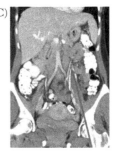

FIGURE 11.1: Contrast CT scans show "nutcracker syndrome" with compressed left renal vein (*blue arrow*) between aorta (*yellow arrow*) and superior mesenteric artery (*red arrow*) in axial scan of the abdomen (*A*); pelvic varices (*yellow arrow*) in axial scan of pelvis (*B*); and dilated ovarian vein (*pink arrow*) in coronal scan of the abdomen (*C*).

volume and increased venous capacity with each term of gestation.[17,18]

Likewise, the pelvic varices develop during pregnancy and continue to progress in size during each term of gestation. Continued venous engorgement predisposes to venous valvular insufficiency. As a result, venous varicosities may be seen internally around the pelvis and sometimes externally at the buttocks, varices extending onto the legs or in the vulvar area under soft tissue, resulting in labial asymmetry.[4] Vulvar or perineal varicosities are reported in more than 10% of the patients with lower extremity superficial venous insufficiency, and these may accompany and reflect ovarian vein insufficiency. These varices can extend over the buttock and posteromedial thigh and communicate with both greater and smaller saphenous veins. They most commonly manifest during pregnancy and regress in the postpartum period. Missed diagnosis of PVI in such cases may explain treatment failure in patients of lower extremity superficial venous insufficiency.[19]

APPLIED CLINICAL ANATOMY

Normal ovarian veins are usually less than five millimeters in diameter and have functional valves.[5,12,13] The left ovarian plexus drains into left ovarian vein, which empties into the left renal at an angle of 90 degrees. The right ovarian plexus drains into the right ovarian vein, which empties usually into the inferior vena cava (IVC) antero-laterally at a 45-degree angle just below the right renal vein. Rarely, the right ovarian vein may drain into the right renal vein. It is important to understand that veins draining the bladder, vagina, uterus, and rectum are interconnected and highly variable. The uterus and vagina drain into the uterine veins and ovarian plexus via the utero-ovarian and salpingo-ovarian veins, and then into branches of the internal iliac veins. Vulvar and perineal veins drain into the internal pudendal vein, then into the inferior gluteal vein, then the external pudendal vein, which drains into the great saphenous vein, or into the circumflex femoral vein, and then into the femoral vein.[20]

The main trunks of ovarian veins have valves, particularly at the terminus of the ovarian vein, to maintain antegrade flow. Most other pelvic venous plexuses and the internal iliac veins are relatively devoid of valves.[18,20] This is an additional contributing factor involved in venous dilation of the pelvic venous anatomy in some patients, even without pregnancy. Congenital absence of venous valves in ovarian veins has been demonstrated in 15% of the PCS patients on the left and 6% on the right.[21] Moreover, valvular incompetency has been recorded in more than one-third of patients, both in the right and in the left ovarian veins.

The development of ovarian/pelvic varices is caused by a combination of factors: (1) valvular incompetence leading to reversal of flow, (2) mechanical venous obstruction, and (3) endocrine/hormonal factors. Of note, all three may play role in the delayed clearance of pelvic venous flow in the utero-ovarian and salpingo ovarian veins, resulting in pelvic venous congestion.

The diagnosis of PCS is defined by the presence of (a) ovarian vein reflux and (b) pelvic varicosities. Ovarian vein reflux can also be present in healthy, asymptomatic, parous women. During pregnancy, pelvic venous capacity increases by 60% due to mechanical compression of the gravid uterus and the vasodilator action of progesterone. Mechanical obstruction caused by the gravid uterus is a main contributing factor in the development of pelvic varicosities. Ovarian vein valvular incompetence leads to reversal of venous flow in the ovarian vein, with dilation of veins in the pelvis and development of ovarian and internal iliac varices. This explains why successive pregnancies may cause venous valves to break down and allow varices to extend to the adjoining pelvic venous plexus; e.g., around uterus (uterovaginalis), bladder (vesicalis), vulva (vulvaris), and rectum (rectalis), and finally the right ovarian vein.[14,22,23]

DIAGNOSTIC IMAGING

Both CT and duplex ultrasound of the pelvis provide excellent resolution of the uterus. A CT scan has greater sensitivity for showing pelvic varicosities; however, duplex ultrasound is increasingly gaining favor as it provides dynamic information about visualized venous blood flow and therefore can be used to evaluate pelvic varicosities, detect venous reflux, and diagnose compression syndromes (e.g., NCS and May-Thurner syndrome). Diagnostic criteria for pelvic duplex sonography include: (1) visualization of enlarged ovarian veins, measuring >6 mm in diameter; (2) the presence of pelvic varicocele (>5 mm; Figure 11.2) and dilated and tortuous myometrial arcuate veins (>5 mm) communicating with pelvic varicose veins/varicocele,

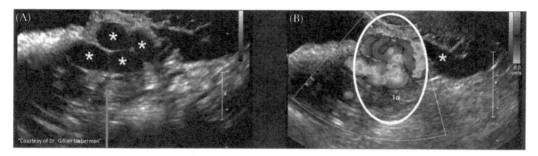

FIGURE 11.2: Sagittal transvaginal ultrasound images of left ovary without (*A*); and with (*B*) Doppler show markedly dilated veins (* *and grey arrow*) adjacent to ovary (+).

bilaterally; and (3) reversed and slow flow (less than 3 cm/s), particularly in the left ovarian vein.[24] Pelvic ultrasonography is a good screening tool, but it can lead to a number of false negative studies due to slow blood flow in pelvic varicosities.[25] Likewise, advanced imaging techniques such as CT and magnetic resonance venography (MRV) can be used to detect dilated pelvic varicosities, areas of venous compression, and rule out other potential etiologies for pelvic pain, especially underlying malignancies. Pelvic MRI typically demonstrates dilated, tortuous, enhancing tubular structures (enlarged pelvic veins) near the uterus and ovary extending to the broad ligament and pelvic sidewall (dilated utero-ovarian and salpingo ovarian veins). Contrast enhancement with gadolinium not only improves visualization, but increases sensitivity if MR sequences are obtained while patients perform a Valsalva maneuver (Figure 11.3). Of note, CT or duplex ultrasound of the pelvis has a relatively lower sensitivity—13 and 20%, respectively—for PCS compared with MRI/MRV (59%) or diagnostic venogram. Diagnostic laparoscopy is sometime used in patients with chronic pelvic pain to rule out other etiologies, especially pelvic endometriosis. Examinations performed in the supine position may not recognize PCS in 80–90% of patients.[20,26,27]

PCS can be a difficult diagnosis to make at primary care level and often requires a referral to a interventional radiologist or vascular surgeon or a pain specialist. One or more imaging modalities may already have been used by the time PCS patients are referred to an interventional radiologist or pain specialist, and usually with the missing diagnosis. The diagnosis of PCS is best made with ovarian venography.[4,5,6] For compete evaluation, left renal, bilateral ovarian, and iliac, including internal iliac, venography is performed. Pressure gradients across the renal (reno-caval) and left common iliac vein are obtained whenever an abnormality is visualized on diagnostic imaging. Even though regarded as the most informative method, ovarian and iliac venography should not be used as first-line diagnostic tests, but rather as means to confirm the findings of non-invasive testing, and should not routinely be performed in patients who do not have severe symptoms of PCS. Most interventional radiologists now prefer MRI/MRV as a primary imaging modality to rule out other potential etiologies for pelvic pain, analyze the severity of the PCS, and assess whether the

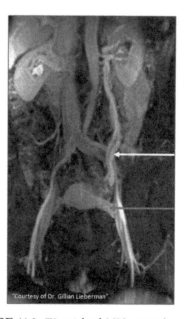

FIGURE 11.3: T2-weighted MRI, coronal maximum intensity projection (MIP) reconstruction shows dilated ovarian veins (*white arrow*) and adnexal vein (*grey arrow*).

patient is a candidate for endovascular treatment. Venographic demonstration of ovarian vein incompetency and pelvic varicosities are the most common clinical signs that should raise suspicion for the diagnosis of PCS (Figure 11.4).

In order to perform venography, the common femoral vein is accessed using a 21-gauge micro-puncture needle. A catheter is then advanced into the inferior vena cava to select and image the ovarian and/or pelvic veins following contrast injection under fluoroscopic guidance. Diagnostic criteria on the selective ovarian and pelvic venography are: (1) ovarian vein measuring >6 mm in diameter (upper limit of normal is considered to be 5 mm); (2) retrograde ovarian or pelvic venous flow; (3) the presence of pelvic varicosities and multiple tortuous, cross-pelvic, venous collaterals from left-to-right/contralateral reflux; (4) stagnation and delayed clearance of contrast in the pelvic veins; and (5) visualization of vulvoperineal or posteromedial thigh varices.[26] De Schepper explained this phenomenon by the so-called "left-to-right" theory of PCS and graded the pelvic varicosities as follows: Grade I = dilated left ovarian vein/plexus; Grade II = the same as I, plus dilated left utero-vaginal vein plexus; and Grade III = the same as II, plus dilated right utero-vaginal plexus and right ovarian vein.[23]

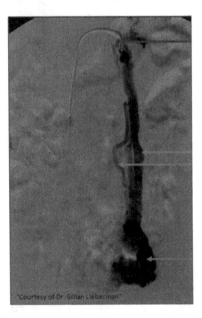

FIGURE 11.4: Left ovarian venogram via a catheter (*top arrow*) shows dilated ovarian (*middle arrows*) and pelvic veins (*bottom arrow*).

The direct relationship between varices and chronic pelvic pain remains difficult to ascertain, indicating that other causes of pelvic pain may coexist with pelvic varicosities.[4,5] Moreover, ovarian veins (the left more commonly than the right) can show reflux in healthy asymptomatic parous women, and no definitive diagnosis is usually made in 60% of patients.[14] This provides a snapshot for classifying patients with PCS as follows: (1) asymptomatic, with incidentally detected pelvic varices; (2) those with unusual vulvar or posteromedial thigh varices, complicating lower extremity superficial venous insufficiency with or without pelvic pain; and (3) PCS with painful pelvic varicosities secondary to PVI.[27]

TREATMENT OPTIONS

PCS has been encountered by physicians in a variety of disciplines and may cause substantial patient morbidity. Pain secondary to PCS is defined as noncyclical pelvic pain for at least six months' duration associated with standing, intercourse, and dilated ovarian, periuterine, or vaginal veins.

Treatment of PCS may be medical, surgical (ligation of ovarian veins, hysterectomy with or without bilateral salpingo-oophorectomy), or minimally invasive endovascular transcatheter embolization. Currently, many minimally invasive therapeutic choices with excellent results are available for these patients. Pain caused by PCS can be managed by analgesics, alone or in combination with drug-producing ovarian suppression (medroxyprogesterone acetate [MPA: 30 mg per day, PO for 6 months] or gonadotropin receptor agonists [GnRH; goserelin to be given parenterally 3.6 mg, monthly x 6 doses]). Chemical ovarian suppression with MPA or GnRH blocks the direct vasodilator effect of estrogen, and thereby provides relief of pelvic congestion and patients' symptoms by reducing venous distention.[27] Failed medical treatment or recurrence of symptoms is an indication for laparoscopic surgery or an endovascular procedure such as ovarian vein coil embolization or embolotherapy using detachable balloons, sclerosing agents such as 3% sodium tetradecyl sulfate (STS) foam, or glue such as enbucrilate. The goal of the interventional treatment is elimination of ovarian vein reflux, with or without direct sclerosis of enlarged pelvic varicosities. Endovascular therapy has been validated with standardized pain assessment surveys before and after embolotherapy and during follow-up using a visual analog scale (VAS). Currently, embolotherapy of ovarian veins with and without internal iliac vein embolization is an effective endovascular treatment for PCS. This should always be performed prior to varicose vein treatment of the lower limb if there are any. Ovarian and internal iliac veins are in close communication; therefore, in some cases, embolization of the iliac veins may also be required. The internal iliac vein embolization is performed after treatment of the ovarian vein. Of note, coils should be avoided in the internal iliac veins because of the risk of their migration to the lungs/heart due to capacious iliac veins: as seen in Cases 11.1 and 11.2, following.

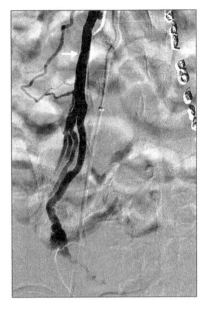

FIGURE 11.5: A 36-year-old female patient with PCS confirmed on ovarian venography. Digital subtraction angiography (DSA) image shows dilated Rt. ovarian vein (*white arrow*) with reverse blood flow.

CASE 11.1

A 36-year-old, female presented with chronic pelvic pain of moderate severity without dyspareunia. Associated symptoms included right lower extremity swelling, and varicose veins over the pubic area for over ten years. She complained of continuous discomfort requiring daily analgesics to get relief, and denied abdominal or urogynecological pain. The patient's past medical history was significant for normal menstrual cycle, two pregnancies via C section, right hip fracture 12 years ago, and deep vein thrombosis (DVT) in the right lower extremity (RLE). Peripheral vascular exam showed normal distal pulses, with gross varicosities over the pubic area extending to the right labia majora, and diffuse swelling of RLE. Initial venous duplex US of the RLE were consistent with normal phasic flow and good augmentation at all levels, incompetent deep venous system with severe reflux involving the popliteal vein, and an incompetent superficial venous system with severe reflux involving the greater saphenous vein.

Based on patient's history of chronic pelvic pain, multi-parous status, and gross varicosities over the pubic area/vulval varices, a diagnosis of PCS was considered.

The patient was scheduled for bilateral ovarian venography under monitored anesthesia care in reverse Trendelenburg position. Venography demonstrated bilateral enlarged ovarian veins measuring greater than 6 mm in diameter. Both veins were individually cannulated and coil embolized (Figures 11.5, 11.6, and 11.7). Postoperative follow-up pelvic duplex imaging of the adnexal vasculature six weeks after the procedure demonstrated no significant change in

the size of the pelvic vasculature with Valsalva. Likewise, during a follow-up office visit, her pain was resolved, and remained asymptomatic as of the two-year post-procedural follow-up.

CASE 11.2

A 32-year-old female was referred to us for the evaluation of recurrent post-phlebitic pelvic and groin pain of moderate severity and dyspareunia requiring narcotic analgesics for over five years. On complete evaluation, she was diagnosed with May-Thurner syndrome, which was managed with left common iliac vein stenting in March of 2004. Due to persistent pelvic pain and swelling in her left thigh, repeat venography was performed that demonstrated a moderate stenosis of the left external iliac vein below the previously placed left common iliac stent. This was treated with percutaneous transluminal angioplasty and stent placement in the left external iliac vein in October 2004.

The patient continued to have persistent mild swelling in the left thigh, left leg pain, and dyspareunia requiring narcotic analgesics. A left renal venogram was performed in July 2007,

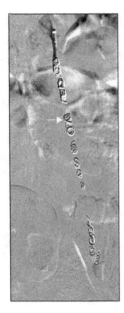

FIGURE 11.6: A 36-year-old female patient with PCS confirmed on ovarian venography. DSA image shows complete coil embolization of Lt. ovarian vein (*white arrow*) without any reflux.

which demonstrated retrograde filling of left ovarian and pelvic veins via collaterals. A left ovarian vein coil embolization was performed at the same outside hospital. The patient's leg

swelling and pain were improved, but pelvic pain and dyspareunia continued.

Due to persistent venous disability with previously stented May-Thurner syndrome and left ovarian vein coil embolization, a pre-procedural diagnosis of incompletely resolved PCS was considered. She was then scheduled for ilio-caval and ovarian venography. Complete procedural steps were recorded as follows: Anterior–posterior spot fluoroscopic imaging of the abdomen was taken in supine position (Figure 11.8). Preliminary iliocaval venography demonstrated patent iliac veins and patent IVC. Next, left renal venogram showed a patent left renal vein without hilar dilatation, and occluded left ovarian vein from previous embolization without any evidence of collaterals (Figure 11.9 and Figure 11.10). Subsequent right ovarian venogram revealed a patent but grossly dilated right ovarian vein (diameter above the iliac crest: 10.4 mm, at iliac crest: 8.9 mm, and below the iliac crest: 10.1 mm—mean: 9.8 mm) with retrograde flow and cross-pelvic collaterals confirming grade III PCS (Figure 11.11). Tornado coils were successfully deployed in the right

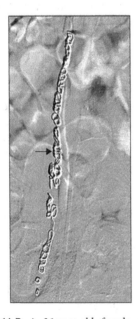

FIGURE 11.7: A 36-year-old female patient with PCS confirmed on ovarian venography. DSA image shows complete coil embolization of Rt. ovarian vein (*black arrow*) without any reflux.

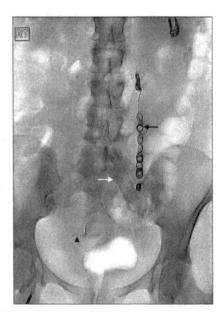

FIGURE 11.8: A 32-year-old multi-parous woman with unresolved incapacitating PCS and history of previous successfully stented May-Thurner syndrome and left ovarian vein embolization. Plain X-ray abdomen shows iliac stenting on the left side (*white arrow*), multiple embolization coils blocking the left ovarian vein (*black arrow*), and an intrauterine contraceptive device in the pelvis (*arrowhead*).

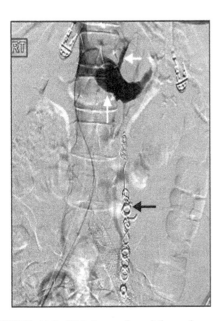

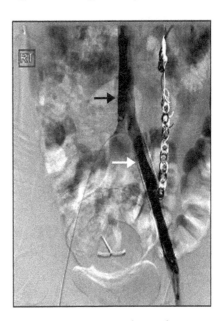

FIGURE 11.9: DSA image from left renal venography demonstrates a patent left adrenal vein (*small white arrow*) and renal vein without distension of its hilar portion as opposed to NCS (*large white arrow*). Multiple embolization coils blocking the left ovarian vein (*black arrow*) with absence of spontaneous retrograde flow in the left ovarian vein or any parapelvic collaterals. Aforementioned findings did not represent NCS (extrinsic left renal vein compression at the aorto-mesenteric fork).

FIGURE 11.10: DSA image from inferior venacavogram and iliac venogram demonstrates patent IVC (*black arrow*) and iliac stents on the left side (*white arrow*) with multiple embolization coils blocking the left ovarian vein.

ovarian vein, starting from lower border of the right iliac crest toward the level of entry of the right ovarian vein into the IVC. Post–coil embolization selective right ovarian venogram demonstrated occlusion of the right ovarian vein (Figure 11.12). Follow-up pelvic duplex images of the adnexal vasculature after two months of the procedure demonstrated no significant change in the size of the pelvic vasculature with Valsalva. Likewise, during a follow-up office visit, her pain was resolved and remained asymptomatic until the two-year post-procedural follow-up. Persistent PCS despite left ovarian vein embolization and iliac venous stentings in the index case was likely due to unrecognized coexisting right ovarian vein incompetency.

TREATMENT RESULTS

Medical treatment suppresses the ovarian function and/or increases venous contraction; several studies have reported both MPA and goserelin to be equally effective, with 71% of

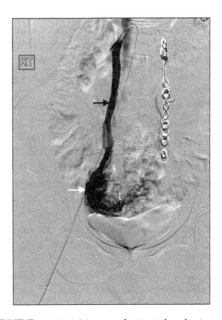

FIGURE 11.11: DSA image during right selective ovarian venography demonstrates the catheter in the patient's right ovarian vein with contrast traversing down into the dilated right ovarian vein (*black arrow*). Note the reversed/caudal flow in the ovarian vein and retrograde filling of varicose veins in the pelvis lying around the ovaries, uterus, bladder, and bowel (*white arrow*).

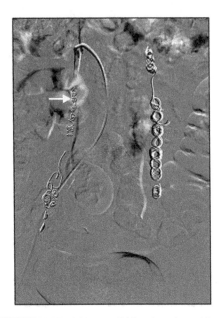

FIGURE 11.12: A 32-year-old female patient with unresolved PCS confirmed on right ovarian venography. Post–coil embolization final DSA image during Valsalva demonstrates sets of embolization coils—all completely blocking the right ovarian vein (*white arrow*) without any reflux.

the women reporting ≥ 50% reduction in pain score at less than one year follow-up.[28] Chemical ovarian ligation is not without adverse effects; estrogen replacement therapy is often required. It is unclear if the benefits of chemical ligation for pelvic varices are long lasting.

Hysterectomy with removal of one or both ovaries was performed, with a response rate of 75%. However, studies reported residual pain in 33% of patients after hysterectomy. This led to the advent of less invasive procedures such as extraperitoneal surgical ligation or resection of ovarian veins, as described by Rundqvist et al.[29] Laparoscopic ligation of bilateral ovarian veins gained popularity, with a response rate of 75%.[30] However, the carbon dioxide insufflations into the peritoneal cavity during laparoscopy cause venous decompression, thus not allowing an accurate estimation of pelvic varices, therefore decreasing procedural efficacy.

Surgical treatment for PCS has evolved dramatically since the 1980s. Successful bilateral ovarian vein embolization using steel endovascular coils was first reported by Edwards et al. in 1993.[31] The procedure is usually performed at the time of diagnostic venography. Recently, Laborda et al., in 2013, analyzed the clinical outcome and

satisfaction surveys for PCS coil embolization in patients with chronic pelvic pain who initially consulted for lower limb venous insufficiency (n = 202; mean age: 43.5 years; range: 27–57; follow-up at 1, 3, and 6 months and every year for 5 years). Patients with lower limb varices and chronic pelvic pain (>6 months), >6 mm pelvic venous caliber in ultrasonography, and venous reflux or presence of communicating veins/collaterals were recruited prospectively.[19] They used coil occlusion alone, and targeted all refluxing veins, including both ovarian and refluxing branches of both internal iliac veins. Pain level was assessed before and after embolotherapy and during follow-up using a visual analog scale (VAS). Technical and clinical success and recurrence of leg varices were recorded as 100%, 93.85% (n = 168) and 12.5% (n = 24), respectively. VAS was 7.34 ± 0.7 preprocedurally, versus 0.78 ± 1.2 at the end of follow-up (P < 0.0001). Complications were reported as follows: groin hematoma (n = 6), coil migration (n = 4), reaction to contrast media (n = 1), and post-procedural pain (n = 23).

In 2008, Gandini et al. reported the use of 3% STS as a sclerosant without using endovascular coils in patients with PVI (n = 38; 2 mL of STS mixed with 8 mL of air). These injected foam until pelvic venous stasis was visualized. Total injection volumes used were 30 mL and 20 mL on the left and right, respectively. Of note, the right-sided incompetency was treated only when varices did not cross the midline from left to right. Clinical success rate was reported in 100% of their cases. Lower procedural cost and less radiation time are the benefits with a sclerosant-only approach over coil embolization.[32]

Kim et al., in 2006, evaluated the long-term clinical outcome of transcatheter embolotherapy in women with PCS caused by ovarian and pelvic varices (n = 131; mean age, 34.0 years +/–12.5). Basal female hormonal levels were obtained before and after the embolotherapy and compared. Percutaneous transfemoral venography confirmed the presence of ovarian varices in 127/131 (97.0%), and all were treated with embolotherapy. Of these, 108/127 (85%) underwent internal iliac embolotherapy. In 97/127 at long-term clinical follow-up (mean 45 months+/–18), the mean pelvic pain level improved significantly, from 7.6 +/–1.8 before embolotherapy to 2.9 +/–2.8 after embolotherapy (P < .0001). Overall, 83% of the patients exhibited clinical improvement at long-term follow-up; 13% had no significant change; and 4% exhibited a worsened condition.

No significant change was noted in hormone levels after embolotherapy, and successful pregnancies were noted in two patients after ovarian and pelvic vein embolotherapy.

Maleux et al., in 2000, reported their results of ovarian vein embolization for the treatment of PCS.[33] In their study, all cases (*n* = 41; mean age, 37.8 years) had pelvic pain and varicosities detected on ovarian venography. Of 41 cases, 32 patients underwent unilateral embolization, and nine patients underwent bilateral embolization. Embolizing material used were the mixture of enbucrilate + lipiodized oil (*n* = 40) and enbucrilate + minicoils (*n* = 1). They reported a technical success rate of 98%, with pain relief in 58.5% of their cases (mean clinical follow-up: 19.9 months). Later, Kwon et al., in 2007, evaluated the therapeutic effectiveness of ovarian vein embolization using coils for PCS.[22] They enrolled 67 patients, all confirmed on ovarian venography, and undertook left ovarian vein embolization (*n* = 64), right ovarian vein embolization (*n* = 1), and bilateral ovarian vein embolization (*n* = 2) using 0.035–0.038 inch coils (5–15 mm; average: 5.8 coils; range: 3–8; COOK, US). Fifty-five of 67 patients (82%) experienced pain reduction with coil embolization alone; all were satisfied, and did not pursue any further treatment (mean follow-up: 44.8 +/– 21 months). Immediate complications of coil migration were recorded in 3% (*n* = 2) of the cases (pulmonary circulation = 1 [retrieved with snare], and left renal vein = 1 [retrieved with snare]).

Results from studies mentioned above have demonstrated that PCS patients who underwent ovarian vein embolization have an acceptable result in reduction of their pelvic pain. Both ovarian veins usually have multiple branches; of note, multiple main trunks off the ovarian vein exist in as many as 40% and 25% on the left and right, respectively; and furthermore, most communicating pelvic venous plexus are devoid of valves.[20,27] Therefore, incomplete embolization of the tributaries often leads to recurrence/clinical failure of the procedures, both endovascular embolization and laparoscopic ligation.

Complications

Complications that have been reported during or following ovarian vein coil embolization are as follows: Bleeding, post-embolization syndrome (up to 80% of cases), ovarian vein thrombophlebitis, coil migration (3–4%) and recurrence of varices (5%).[10,11,12,14] Kwon et al., in their study, reported

that coil migration occurred in 3% (*n* = 2) of the cases (pulmonary circulation = 1 [retrieved with snare], and left renal vein = 1 [retrieved with snare]). Coil migration in rare circumstances can occur partly because of disparity between the size of coils and the size of dilated ovarian veins, which can change in their diameters, depending on pelvic venous hemodynamics. A guide catheter can be used to provide additional stability and support for coil delivery. However, in the setting of incompetent veins, assessing the true diameter of the dilated vein can be a difficult task.

CONCLUSIONS

Most PCS patients are asymptomatic. In the recent past, an equivocal diagnosis of PCS/chronic pelvic pain left many patients untreated, leading to inappropriate use of opiate and non-opiate analgesics. Diagnosis of PCS is made by clinical history, physical examination findings, and imaging that demonstrates ovarian and pelvic varicosities.

Patients with severe venous disability symptoms may benefit from an endovascular intervention after conservative medical treatment has failed. In addition to being less expensive than surgery, endovascular ovarian vein embolization offers a safe, effective, minimally invasive treatment option that restores patients to their normal quality of life. The procedure is highly successful in blocking the retrograde blood flow, with technical success rate of 95--100%. Overall, 85–95% of women have demonstrated improvement in their pain symptoms after the procedure.

REFERENCES

1. Taylor HC. Vascular congestion and hyperemia: their effect on function and structure in the female reproductive organs. Part I. Physiological basis and history of the concept. *Am J Obstet Gynecol.* 1949;57:211–230.
2. Taylor HC. Vascular congestion and hyperemia: their effect on function and structure in the female reproductive organs. Part II. Clinical concepts of the congestion-fibrosis syndrome. *Am J Obstet Gynecol.* 1949;57:637–653.
3. Taylor HC. Vascular congestion and hyperemia: their effect on function and structure in the female reproductive organs. Part III. Etiology and therapy. *Am J Obstet Gynecol.* 1949;57:654–668.
4. Mathias SD, Kuppermann M, Liberman RF, Lipschutz RC, Steege JF. Chronic pelvic pain: prevalence, health-related quality of life, and economic correlates. *Obstet Gynecol.* 1996;87(3):321–327.

5. Rudloff U, Holmes RJ, Prem JT, Faust GR, Moldwin R, Siegel D. Mesoaortic compression of the left renal vein (nutcracker syndrome): case reports and review of the literature. *Ann Vasc Surg.* 2006;20(1):120–129.

6. Barsoum MK, Shepherd RF, Welch TJ. Patient with both Wilkie syndrome and nutcracker syndrome. *Vasc Med.* 2008;13(3):247–250.

7. Fu WJ, Hong BF, Xiao YY, et al. Diagnosis of the nutcracker phenomenon by multislice helical computed tomography angiography. *Chin Med J (Engl).* 2004;117(12):1873–1875.

8. Scultetus AH, Villavicencio JL, Gillespie DL. The nutcracker syndrome: its role in the pelvic venous disorders. *J Vasc Surg.* 2001;34(5):812–819.

9. Rogers A, Beech A, Braithwaite B. Transperitoneal laparoscopic left gonadal vein ligation can be the right treatment option for pelvic congestion symptoms secondary to nutcracker syndrome. *Vascular.* 2007;15(4):238–240.

10. Hartung O, Grisoli D, Boufi M, et al. Endovascular stenting in the treatment of pelvic vein congestion caused by nutcracker syndrome: lessons learned from the first five cases. *J Vasc Surg.* 2005;42(2):275–280.

11. Farquhar CM, Rogers V, Franks S, Pearce S, Wadsworth J, Beard RW. A randomized controlled trial of medroxyprogesterone acetate and psychotherapy for the treatment of pelvic congestion. *Br J Obstet Gynaecol.* 1989;96(10):1153–1162.

12. Park SJ, Lim JW, Ko YT, et al. Diagnosis of pelvic congestion syndrome using transabdominal and transvaginal sonography. *AJR Am J Roentgenol.* 2004;182(3):683–688.

13. Park YB, Lim SH, Ahn JH, et al. Nutcracker syndrome: intravascular stenting approach. *Nephrol Dial Transplant.* 2000;15(1):99–101.

14. Rozenblit AM, Ricci ZJ, Tuvia J, Amis ESJr. Incompetent and dilated ovarian veins: a common CT finding in asymptomatic parous women. *AJR Am J Roentgenol.* 2001;176(1):119–122.

15. Kurklinsky AK, Rooke TW. Nutcracker phenomenon and nutcracker syndrome. *Mayo Clin Proc.* 2010 Jun;85(6):552–559.

16. Stones RW. Pelvic vascular congestion—half a century later. *Clin Obstet Gynecol.* 2003 Dec;46(4):831–836. Review.

17. Hodgkinson CP. Physiology of the ovarian veins during pregnancy. *Obstet Gynecol.* 1953;1(1):26–37.

18. Viala JL, Flandre O, Girardot B, Maamer M [Histology of the pelvic vein. Initial approach]. *Phlebologie.* 1991;442369:372.372; discussion, 373.

19. Laborda A, Medrano J, de Blas I, Urtiaga I, Carnevale FC, de Gregorio MA. Endovascular treatment of pelvic congestion syndrome: visual analog scale (VAS) long-term follow-up clinical evaluation in 202 patients. *Cardiovasc Intervent Radiol.* 2013;36(4):1006–1014.

20. Durham JD, Machan L. *Semin Intervent Radiol.* 2013 Dec;30(4):372–380. doi: 10.1055/s-0033-1359731

21. Belenky A, Bartal G, Atar E, Cohen M, Bachar GN. Ovarian varices in healthy female kidney donors:incidence, morbidity, and clinical outcome. *AJR Am J Roentgenol.* 2002;179(3):625–627.

22. Kwon SH, Oh JH, Ko KR, Park HC, Huh JY. Transcatheter ovarian vein embolization using coils for the treatment of pelvic congestion syndrome. *Cardiovasc Intervent Radiol.* 2007;30(4):655–661.

23. d'Archambeau O, Maes M, De Schepper AM. The pelvic congestion syndrome: role of the "nutcracker phenomenon" and results of endovascular treatment. *JBR-BTR.* 2004 Jan–Feb;87(1):1–8.

24. Park SJ, Lim JW, Ko YT. et al. Diagnosis of pelvic congestion syndrome using transabdominal and transvaginal sonography. *AJR Am J Roentgenol.* 2004; 182(3):683–688.

25. Kim HS, Malhotra AD, Rowe PC, Lee JM, Venbrux AC. Embolotherapy for pelvic congestion syndrome: long-term results. *J Vasc Interv Radiol.* 2006;17(2, Pt 1):289–297.

26. Beard RW, Highman JH, Pearce S, Reginald PW. Diagnosis of pelvic varicosities in women with chronic pelvic pain. *Lancet.* 1984;2(8409):946–949.

27. Venbrux AC, Sharma GK Jackson ET, et al. Pelvic varices embolization. *Women Health Intervent Radiol.* 2012;16:37–59.

28. Soysal ME, Soysal S, Vicdan K, et al., A randomized controlled trial of goserelin and medroxyprogesterone acetate in the treatment of pelvic congestion. *Hum Reprod.* 2004 Jan;19(1):160–167.

29. Rundqvist E, Sandholm LE, Larsson G. Treatment of pelvic varicosities causing lower abdominal pain with extraperitoneal resection of the left ovarian vein. *Ann Chir Gynaecol.* 1984;73(6):339–341.

30. Carter JE. Surgical treatment for chronic pelvic pain. *Journal of the Society of Laparoendoscopic Surgeons.* 1998 Apr–Jun;2(2):129–139. Review.

31. Edwards RD, Robertson IR, MacLean AB, Hemingway AP. Case report: pelvic pain syndrome—successful treatment of a case by ovarian vein embolization. *Clin Radiol.* 1993 Jun;47(6):429–431.

32. Gandini R, Chiocchi M, Konda D, et al. Transcatheter foam sclerotherapy of symptomatic female varicocele with sodium-tetradecyl-sulfate foam. *Cardiovasc Intervent Radiol.* 2008 Jul–Aug;31(4):778–784. doi:10.1007/s00270-007-9264-6

33. Maleux G, Stockx L, Wilms G, et al. Ovarian vein embolization for the treatment of pelvic congestion syndrome: long-term technical and clinical results. *JVIR,* 2000;11:859–864.

12

Male Pelvic Pain

MICHEL A. PONTARI AND EMMANUEL A. GHORMOZ

Chronic prostatitis/chronic pelvic pain syndrome (CP/CPPS) is a symptom complex characterized by pelvic pain, with or without voiding symptoms. CP/CPPS is included in the NIH classification of prostatitis as category III.[1] The term "prostatitis" may be confusing for this condition. The pain of CFP/CPPS may have nothing to do with inflammation. In comparing a large group of men with CP/CPPS to asymptomatic age matched controls, both groups had similar amounts of inflammation in either expressed prostatic fluid (EPS), post prostate massage urine (VB3), or seminal plasma.[2] The term prostatitis is a holdover from a time when it was assumed that men with pelvic pain had prostate inflammation as the cause of the symptoms. Category III is still subdivided as category IIIA, inflammatory, with the presence of white blood cells in EPS, VB3 or seminal plasma, or IIIB, non-inflammatory, without the inflammatory cells.[1] To date, there have been no clinically significant differences demonstrated between these two subclasses.

The NIH definition of CP/CPPS is genitourinary pain in the absence of uropathogenic bacteria detected by standard microbiological methods. This also implies the absence of other diseases which can produce pelvic pain such as bladder cancer, trauma, etc.[1] The diagnosis and treatment of CPPS has evolved. Many years (and not so long ago also) it was thought to be just an infection and treated by antibiotics. Now it is considered a multifaceted chronic pain syndrome with varied presentations, diagnostic challenges and treatments. CP/CPPS can present a challenge as these aspects include areas outside of the usual scope of Urology, including neurological, immunological and psychological factors that influence the disease process.[3]

EPIDEMIOLOGY

A recent review for the International Consultation on Urological Disease (ICUD) and Societe International d'Urologie indicated that prevalence of prostatitis-like symptoms ranged from 2.2% to 16%, with a median prevalence rate approximating 7.1% for chronic prostatitis/chronic pelvic pain syndrome.[4] Given that this condition is found in a relatively consistent rate across continents, it may be that this develops independent of environmental factors specific to a given society. Prostatitis results in a substantial number of physician visits. The Urological Disease in America study reported an annualized visit rate of 1798/100,000 population for prostatitis.[5]

ETIOLOGY

The etiology and much of the pathogenesis of CP/CPPS are unknown. However, there is evidence to support a possible role for infection, neurological causes, inflammatory/autoimmune and psychological factors.

Infection

The symptoms of CP/CPPS are similar to that of a true prostatic infection. Therefore, infection has been commonly assumed by patients and clinicians alike to be the cause of the symptoms. In a study of 30,000 male health professionals, men who reported a history of sexually transmitted disease were found to have 1.8-fold higher odds of prostatitis.[6] In the NIH sponsored Chronic Prostatitis Collaborative Research Network study (CPCRN), patients with CP/CPPS were found to have a significantly greater history of urethritis compared to age-matched controls.[7] While a history of STD seems to lead to greater risk of CP/CPPS, there is no evidence of an active STD in these men.[8] Thus, STD could be a first step, with symptoms persisting after the infection resolves. There is also no difference in the routine cultures of men with CP/CPPS and asymptomatic controls from urine, prostatic fluid and post prostate massage urine or seminal plasma.[2] Eight percent of men had uropathogenic bacteria and roughly 70% had some form of bacteria in each group. This indicates that asymptomatic men appear to routinely have bacteria in the prostate, but may not by themselves produce disease or symptoms. What may be of importance are the specific characteristics of the bacteria. Not all E coli will produce the same infection or symptoms. Uropathogenic bacteria including uropathogenic E coli (UPEC) express virulence factors that produce the ability to infect.[9] In an animal model, a strain of bacteria called CP1 from a man with CP/CPPS induced and sustained chronic pelvic pain that persisted after bacterial clearance from the genitourinary tract. Interestingly the pelvic pain was produced in the NOD strain of mice but not C57BL/6J mice, although infection was established in both types of mice.[10] Thus, it may be that certain bacteria in certain individuals can produce pelvic pain.

Inflammation

The term prostatitis implies inflammation of the prostate gland. However, it is clear that not all men with CPPS have inflammation related to the prostate. Only about one third of men with clinical CPPS have been found to have prostatic inflammation on biopsy.[11] In those with inflammation the degree of that inflammation does not correlate with symptoms.[12,13] Data looking at individual cytokines varies widely and is not conclusive. Some men with CP/CPPS have an increased T cell response to seminal plasma compared to controls.[14] Men with CPPS demonstrate an increased lymphoproliferative response to prostate antigens compared to controls.[15] A region of the PAP molecule, 173–192, results in greater activation of CD4 cells and release of interferon-γ in men with CPPS than controls.[16] Men with CP/CPPS have also been reported to have autoantibodies against human SVS2, seminal vesicle secretory protein 2, which in mice deficient in the autoimmune regulator gene (aire), develop B and T cell immune responses to this protein.[17] These data indicate the likelihood of autoimmunity in some men with CPPS.

Neurological Causes

Men with CP/CPPS were 5 times more likely to self-report a history of nervous system disease compared to asymptomatic age matched controls in the chronic prostatitis collaborative research network (CPCRN) study.[7] In this NIH cohort, the symptom that most contributed to

the difference in neurological disease was numbness and tingling in the limbs. Also significant was a history of vertebral disc disease/surgery. There is evidence for differences in the nerve function of men with CP/CPPS compared to controls. Thermal sensitivity tests given to the perineum and anterior thigh in a much larger group of men with CP/CPPS and controls confirmed pilot data and again showed that men with CP/CPPS were more sensitive to heat in the perineum but not the anterior thigh compared to controls[18]. This indicates alterations in the afferent autonomic nervous system. Studies on the efferent side showed that when on 5 minute resting supine and standing blood pressure measurements, men with CP/CPPS showed alterations in the heart rate variability compared to controls. Whereas measures of parasympathetic activity decreased in the controls, there was little change in men with CPPS, and sympathetic activity increased in the controls and decreased in men with CP/CPPS.[19] Both these studies support central sensitization (or centralization) of the nerves. An informative animal model that provides a mechanistic demonstration is that of chemical irritation of rat prostate or bladder. Irritation of either organ causes c-fos expression at spinal cord levels L6 and S1 along with plasma extravasation at the identical L6 and S1 dermatomes, and inflammation in the other organ, underscoring the overlap of afferent nerve fiber distribution.[20] FMRI studies of the brain have shown differences in the relationship of gray and white matter in men with CPPS compared to controls.[21] It is not known if changes in the CNS are as a result of the chronic pain, or are abnormalities that lead to pain in the first place. The findings in men with CPPS differ from those in other pain conditions including low back pain.[22]

Pelvic Floor Dysfunction

Neurological abnormalities are postulated to also cause spam in the pelvic floor.[23] Men with CPPS are noted on urodynamic studies to have detrusor sphincter dyssynergy in 73% of cases. This is normally seen in patients with suprasacral spinal cord lesions.[24] In the study by Zermann et al., CPPS patients were found to have pathological tenderness of the striated pelvic floor muscle and poor to absent function in ability to relax the pelvic floor efficiently with a single or repetitive effort.[23] An EMG study of the pelvic floor in men with CPPS showed that compared to controls, men with CPPS had (1) greater preliminary resting hypertonicity and instability and (2) lowered voluntary endurance contraction amplitude.[25] Men with CPPS also have more tender points in areas outside of the pelvis as compared to controls.[26]

Psychosocial Factors

The same biological nociceptive process will result in a different pain experience in different individuals on the basis of the psychosocial context of that process. The term "stress prostatitis" was used in the late 1980's to describe CP/CPPS given the common association of psychological stress and symptoms. Later studies have confirmed this association. Ullrich and colleagues used measures of perceived stress in a study of men with CPPS and found that greater perceived stress during the 6 months after the health care visit was associated with greater pain intensity (p = .03) and disability (p = .003) at 12 months, even after controlling for age, symptom duration, and pain and disability during the first 6 months.[27] It is known that stress has physiological consequences, as in addition to many other stimuli such as cytokines, bacterial toxins and hypoxia, mast cells release their contents in response to stress[28]. Chronic stress also changes DNA by epigenetic modifications, in which biochemical changes alter the DNA and effect function.[29] Some of these changes are reversible and some are not.[29]

In the CPCRN study, men with CP/CPPS self-reported a history of anxiety or depression twice as often as age matched controls with no pain.[7] Further detailed investigation of psychological variables in this cohort showed that helplessness/catastrophizing predicted overall pain along with urinary symptoms and depression.[30] The helplessness subscale of catastrophizing also predicts the mental subscale scores on the SF-12 in these patients.[31] It is postulated that catastrophizing may activate central attention centers and inhibit the suppression of significant pain leading to chronic pain.[32]

EVALUATION

Symptoms

Pain and Voiding Symptoms

National Institutes of Health Chronic Prostatitis Symptom Index (NIH-CPSI) is helpful to assess pain location, frequency, severity and effect on quality of life.[33] A more detailed assessment of voiding symptoms can be obtained from the AUA symptom score.[34] One limitation to the NIH CPSI is that it does not have questions about pain thought to be related to the bladder. Interstitial cystitis or painful bladder syndrome (IC/PBS) is another symptom based syndrome whose current diagnosis is made when there is pain with bladder filling, and/or pain relieved by bladder emptying in the absence of other pathological conditions.[35] There are no pathognomonic biological markers or pathology for either CP/CPPS or IC/PBS, as both are symptom complexes. The same symptoms may co-exist in one individual. The clinical importance is to remember to assess for symptoms of bladder pain in men who present with pelvic pain.

Sexual Dysfunction

We have come to recognize the prevalence of sexual dysfunction in even young men with CPPS.[36] A case control study of a large Taiwanese health database showed that men with a diagnosis of ED were more likely to have been previously diagnosed with CP/CPPS.[37] This both emphasizes the need for the assessment of sexual function in these men, but also raises the questions about what common mechanisms may be present in both conditions.

Non-urological Symptoms

Neurological

The possibility of lumbar-sacral disk disease should be assessed by history and physical exam. A complaint of back pain with numbness or pain radiating down the legs should prompt an evaluation with a lumbosacral MRI.

GI

Men with CP/CPPS are more likely to have other chronic pain conditions such as irritable bowel syndrome, Fibromyalgia and Chronic fatigue syndrome.[3] There is overlapping innervation of the bowel and bladder.[38] Irritation of one in experimental models results in inflammation of the other.[39] The evaluation therefore of men with CP/CPPS needs to assess problems such as constipation, diarrhea, and the relation of discomfort to bowel movements. If any such symptoms are present he should see a gastroenterologist.

Rheumatological

Men with CP/CPPS may be at higher risk for systemic chronic pain syndromes.[3] Fibromyalgia manifests as pain in many areas of the body. Pain with significant fatigue may indicate chronic fatigue syndrome. These conditions should be further evaluated by a rheumatologist.

Cardiovascular

Men in the CPCRN study were six times more likely to self-report a history of cardiovascular disease, especially hypertension.[7] A recent report indicates that men with CPPS also have alterations in arterial stiffness and lower reactive hyperemia index, measures of cardiovascular dysfunction.[40] Whether this is related to autonomic dysfunction and/or localized to the endothelium is unclear. Even in young men, note should be taken of the blood pressure, and referral made for untreated hypertension.

Psychological Symptoms

There are no published criteria for the psychological evaluation of men with CP/CPPS. However, men should be queried about significant anxiety, depression, and symptoms of obsessive compulsive behavior. Untreated mental health issues make treatment of chronic pain very difficult.

UPOINT Classification

It has become clear that the phenotype of patients meeting the criteria for CPPS is variable and can include several different types of symptoms. This has been well outlined by Shoskes and colleagues in the UPOINT classification.[41] This includes the categories of Urinary, Psychosocial, Organ-Specific, Infection, Neurological/Systemic and Tenderness of skeletal muscle. This classification is a convenient way to remember the assessment and is also available online.

Lab Tests

Men should have a urinalysis to look for signs of infection, or unevaluated hematuria. The diagnosis of hematuria should be suspected by a positive urine dip but is confirmed by finding 3 or more RBC per hpf on a microscopic evaluation of the urine.[42] Post void residual urine should be checked to rule out urinary retention as a cause of pelvic pain.

TREATMENT

Antibiotics

Although the definition of CPPS is the absence of a uropathogenic source, many symptoms of CP/CPPS overlap with those of prostatic infection. Bacteria classically accepted as uropathogenic and implicated in true chronic bacterial prostatitis prostatitis (category II) include gram-negative enteric bacteria such as *E. coli* (the most prevalent gram negative pathogen), *Klebsiella pneumonia, Proteus mirabilis, and Pseudomonas aeruginosa.* In recent years, it has become accepted that the gram-positive *Enterococcus faecalis* can probably also be included on the list of uropathogenic bacteria. Other organisms thought to be potentially pathogenic include *S. saprophyticus, S. aureus, S. epidermidis, Mycoplasma genitalium, Ureaplasma urealyticum, and C. trachomatis.*[43]

Small, uncontrolled studies have lent credence to the efficacy of antibiotic therapy in ameliorating patients' symptoms, but large randomized, placebo-controlled studies have failed to consistently show meaningful benefit. Fluoroquinolones have demonstrated improvement in CPSI score vs. placebo (-5.6 vs. -3.1 point reductions at 12 weeks follow-up), but no statistical or clinical difference was found at end of treatment or end of follow-up.[44] A 2012 meta-analysis of 35 studies examining all treatments for CP/CPPS found that total NIH-CPSI symptom scores decreased by 1.8 with antibiotic treatment. When broken down into the individual NIH-CPSI domains, antibiotics were associated with a decrease of 0.38 points in the pain domain, a decrease of 0.04 points in the voiding domain, and a decrease of 0.7 points in the quality of life domain. These findings were determined to be both statistically and clinically insignificant and recommendations against their use could be inferred.[45] It is important to note that in all studies of antibiotics examined in this meta-analysis, patients had an average duration of symptoms measurable in years, and had been heavily pre-treated with antibiotics.[46]

One study of importance looked specifically at patients with average symptom duration of 8 weeks and only 41% of patients having previously been treated with antibiotics. This study compared patients with prostatitis-like symptoms and uropathogenic (Group 1) vs. non-uropathogenic (Group 2) bacteria localized to the prostate. At 6 months of follow-up, 70.5% and 72.8% in groups 1 and 2, respectively, had positive clinical response.[47] Another study quotes up to a 75% response rate in patients who are culture positive for non-uropathogenic as well as uropathogenic bacteria with short symptom duration (mean 4 weeks) and without previous antibiotic treatment.[48] Subsequent meta-analyses have been optimistic as well, finding a small statistically significant overall benefit (reduction in symptom score) to antibiotic treatment, although they admit that this may or may not translate to clinically meaningful benefit to patients.[48]

The recommendations at this point in our understanding can be summarized as follows: antibiotics are not recommended in patients who have a long duration of symptoms or in those who have failed previous antibiotic treatment.[48] They may, however, be useful in patients who are antibiotic-naïve and in those with short duration of symptoms, particularly in combination with alpha-blockers.[49] An empiric four week course of antibiotics is an accepted initial therapy.[49] If there is no response at this time, treatment should be stopped. If a response is noted, treatment should be carried out for an addition 2–4 weeks.[50] A repeated course of antibiotics in the absence of a positive urine culture is not accepted therapy.

Fluoroquinolones have been shown to be effective and are recommended in category III prostatitis for patients who are antibiotic-naïve and those with short duration of symptoms. In addition to the evidence presented above, their spectrum of activity (which includes both uropathogenic and non-uropathogenic bacteria) as well as their pharmacokinetic properties allowing for high prostatic concentration make this class of antibiotic a good treatment option.[43] The case has also been made that macrolides and tetracyclines may be used as second-line agents in treating chronic prostatitis associated with chlamydia (macrolides and tetracyclines) and Mycoplasma (tetracyclines).[50] These drugs are not recommended in cases associated with typical pathogens.

One question that has consistently been raised in regard to these recommendations as it relates to category III prostatitis is: If there is no evidence of bacterial invasion or no inflammation of the prostate, how can we explain the benefit we see in certain studies of antibiotic therapy? First, antibiotics may have a significant placebo effect.[51] Antibiotics may also be effective by removing bacteria not considered uropathogenic or not routinely cultured or culturable from prostate specimens. Finally, certain antibiotics, especially fluoroquinolones, have been shown to have an anti-inflammatory effect that may be responsible, at least in part, for the response seen in patients without culture proof of bacterial localization.[51]

Anti-inflammatory Agents

In a met-analysis of treatment trials, anti-inflammatory medications were noted to produce an improvement in symptoms compared to placebo, with a risk ration of 1.7 (95% CI 1.4–2.1). Whether this is clinically significant is not clear, and the authors of the analysis concluded that anti-inflammatories should be used as part of mutli-modal therapy.[52]

Alpha Blockers

Nickel reviewed clinical evidence on alpha blockers for treatment of CP/CPPS and found mixed results.[49] The conclusion was however that alpha blockers appear to achieve improvement in symptoms compared to placebo. The most recent randomized trial used the alpha blocker silodosin for treatment of CPPS in 151 alpha blocker naïve men. There was a significant response rate according to change in CPSI score.[53] Alpha blockers certainly can play a part of therapy in men with CP/CPPS. One limitation is the side effect of retrograde ejaculation usually seen in using Tamsulosin or Silodosin. Men must be counseled about this possibility, especially if they are younger and still in their reproductive years.

PDE5 Inhibitor

Tadalafil can treat lower urinary tract symptoms, erectile dysfunction and possible the symptoms of CP/CPPS as well.[54,55]

5 Alpha Reductase Inhibitor (ARI)

In older men with larger prostates, the use of a 5-alpha reductase inhibitor may help reduce pain and urinary symptoms.[56] The proposed mechanism of action of hormonal agents like finasteride and dutasteride involve regression of glandular tissue, improved voiding parameters and reduced intraprostatic ductal reflux. REDUCE is a 4 year, randomized, double-blind, placebo controlled study of prostate cancer risk reduction using 0.5 mg dutasteride versus placebo in men at risk (age 50–75, PSA 2.5–10 ng/ml with negative TRUS). The NIH-CPSI survey was used to measure baseline and change in symptom severity. Of 5,379 men, 12.6% had prostatitis like pain. After 48 months, the dutasteride group noted a significant decrease in CPSI total score.[56]

Medications for Neuropathic Pain

Patients with suspected neuropathic pain can be started on meds such as tricyclic antidepressants or anti convulsants. Amitriptyline has been widely used in women with Interstitial cystitis[57] but data in men with CPPS are lacking. In the IC studies, a better response was seen if the dose was increased up to 50 mg.[58] The dose should start low, usually 10 mg po qhs and then titrate up as needed and as tolerated. A study of pregabalin, an anti convulsant that is approved for neuropathic pain in other conditions including post herpetic neuralgia, diabetic neuropathy and fibromyalgia.[59] A randomized placebo controlled trial of pregabalin in men with CPPS showed an effect that approached significance but did not reach the primary endpoint.[60] However, several secondary endpoints were significantly improved. This suggests that in a subset of men with CPPS, pregabalin may be effective. Although some men with CP/CPPS responded to 150 mg per day, higher doses of 300 mg per day have been used for diabetes and up to 450 mg per day for fibromyalgia.[61] Therefore, the dosage needed may vary.

Treatment of Pelvic Floor Dysfunction

One area that has seen the greatest improvement in diagnosis and treatment has been in pelvic floor dysfunction. Tight muscles in the pelvic floor lead to tender areas. The group from Stanford has made significant contributions to this area with their studies on myofascial release and treatment of pelvic floor dysfunction [62, 63]. One of the difficulties in assessing the effects of pelvic floor physical therapy is how to control the study. A study from the NIH sponsored UPPCRN group showed the feasibility of using global massage as a control for patients undergoing myofascial physical therapy.[64] Although not powered or designed to be a definitive outcome study, patients undergoing myofascial therapy had a significantly greater response on global assessment response than the therapeutic massage group, 57% to 21% (P = 0.03). Referral to a physical therapist who is familiar with pelvic floor physical therapy techniques is an important part of the treatment of many men with CPPS. Pelvic floor PT can also be combined with the use of skeletal muscle relaxant medications such as Tizanidine or valium, orally or as a rectal suppository. The use of perineal injection of Botulinum toxin has also been reported to relax tender muscle/trigger points.[65]

Psychological Therapy

It has been well documented in recent studies the effect of psychological variables on the pain experience and quality of life in men with CPPS.[66] A prospective, population based study by Chung et al examines the relationship between CP/CPPS and risk of subsequent depressive disorder over a three year follow up in 18,306 patients. After adjusting for age, gender, geographic region, monthly income, BPH and incontinence, CP was a significant predictor for development of Depressive Disorder with a hazard ratio of 1.63 (95% CI = 1.36–1.96).[67] CP is already a disease prevalent in young men, but those <30 are at greatest risk of subsequent depressive disorder with a hazard ratio of 2.50 (95% CI = 1.18–4.51). Recognizing signs of depressive disorder and catastrophizing (helplessness and hopelessness about the condition) can prompt routing psychological assessment. Options for our patients with these psychological factors include traditional therapy with a psychologist or psychiatrist. Some researchers are developing cognitive based therapy to address these issues.[68]

Alternative Treatments

Several recent publications looked at the effect of acupuncture. The mechanism of the improvement in CPPS symptoms after acupuncture is unknown, but can be postulated to have an ameliorating effect on neuropathic pain. Krieger and colleagues performed a sham acupuncture procedure in the setting of a randomized, controlled clinical trial.[69] For the sham, needles shorter than standard were placed 0.5 cm away from the true acupuncture sites. After 10 weeks, 73% of the true acupuncture group had a clinical response, compare to 47% of the sham group (p = 0.017). Beta endorphin and leucine encephalin levels were both higher in the acupuncture group (p < 0.01). The use of electrical stimulation in addition to needle placement has also been used and shown to be superior to sham and advice and exercise alone in men with CPPS.[70] A systematic review of trials of acupuncture in the treatment of CPPS identified 9 clinical trials involving 890 patients that met criteria for inclusion. The authors concluded that the evidence for the efficacy of acupuncture for treating CPPS was encouraging, but the quantity and quality of the available evidence precluded making firm conclusions in favor of acupuncture.[71] In clinical practice, given the relatively few side effects of acupuncture, it can be suggested to individuals who do not respond to first line medical therapy, or to those who would prefer to not take medications for their discomfort.

There is limited data on specific phytotherapy but there is some data to suggest that Quercitin, an anti-oxidant and anti-inflammatory could be effective in some patients.[72] Another suggestion we have been making to our patients is to increase their aerobic exercise if possible. The benefit of exercise has been demonstrated in other chronic pain syndromes like Fibromyalgia.[73]

Treatment Summary and Approach

For the approach to treatment the UPOINT classification can also help us to remember to treat as many aspects of the patient's problem as possible, not just one area. Although a formal placebo controlled trial for every combination is impossible, basing therapy on these categories of symptoms appears to be superior to treating individual symptoms alone[74]. The symptoms present in individual patients will vary widely as well and there certainly is no one treatment fits all approach to CP/CPPS. As important to using combination treatment is also providing counseling and a realistic timeframe for improvement of symptoms. Our experience is symptoms do improve in the majority of men. The usual pattern is that of going from all "bad" days to some "good" days, which eventually outnumber the more painful days. Eventually the pain level on the more painful days decreases and the exacerbation of pain or "flares" gets farther apart. This can take many months, especially n men with long standing pain. We have found that giving a truthfully optimistic yet realistic as to the timeframe of improvement helps prevent the anxiety of worrying that (1) he may never get better and (2) that it will happen in a rapid time frame. Finally, many if not most patients need to see more than one type of specialist. This often involves neurology, gastroenterology, pain management, psychiatry, physical medicine and rehabilitation in addition to Urology. Each individual is truly different and a unique case.

REFERENCES

1. Krieger JN, Nyberg LJr, Nickel JC. NIH consensus definition and classification of prostatitis. *JAMA.* 1999;282:236.
2. Nickel JC, Alexander RB, Schaeffer AJ, et al. Leukocytes and bacteria in men with chronic prostatitis/chronic pelvic pain syndrome compared to asymptomatic controls. *J Urol.* 2003; 170:818.
3. Rodriguez MA, Afari N, Buchwald DS, et al. Evidence for overlap between urological and nonurological unexplained clinical conditions. *J Urol.* 2009;182:2123.
4. Nickel J, Wagenlehner F, Pontari M et al: Male chronic pelvic pain syndrome (CPPS). In: *Male Lower Urinary Tract Symptoms (LUTS); An International Consultation on Male LUTS.* Ed. Christopher Chapple and Paul Abrams Montreal, Canada: Societe Internationale d'Urologie (SIU) 2013;331–372.
5. Pontari MA, Joyce GF, Wise M, et al. Prostatitis. *J Urol.* 2007;177:2050.
6. Collins MM, Meigs JB, Barry MJ, et al. Prevalence and correlates of prostatitis in the health professionals follow-up study cohort. *J Urol.* 2002; 167:1363.
7. Pontari MA, McNaughton-Collins M, O'leary MP, et al. A case-control study of risk factors in men with chronic pelvic pain syndrome. *BJU Int.* 2005;96:559.
8. Weidner W, Schiefer HG, Krauss H, et al. Chronic prostatitis: a thorough search for etiologically involved microorganisms in 1,461 patients. *Infection.* 1991;19:S119.
9. Johnson JR. Microbial virulence determinants and the pathogenesis of urinary tract infection. *Infect Dis Clin North Am.* 2003;17:261.
10. Rudick CN, Berry RE, Johnson JR, et al. Uropathogenic *Escherichia coli* induces chronic pelvic pain. *Infect Immun.* 2011;79:628.
11. True LD, Berger RE, Rothman I, et al. Prostate histopathology and the chronic prostatitis/chronic pelvic pain syndrome: a prospective biopsy study. *J Urol.* 1999;162:2014.
12. Nickel JC, Roehrborn CG, O'Leary MP, et al. The relationship between prostate inflammation and lower urinary tract symptoms: examination of baseline data from the REDUCE trial. *Eur Urol.* 2008;54:1379.
13. Schaeffer AJ, Knauss JS, Landis JR, et al. Leukocyte and bacterial counts do not correlate with severity of symptoms in men with chronic prostatitis: the National Institutes of Health Chronic Prostatitis Cohort Study. *J Urol.* 2002;168:1048.
14. Alexander RB, Brady F, Ponniah S. Autoimmune prostatitis: evidence of T cell reactivity with normal prostatic proteins. *Urology.* 1997;50:893.
15. Motrich RD, Maccioni M, Riera CM, et al. Autoimmune prostatitis: state of the art. Scand J Immunol. 2007;66:217.
16. Kouiavskaia DV, Southwood S, Berard CA, et al. T-cell recognition of prostatic peptides in men with chronic prostatitis/chronic pelvic pain syndrome. *J Urol.* 2009;182:2483.
17. Hou DS, Long WM, Shen J, et al. Characterisation of the bacterial community in expressed prostatic secretions from patients with chronic prostatitis/chronic pelvic pain syndrome and infertile men: a

preliminary investigation. *Asian J Androl.* 2012; 14:566.

18. Yang CC, Lee JC, Kromm BG, et al. Pain sensitization in male chronic pelvic pain syndrome: why are symptoms so difficult to treat?. *J Urol.* 2003; 170:823.

19. Yilmaz U, Liu YW, Berger RE, et al. Autonomic nervous system changes in men with chronic pelvic pain syndrome. *J Urol.* 2007;177:2170.

20. Ishigooka M, Zermann DH, Doggweiler R, et al. Similarity of distributions of spinal c-Fos and plasma extravasation after acute chemical irritation of the bladder and the prostate. *J Urol.* 2000; 164:1751.

21. Farmer MA, Chanda ML, Parks EL, et al. Brain functional and anatomical changes in chronic prostatitis/chronic pelvic pain syndrome. *J Urol.* 2011;186:117.

22. Baliki MN, Schnitzer TJ, Bauer WR, et al. Brain morphological signatures for chronic pain. *PLoS ONE* [Electronic Resource]. 2011;6:e26010.

23. Zermann DH, Ishigooka M, Doggweiler R, et al. Neurourological insights into the etiology of genitourinary pain in men. *J Urol.* 1999;161:903.

24. Blaivas JG, Sinha HP, Zayed AA, et al. Detrusor-external sphincter dyssynergia. *J Urol.* 1981;125:542.

25. Hetrick DC, Glazer H, Liu YW, et al. Pelvic floor electromyography in men with chronic pelvic pain syndrome: a case-control study. *Neurourol Urodynam.* 2006;25:46.

26. Berger RE, Ciol MA, Rothman I, et al. Pelvic tenderness is not limited to the prostate in chronic prostatitis/chronic pelvic pain syndrome (CPPS) type IIIA and IIIB. comparison of men with and without CP/CPPS. BMC *Urology.* 2007;7:17.

27. Ullrich PM, Turner JA, Ciol M, et al. Stress is associated with subsequent pain and disability among men with nonbacterial prostatitis/pelvic pain. *Ann Behav Med.* 2005;30:112.

28. Spanos C, Pang X, Ligris K, et al. Stress-induced bladder mast cell activation: implications for interstitial cystitis. *J Urol.* 1997;157:669.

29. Babenko O, Golubov A, Ilnytskyy Y, et al. Genomic and epigenomic responses to chronic stress involve miRNA-mediated programming. *PLoS ONE* [Electronic Resource]. 2012;7:e29441.

30. Tripp DA, Nickel JC, Wang Y, et al.; National Institutes of Health–Chronic Prostatitis Collaborative Research Network (NIH-CPCRN) Study Group. Catastrophizing and pain-contingent rest predict patient adjustment in men with chronic prostatitis/chronic pelvic pain syndrome. *J Pain.* 2006;7:697.

31. Nickel JC, Tripp DA, Chuai S, et al. Psychosocial variables affect the quality of life of men diagnosed

with chronic prostatitis/chronic pelvic pain syndrome. *BJU Int.* 2008;101:59.

32. Seminowicz DA, Davis KD. Cortical responses to pain in healthy individuals depends on pain catastrophizing. *Pain.* 2006;120:297.

33. Litwin MS, McNaughton-Collins M, Fowler FJJr, et al. The National Institutes of Health chronic prostatitis symptom index: development and validation of a new outcome measure. Chronic Prostatitis Collaborative Research Network. *J Urol.* 1999; 162:369.

34. Barry MJ, Fowler FJJr, O'Leary MP, et al. The American Urological Association symptom index for benign prostatic hyperplasia. The Measurement Committee of the American Urological Association. *J Urol.* 1992;148:1549.

35. Hanno PM, Burks DA, Clemens JQ, et al.; and Interstitial Cystitis Guidelines Panel of the American Urological Association Education and Research. AUA guideline for the diagnosis and treatment of interstitial cystitis/bladder pain syndrome. *J Urol.* 2011;185:2162.

36. Shoskes DA. The challenge of erectile dysfunction in the man with chronic prostatitis/chronic pelvic pain syndrome. *Curr Urol Rep.* 2012;13:263.

37. Chung SD, Keller JJ, Lin HC. A case-control study on the association between chronic prostatitis/chronic pelvic pain syndrome and erectile dysfunction. *BJU Int.* 2012;110:726.

38. Christianson JA, Liang R, Ustinova EE, et al. Convergence of bladder and colon sensory innervation occurs at the primary afferent level. *Pain.* 2007;128:235.

39. Pezzone MA, Liang R, Fraser MO. A model of neural cross-talk and irritation in the pelvis: implications for the overlap of chronic pelvic pain disorders. *Gastroenterology.* 2005;128:1953.

40. Shoskes DA, Prots D, Karns J, et al. Greater endothelial dysfunction and arterial stiffness in men with chronic prostatitis/chronic pelvic pain syndrome--a possible link to cardiovascular disease. *J Urol.* 2011;186:907.

41. Shoskes DA, Nickel JC, Rackley RR, et al. Clinical phenotyping in chronic prostatitis/chronic pelvic pain syndrome and interstitial cystitis: a management strategy for urologic chronic pelvic pain syndromes. *Prostate Cancer P D.* 2009;12:177.

42. Davis R, Jones JS, Barocas DA, et al. Diagnosis, evaluation and follow-up of asymptomatic microhematuria (AMH) in adults: AUA guideline. *J Urol.* 2012;188:2473.

43. Nickel JC, Moon T. Chronic bacterial prostatitis: an evolving clinical enigma. *Urology.* 2005; 66:2.

44. Nickel JC, Downey J, Clark J, et al. Levofloxacin for chronic prostatitis/chronic pelvic pain syndrome

in men: a randomized placebo-controlled multi-center trial. *Urology.* 2003;62:614.

45. Cohen JM, Fagin AP, Hariton E, et al. Therapeutic intervention for chronic prostatitis/chronic pelvic pain syndrome (CP/CPPS): a systematic review and meta-analysis. *PLoS ONE* [Electronic Resource]. 2012;7:e41941.

46. Nickel JC. The three As of chronic prostatitis therapy: antibiotics, alpha-blockers and anti-inflammatories. What is the evidence? *BJU Int.* 2004; 94: 1230.

47. Nickel JC, Xiang J. Clinical significance of non-traditional bacterial uropathogens in the management of chronic prostatitis. *J Urol.* 2008;179:1391.

48. Nickel JC. Treatment of chronic prostatitis/chronic pelvic pain syndrome. *Int J Antimicrob Agents.* 2008;31:S112.

49. Anothaisintawee T, Attia J, Nickel JC, et al. Management of chronic prostatitis/chronic pelvic pain syndrome: a systematic review and network meta-analysis. *JAMA.* 2011;305:78.

50. Perletti G, Skerk V, Magri V, et al. Macrolides for the treatment of chronic bacterial prostatitis: an effective application of their unique pharmacoki-netic and pharmacodynamic profile (review) *Mol Med Rep.* 2011;4:1035.

51. Nickel JC, Downey J, Johnston B, et al. Predictors of patient response to antibiotic therapy for the chronic prostatitis/chronic pelvic pain syndrome: a prospective multicenter clinical trial. *J Urol.* 2001;165:1539.

52. Thakkinstian A, Attia J, Anothaisintawee T, et al. alpha-blockers, antibiotics and anti-inflammatories have a role in the management of chronic prostatitis/chronic pelvic pain syndrome. *BJU Int.* 2012;110:1014.

53. Nickel JC, O'Leary MP, Lepor H, et al. Silodosin for men with chronic prostatitis/chronic pelvic pain syndrome: results of a phase II multicenter, double-blind, placebo controlled study. *J Urol.* 2011;186:125.

54. Oelke M, Giuliano F, Mirone V, et al. Monotherapy with tadalafil or tamsulosin similarly improved lower urinary tract symptoms suggestive of benign prostatic hyperplasia in an international, ran-domised, parallel, placebo-controlled clinical trial. *Eur Urol.* 2012;61:917.

55. Grimsley SJ, Khan MH, Jones GE. Mechanism of Phosphodiesterase 5 inhibitor relief of prostatitis symptoms. *Med Hypotheses.* 2007;69:25.

56. Nickel JC, Roehrborn C, Montorsi F, et al. Dutasteride reduces prostatitis symptoms compared with placebo in men enrolled in the REDUCE study. *J Urol.* 2011;186:1313.

57. van Ophoven A, Hertle L. Long-term results of amitriptyline treatment for interstitial cystitis. *J Urol.* 2005;174:1837.

58. Foster HE,Jr, Hanno PM, Nickel JC, et al. Effect of amitriptyline on symptoms in treatment naive patients with interstitial cystitis/painful bladder syndrome. *J Urol.* 2010;183:1853.

59. Boyle J, Eriksson ME, Gribble L, et al. Randomized, placebo-controlled comparison of amitriptyline, duloxetine, and pregabalin in patients with chronic diabetic peripheral neuropathic pain: impact on pain, polysomnographic sleep, daytime functioning, and quality of life. *Diabetes Care.* 2012; 35:2451.

60. Pontari MA, Krieger JN, Litwin MS, et al. Pregabalin for the treatment of men with chronic prostatitis/chronic pelvic pain syndrome: a randomized controlled trial. *Arch Intern Med.* 2010; 170:1586.

61. Crofford LJ, Rowbotham MC, Mease PJ, et al. Pregabalin for the treatment of fibromyalgia syndrome: results of a randomized, double-blind, placebo-controlled trial. *Arthritis Rheum.* 2005; 52:1264.

62. Anderson RU, Sawyer T, Wise D, et al. Painful myofascial trigger points and pain sites in men with chronic prostatitis/chronic pelvic pain syndrome. *J Urol.* 2009;182:2753.

63. Anderson RU, Wise D, Sawyer T, et al. Integration of myofascial trigger point release and paradoxical relaxation training treatment of chronic pelvic pain in men. *J Urol.* 2005;174:155.

64. Fitzgerald MP, Anderson RU, Potts J, et al. Randomized multicenter feasibility trial of myofascial physical therapy for the treatment of urological chronic pelvic pain syndromes. *J Urol.* 2013;189:S75.

65. Gottsch HP, Yang CC, Berger RE. A pilot study of botulinum toxin A for male chronic pelvic pain syndrome. *Scand J Urol Nephrol.* 2011;45:72.

66. Tripp DA, Nickel JC, Wang Y, et al. National Institutes of Health-Chronic Prostatitis Collaborative Research Network (NIH-CPCRN) Study Group: Catastrophizing and pain-contingent rest predict patient adjustment in men with chronic prostatitis/chronic pelvic pain syndrome. *J Pain.* 2006;7:697.

67. Chung SD, Huang CC, Lin HC. Chronic prostatitis and depressive disorder: a three year population-based study. *J Affect Disord.* 2011; 134:404.

68. Nickel JC, Mullins C, Tripp DA. Development of an evidence-based cognitive behavioral treatment program for men with chronic prostatitis/chronic pelvic pain syndrome. *World J Urol.* 2008; 26:167.

69. Lee SW, Liong ML, Yuen KH, et al. Validation of a sham acupuncture procedure in a randomised, controlled clinical trial of chronic pelvic pain treatment. *Acupunct Med.* 2011;29:40.

70. Lee SH, Lee BC. Electroacupuncture relieves pain in men with chronic prostatitis/chronic pelvic pain syndrome: three-arm randomized trial. *Urology.* 2009;73:1036.

71. Posadzki P, Zhang J, Lee MS, et al. Acupuncture for chronic nonbacterial prostatitis/chronic pelvic pain syndrome: a systematic review. *J Androl.* 2012;33:15.

72. Shoskes DA, Nickel JC. Quercetin for chronic prostatitis/chronic pelvic pain syndrome. *Urol Clin North Am.* 2011;38:279.

73. Sanudo B, Carrasco L, de Hoyo M, et al. Effects of exercise training and detraining in patients with fibromyalgia syndrome: a 3-yr longitudinal study. *Am J Phys Med Rehabil.* 2012;91:561.

74. Shoskes DA, Nickel JC, Kattan MW. Phenotypically directed multimodal therapy for chronic prostatitis/chronic pelvic pain syndrome: a prospective study using UPOINT. *Urology.* 2010;75:1249.

13

Musculoskeletal Causes of Chronic Pelvic Pain

CHRIS R. ABRECHT, LESLEY E. BOBB, AND ASSIA T. VALOVSKA

Musculoskeletal disorders should be considered in all patients presenting with chronic pelvic pain, not only those who have already undergone an exhaustive, unrevealing workup. Furthermore, given the often-multifactorial etiology of chronic pelvic pain, it should also be considered as a possible comorbid condition in patients with known causes of pelvic pain, such as endometriosis, ovarian cysts, or pregnancy. Musculoskeletal disorders are also a frequent cause of pelvic pain: according to one study examining female pelvic pain patients presenting for evaluation at an academic chronic pelvic pain clinic, dysfunctions of the piriformis and levator ani muscles were found to occur at rates of 14% and 22%, respectively.[1] While many of the physicians to whom these patients present may not be well trained in the diagnosis and treatment of problems of the muscle, fascia, and connective tissue, the approach is relatively straightforward. After obtaining a detailed medical history, including a history of trauma or athletic injuries, the clinician must perform a thorough physical examination. This exam should include the following: observing the patient's gait and posture while seated, visualizing and palpating the spine and pelvic joint, and testing muscle strength, sensation, and reflexes. Additional imaging studies such as ultrasound, CT scans, and MRIs are often not required to make the diagnosis of most musculoskeletal disorders. This chapter will provide a brief overview of some of the common musculoskeletal disorders causing pelvic pain. It will emphasize presenting symptoms, physical exam findings, and useful treatment modalities.

SPINE

Disorders of the spine may manifest as pelvic pain. Three such important disorders are discogenic pain, radicular pain, and lumbar plexopathy, which may be the result of myriad conditions, such as degenerative joint disease, trauma, tumor, or radiation. According to the International Association for the Study of Pain, lumbar discogenic pain stems from a lumbar intervertebral disk, with or without referred pain.[2] Lumbar radicular pain, in turn, stems from insult to the lumbar nerve root; lumbar plexopathy stems from insult to the lumbosacral plexus (L1–S4). In all cases, patients may experience pain in the lower back, buttock, thigh, groin, or pelvis. Initial evaluation of these disorders should be via history and a physical exam, looking in particular at range of motion, muscle strength, and sensory changes in a dermatomal distribution. The straight leg raise, described in Figure 13.1, may be used to evaluate for nerve root compression, as occurs from herniated intervertebral discs. The initial treatment of these conditions is usually physical therapy and anti-inflammatory medications (e.g., NSAIDs). Saddle anesthesia, rapidly worsening weakness, and incontinence of the bladder, however, should prompt urgent imaging of the lumbar spine and possibly neurosurgical evaluation.

HIP

Hip pathology may manifest as pain in a variety of territories, including the groin, posterior pelvis, and thigh.[3] Some of the conditions that may result in such pain are congenital or developmental hip dysplasia and femoroacetabular impingement, in which bony abnormalities result in abnormal stresses in the hip joint. The result of these conditions is often osteoarthritis, in which loss of the protective cartilage in the hip joint results in pain that is usually worse in the morning and with weight-bearing activities. Diagnosis of bone abnormalities, fractures, and osteoarthritis can often be achieved with simple radiographs. Management of osteoarthritis

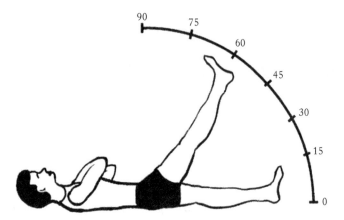

FIGURE 13.1: Straight leg raise test: To perform the straight leg raise, the patient is positioned supine. A single leg is then raised by the clinician. Reproduction of radicular pain at an angle of 30–70 degrees is a positive result, indicating possible compression of the L4–S1 nerve roots. A meta-analysis found that the sensitivity of this test in a population with a high prevalence of disc herniation was 0.92. The specificity varied widely, from 0.1 to 1.

Van der Windt DA, Simons E, Riphagen II, et al. Physical examination for lumbar radiculopathy due to disc herniation in patients with low-back pain. *Cochrane Database Syst Rev.* 2010;(2):CD007431. Image courtesy of James Bell.

includes physical therapy and anti-inflammatory agents (e.g., NSAIDs).[4]

PUBIS

Another possible cause of pain localizing to the pubic area is osteitis pubis, defined as inflammation of the pubic symphysis and the abdominal muscles that attach distally to it. This pain may be worse with physical activity such as kicking, lying on one side, running, walking, or climbing stairs. These patients may also present with fever or chills, which, if present, should prompt an evaluation to rule out osteomyelitis. The direct spring test is the most specific test for diagnosis: in this test, pain produced by direct pressure on the pubic rami is considered a positive result. Another test is the pubic symphysis gap test in which the patient flexes the knees and hips at 90 degrees and then performs isometric adductor contraction against the examiner's fist. A positive pubic symphysis gap test consists of pain upon performance of this procedure. The mainstay of treatment for this condition is conservative management, including physical therapy.[5]

Stress fractures of the pelvis may also result in pelvic pain, often marked by a prolonged onset. In females, the gender more frequently affected by this condition, the pain may manifest in the perineum, buttock, or thigh.[6] In males, the pain may manifest in the abdomen, perineum, or scrotum. On physical examination, there will be tenderness with palpation of the pubic symphysis

and the insertion site of the adductors.[6] Given the propensity of athletes to acquire this injury, it is important upon exam to inquire about repetitive activities and "the female triad" of amenorrhea, osteopenia/osteoporosis, and eating disorders.[7] MRI may be used for diagnosis and staging of fractures. Conservative management is the mainstay of treatment.

COCCYX

Another possible source of pelvic pain is the coccyx, which, along with the ischial tuberosities, provides weight-bearing support in the seated position. The etiology of coccydynia may be hypermobility or hypomobility of the joint, degenerative joint disease, neoplasm, or trauma leading to bruising, dislocation, or fracture. Coccydynia occurs approximately five times more often in women than in men and requires a thorough work-up to rule out referred pain from the spine. X-ray or MRI may assist in this diagnosis. Treatment involves physical therapy to correct poor posture and for pelvic floor rehabilitation, as well as the administration of non-steroidal anti-inflammatory drugs (NSAIDs). Surgical repairs of coccyx fractures have been attempted, but no randomized controlled trials have evaluated this intervention.[8]

SACROILIAC JOINT

Sacroiliac joint dysfunction, often resulting from arthritic changes at the sacroiliac joint, may result in sacroiliitis. This pain is often described as in the lower back, radiating into the buttocks and groin, but not past the knee. It may be worsened by prolonged sitting or standing and may be either unilateral or bilateral. To make this diagnosis, the patient should complain of this manner of pain around the sacroiliac joint and should report worsening of pain with provocative physical exam tests, such as Patrick's or the FABER test (**f**lexion, **ab**duction, **e**xternal **r**otation of the hip).[2] Figure 13.2 depicts the Patrick's test. Imaging is generally unrevealing, showing either a normal-appearing joint or non-specific arthritic changes; it is not a requirement for diagnosis but should of course be considered to rule out other pathologies such as infection or tumor. Treatment consists of an injection with local anesthetic and steroid, a procedure often performed under fluoroscopy by interventional pain management physicians.

PELVIC FLOOR
The musculature of the pelvic floor is another possible cause of chronic pelvic pain and may

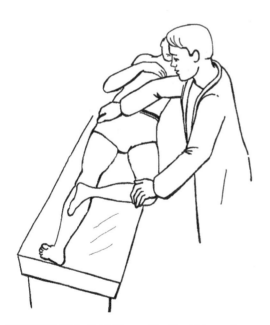

FIGURE 13.2: Patrick's test: The Patrick's test is performed with the patient supine. The patient's foot is positioned as depicted below the patient's contralateral knee. Pressure is then applied to the patient's knee and contralateral hip. A positive test will result in reproduction of the patient's sacroiliac joint pain.

Image modified from neckandback.com, courtesy of Angela Mark.

manifest as a myofascial pain syndrome or pelvic floor hypertonicity. Myofascial pain syndrome is thought to result from acute macrotrauma or chronic microtrauma to muscles, resulting in classic "tender points" of muscle knots, which, when palpated, result in referred pain. While better known for causing chronic, aching, cramplike pain in the trapezius and lumbar paraspinous muscles, myofascial pain syndrome may also present in the pelvic musculature. One study of patients with chronic pelvic pain found, for instance, a 71% prevalence of tender points involving the levator ani, obturator internus, and piriformis muscles.[9] Identification and cessation of the initiating trauma and trigger-point injections consisting of the injection of local anesthetic into these muscle bands are the treatment standard.

Hypertonicity of the pelvic musculature may be the result of pelvic or systemic disorders or could be a primary problem. Regardless of the cause of the hypertonicity, a variety of symptoms may be present due to the important roles these muscles play in maintaining urinary and fecal continence, posture, and normal sexual function. The myriad associated symptoms therefore include, but are not limited to, urinary or bowel incontinence, lower back pain, and dyspareunia. Commonly involved muscles include the levator ani resulting in pain in the coccyx, hip, and back, as well as pain with bowel movements, and pain in the perineum when sitting. Another commonly involved muscle is the obturator internus, resulting in pain in the posterior thigh as well as rectal fullness.[10] Diagnosis is usually achieved based on history and physical exam, with tender, high-tone muscles noted during the pelvic exam. In some cases, electromyography may be obtained for confirmation. Treatment usually starts with behavior changes, such as avoidance of triggers; and physical therapy, which can include biofeedback, soft-tissue therapy, and ultrasound therapy. If those are unsuccessful, additional available interventions include pharmacological therapy with amitriptyline, tizanidine, or baclofen suppositories.[11]

PIRIFORMIS MUSCLE
Piriformis syndrome, a condition affecting females more than males, is yet another possible cause of pelvic pain. The piriformis is a muscle that is flat, banded, and located deep to the gluteus maximus with attachments at the sacrum and the greater trochanter of the femur.

There are two types of piriformis syndrome. In type one, the sciatic nerve is compressed due to a split piriformis muscle, a split sciatic nerve, or an alternative nerve path. Type two is secondary to trauma or ischemia. Patients may present with pain starting in the buttock and sacroiliac joint and progressing to symptoms resembling sciatica. The onset may be gradual or sudden. Symptoms may be initiated or worsened by sitting for long periods of time (particularly with legs crossed), climbing stairs, or applying pressure directly over the muscle. Prior to accepting a diagnosis of piriformis syndrome, other causes of sciatica such as degenerative disc disease must be ruled out. The "Lasegue sign" refers to tenderness to palpation of the piriformis muscle, indicating some impingement of the sciatic nerve by the muscle.[12] The "Freiberg sign" refers to pain with passive internal rotation of the hip. The "Beatty test" refers to placing the patient on the unaffected side while holding the superior knee approximately four inches off the table. If sciatic symptoms are produced with this maneuver, then the test is positive, and piriformis syndrome is more likely.[13] Prevention includes using proper form when performing repetitive activities such as running. Treatment includes rest, physical therapy, heating or icing, and anti-inflammatory medications.

ILIOPSOAS MUSCLE

Another muscle sometimes responsible for pelvic pain is the iliopsoas, a muscle composed of the distal ends of the psoas and iliacus muscles, and which functions as a hip flexor. Two painful conditions associated with this muscle are iliopsoas tendonitis and iliopsoas bursitis. In iliopsoas tendonitis, pain, typically of gradual onset, develops in the hip and groin, with occasional radiation to the knee. These symptoms may persist for years and be associated with a snap or click of the hip or groin. On exam there may be tenderness to palpation of the lesser trochanter deep to the gluteus maximus. One of the tests indicative of iliopsoas tendonitis is Ludloff's sign, in which the patient sits with knees extended and then raises the leg approximately 15 degrees. Pain with this maneuver is a positive Ludloff's sign. Treatment includes resting, stretching, and anti-inflammatory medications.[14,15] Iliopsoas bursitis, in turn, is inflammation of the iliopsoas bursa, which lies deep to the iliopsoas muscle. This condition may be seen in athletes, patients with acute trauma, or those with rheumatoid arthritis. Symptoms are similar to those of iliopsoas tendonitis. The snapping hip maneuver may help diagnose iliopsoas syndrome. In this maneuver, the patient lies supine and the examiner places one hand on the inguinal crease while passively flexing, abducting, and externally rotating the hip. A click in the last portion of the maneuver is a positive test. (See Figure 13.3.) Treatment includes physical therapy and anti-inflammatory medications. In some cases, intrabursal injections or even surgical lengthening have been required.[15]

NEUROPATHIES

Along with musculoskeletal disorders, neuropathies deserve consideration when evaluating

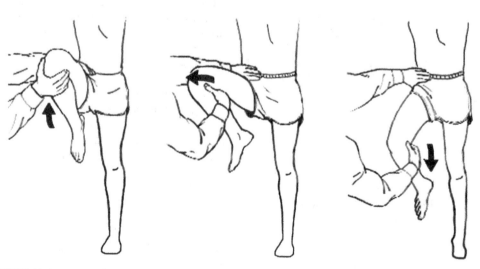

FIGURE 13.3: Snapping hip maneuver.
Image courtesy of James Bell.

a patient with pelvic pain. The causes of nerve injury resulting in a painful neuropathy are varied and include stretching, blunt trauma, surgical trauma, fibrosis, and compression with hypoxia.[16] By far the most important neuropathy related to pelvic pain is that of the pudendal nerve, a mixed sensory and motor nerve originating from S2–S4, which is discussed in detail in a separate chapter. Other important neuropathies include the closely related ilioinguinal, genitofemoral, iliohypogastric, and obturator neuralgias, as described in Table 13.1. The similarity of the anatomical territories affected by these blocks may require a diagnostic and therapeutic procedure to correctly identify the affected nerve. Either ilioinguinal or genitofemoral neuralgia may, for instance, be the culprit in a patient with neuropathic pain in the inner thigh and groin. Ultrasound-guided block with local anesthetic and steroid of the causative nerve will result in pain relief. In a similar vein, a paravertebral block at T12–L1 may provide relief in ilsiohypogastric neuralgia, but less so for illoginguinal or genitofemoral neuralgia. In addition, isolated muscle weakness may narrow the diagnosis: lack of a cremasteric relief may suggest genitofemoral neuropathy, and diminished thigh adduction may suggest obturator neuropathy.[17]

Nerve entrapment syndromes are an important cause of neuropathic pain. "Abdominal cutaneous nerve entrapment syndrome" (ACNES) refers to entrapment of the thoracoabdominal nerves terminating as the cutaneous nerves supplying sensation to the abdominal wall. The thoracic corollary to this condition is intercostal neuralgia. In ACNES, the most common entrapment site is at the lateral border of the rectus muscle, where the nerve passes through a fibrous ring and may be compressed, causing ischemia. This pain is usually well localized and affects only one side; patients are often able to indicate with a single finger the painful site at the lateral border of the rectus muscle from which the pain originates. Nerve blocks with local anesthetic and steroid at these sites may be both diagnostic and therapeutic.[18] Another entrapment syndrome involves the posterior femoral cutaneous nerve, originating from S1–S3 and terminating as the inferior cluneal nerves, which supplies sensation to the caudal buttock and the perineum. Here, compression at the insertions of the gluteus maximus and hamstring muscles may result in a neuropathy.[19]

A related nervous system disorder in which compression of nerve roots may result in pelvic pain is the Tarlov cyst. These cysts, also known as perineurial cysts, are dilations of the meninges between the perineurium and endoneurium in the posterior nerve roots which may grow large enough to impinge on other neural structures. See Figure 13.4 for an anatomical illustration. The etiology of these cysts is unclear; theories include inflammatory cells in the cyst walls, congenital malformation, or increased hydrostatic pressure in the cyst walls. When symptomatic, these cysts may cause radiculopathy, pelvic paresthesias, and incontinence of the bowel or bladder. Treatment includes anti-inflammatory medical management and physical therapy. In refractory or severe cases, surgical treatment, including cyst resection at the neck and surgical cyst fenestration, are available options.[20]

CONCLUSION

Musculoskeletal and related nervous system disorders should be considered in all patients presenting with chronic pelvic pain, as the primary or as a contributing cause of their discomfort. An anatomically structured approach may be useful in narrowing a differential in these

---

TABLE 13.1 PERIPHERAL NEUROPATHIES ASSOCIATED WITH PELVIC PAIN

Somatic nerve	Origins	Sensory component	Motor component
Ilioinguinal nerve	L1–L2	Inner thigh, groin, mons, labia, penis, scrotum	
Genitofemoral nerve	L1–L2	Inner thigh, mons, labia, scrotum	Cremasteric reflex
Iliohypogastric nerve	T12–L1	Groin, symphysis pubic	Transversus abdominus, internal oblique
Obturator nerve	L2,L3,L4	Medial thigh, groin	Adductor longus, gracilis, adductor brevis

(A)

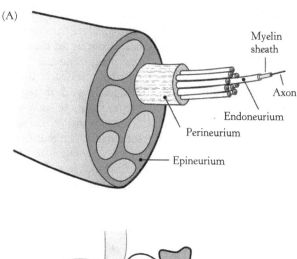

Myelin sheath

Axon

Endoneurium

Perineurium

Epineurium

(B)

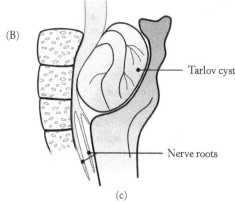

Tarlov cyst

Nerve roots

(c)

FIGURE 13.4: Tarlov cyst: *A.* Tarlov or perineural cysts are dilations in the space between the perineurium and endoneurium. *B.* These cysts may grow quite large, compressing adjacent neurovascular structures.

Image courtesy of Angela Mark.

patients. Consider disorders of bone (spine, hip, sacroiliac joint, pubis, coccyx), pelvic floor musculature, and pelvic neuropathies. Such an approach may identify important musculoskeletal causes of pelvic pain and spare the patient unnecessary, invasive, and unrevealing tests.

REFERENCES

1. Tu FF, As-Sanie S, Steege JF. Prevalence of pelvic musculoskeletal disorders in a female chronic pelvic pain clinic. *J Reprod Med.* 2006;51:185–189.

2. Merskey H, Bogduk N. *Classification of Chronic Pain: Descriptions of Chronic Pain Syndromes and Definitions of Pain Terms.* 2nd ed. Seattle, WA: IASP Press; 1994.

3. Lesher JM, Dreyfuss P, Hager N, et al. Hip joint pain referral patterns: a descriptive study. *Pain Med.* 2008;9(1):22–25.

4. Prather H, Camacho-Soto A. Musculoskeletal etiologies of pelvic pain. *Obstet Gynecol Clin N Am.* 2014;41:433–442.

5. Rodriguez C, Miguel A, Lima H, Heinrich's K. Osteitis pubis syndrome in the professional soccer athlete: a case report: *Journal of Athletic Training.* Oct–Dec 2001;36(4):437–440.

6. Hosey RG, Fernandez, MMF, Johnson DL. Evaluation and management of stress fractures of the pelvis and sacrum. *Orthopedics.* 2008 April; 31(4):383–385.

7. Pepper M, Akuthota V, McCarty E. The pathophysiology of stress fractures. *Clin Sports Med.* 2006;25:1–16.

8. Lirette LS, Chaiban G, et al. Coccydynia: an overview of the anatomy, etiology, and treatment of coccyx pain. *Ochsner J.* 2014;14(1):84–87.

9. Gyang A, Hartman M, Lamvu G. Musculoskeletal causes of chronic pelvic pain: What a gynecologist should know. *Obstet Gynecol.* 2013;121(3): 645–650.

10. Prendergast SA, Weiss JM. Screening for musculoskeletal causes of pelvic pain. *Clin Obstet Gynecol.* 2003;46(4):773–782.

11. Butrick CW. Pelvic floor hypertonic disorders: identification and management. *Obstet Gynecol Clin N Am.* 2009;36:707–722.

12. Boyajian-O'Neill LA, McClain RL, et al. Diagnosis and management of piriformis syndrome: an osteopathic approach. *J Am Osteopath Assoc.* 2008; 108(11):657–664.

13. Robinson DR. Pyriformis syndrome in relation to sciatic pain. *Am J Surg.* 1947;73:355–358.

14. Margo K, Drezner J, Motzkin, D. Evaluation and management of hip pain: an algorithmic approach. *J Fam Pract.* 2003;52(8):607–617.

15. Tibor LM, Sekiya JK. Differential diagnosis of pain around the hip joint. *Arthroscopy.* 2008;24(12):1407–1421.

16. Perry CP. Peripheral neuropathies and pelvic pain: diagnosis and management. *Clin Obstet Gynecol.* 2003;46(4):789–796.

17. Tipton JS. Obturator neuropathy. *Curr Rev Musculoskel Med.* 2008;1(3):234–237.

18. Applegate WV. Abdominal cutaneous nerve entrapment syndromes (ACNES): a commonly overlooked cause of abdominal pain. *Permanente J.* 2002;6(3):20–27.

19. Darnis B, Robert R, Labat JJ, et al. Perineal pain and inferior cluneal nerves: anatomy and surgery. *Surg Radiol Anat.* 2008;30:177–183.

20. Acosta FL, Quinones-Hinjosa A, Schmidt MC, Weinstein PR. Diagnosis and management of sacral Tarlov cysts. *Neurosurg Focus.* 2003;15(2):1–7.

14

Pelvic Cancer Pain

JONATHAN SNITZER, YURY KHELEMSKY, AND KARINA GRITSENKO

EPIDEMIOLOGY

There is a variety of cancers involving both the viscera and the musculoskeletal structures of the pelvis, and these cancers can be either gender-specific or gender-neutral. Some of the cancers occurring in both sexes include bladder, anal, rectal, colon, chondrosarcoma and osteosarcoma. Gender-specific cancers include prostate and testicular cancer in men, and uterine, cervical, ovarian, and vaginal cancer in women. Cancers involving the pelvis are extremely common and carry significant morbidity and mortality. For example, colorectal cancer is responsible for 10% of all cancers in the United States, with approximately 147,000 new cases in 2009.[1] More recently, in the United States, there were 40,000 new cases of rectal cancer, 6,230 of anal cancer, 73,510 of bladder cancer, 241,740 of prostate cancer, and 12,170 of cervical cancer in 2012. Additionally there are approximately 46,000 new cases of uterine cancer each year.[2]

The neoplasm itself, secondary to compression of surrounding structures, or invasion of surrounding tissue, may cause pelvic cancer pain. Pain may also occur as a result of treatment (e.g., surgery, radiation, or chemotherapy). Specific agents known to cause neuropathies include oxaliplatin, carboplatin, cisplatin, paclitaxel, docetaxel, bortezomib, lenalidomide, thalidomide, epothilone, and the vinca alkaloids.[3] In one study, inpatients were found to have pain directly attributable to the tumor 78% of time, and only 19% of the time was the pain considered to be secondary to their treatment. In outpatients with cancer, the pain was attributed to the neoplasm 62% of time and 25% of time as an adverse effect of treatment.[4] Pain is extremely common in cancer and occurs in over 50% of patients.[5] Patients with cancer had pain as their presenting symptom 20–50% of the time.[5] The prevalence of pain varies significantly, depending on one's course in treatment or stage of disease. Patients undergoing treatment for cancer had a lower prevalence of pain, 59% compared to 64% of patients with more advanced disease.[6] Both groups, however, had significantly higher rates of pain than patients who were successfully treated for cancer (33%).

Cancer pain has also been associated with emotional distress. Patients with depression have higher levels of pain than those who do not suffer from depression.[7] Additionally, higher pain scores are associated with significant cognitive impairment.[8] Improving one's mental health is directly correlated to treatment of the pain.[8,9] Untreated pain lowers one's quality of life.[10,11] Additionally, there is evidence that earlier and comprehensive pain control may actually prolong life.[12] Ultimately, appropriate management of a patient's pain is essential to the overall success of therapy.

There are three general forms of pain that occur in cancer patients: somatic, visceral, and neuropathic. Somatic pain is due to direct stimulation of nociceptors located in the skin and deeper musculoskeletal tissues. The pain is localized and is achy, throbbing, or sharp. Visceral pain is due to abnormal distension, contractions, ischemia, or inflammation of viscera. The pain, which is carried by autonomic fibers, is typically vague, dull, and poorly localized. Neuropathic pain is due to compression of a nerve, direct invasion of a nerve by the neoplasm, or neurotoxic effects of medical treatments. The pain that is described as shooting, electrical, and burning, is due to injury to the nerve itself.

PELVIC ANATOMY

The anatomical pelvis is formed by the musculoskeletal components of pelvis and contains the pelvic viscera (e.g. bladder, urethra, vagina, adnexa, and rectum). The bony structure of the pelvis consists of the hip bones made up of the ilium, ischium, and pubis, and the sacrum and coccyx. Anteriorly, the pubic bones articulate with each other, forming the pubic symphysis. The sacrum and ilium articulate, forming the sacroiliac joint. Both of these joints are extremely crucial in stabilization of the pelvis. The pelvis consists of multiple foramina. The obturator foramen located between the ischium and pubis allows the passage of the obturator neurovascular bundle. Posteriorly, the sacrospinous and sacrotuberous ligaments delineate the greater and lesser sciatic foramina. The greater sciatic foramen allows passage of the sciatic nerve, sacral plexus, piriformis muscle, and internal pudendal and inferior gluteal vessels. The pudendal nerve and obturator internus tendon travel through the lesser sciatic foramen.

The posterior border of the anatomical pelvis is created by the sacrum, coccyx, and both the coccygeus and piriformis muscles. The hip bones and obturator internus muscle form the lateral border. The inferior border of the pelvis is formed by the pelvic diaphragm. The pelvic diaphragm is composed of the levator ani and coccygeus muscles. These muscles are extremely important in supporting the pelvic viscera. The anterior border of the pelvis is defined by the pubococcygeus muscle and the pubic symphysis.

The pelvic viscera are supplied by both the sympathetic and parasympathetic systems and have both afferent and efferent nerve fibers. The sympathetic nerves originate in the thoracic and lumber regions of the spinal cord from ganglia that are located just anterolateral to the spinal cord. Parasympathetic innervation is supplied by the cranial nerves and the sacral segment of the spinal cord. Unlike the sympathetic ganglia, the parasympathetic ganglia are located close to the pelvic organs. The two main nerve plexi of the pelvis are the superior and inferior hypogastric. The superior hypogastric plexus is the extension of the aortic and inferior mesenteric plexi. The plexus is located inferior to the aortic bifurcation and extends from L4 to the sacrum. The superior plexus divides to form the left and right hypogastric nerves and continues to form the inferior hypogastric plexus. The superior hypogastric plexus also provides the ureteral, testicular, and ovarian plexi. Both sympathetic and parasympathetic fibers and nociceptive impulses from the uterus, cervix, distal transverse colon, and descending colon travel through the plexus.

In addition to its supply from the superior hypogastric plexus, the inferior plexus receives contributions from the sacral sympathetic trunk via the sacral splanchnic nerves and the pelvic splanchnic nerves. The inferior hypogastric plexus travels with branches of the internal iliac artery and provides innervation to the rectum, urinary bladder, prostate, uterus, and vagina. The sacral sympathetic trunk runs posterior to the common iliac arteries and unites to form the ganglion impar just anterior to the coccyx. The trunk provides sympathetic fibers to the inferior hypogastric plexus. The pelvic splanchnic nerves are located just inferior to the bifurcation of the common iliac artery and carry parasympathetic and visceral afferents back and forth from the inferior hypogastric plexus.

The bladder receives parasympathetic motor fibers from S2–4 and sympathetic fibers from the inferior and superior hypogastric plexus originating at T10–L2. The ureter has a complex nerve supply and ultimately is innervated by the aortic, renal, superior hypogastric, and inferior hypogastric plexuses. These fibers originate from T10–12, L1, and S2–4. Pain is commonly referred to the groin and may extend to the scrotum or labia. The pelvic diaphragm receives innervation from S2–4 via the pudendal nerve.

The uterus, ovaries, and fallopian tubes receive sympathetic innervation from the uterovaginal plexus or Frenkenhauser ganglion, a division of the inferior and superior hypogastric plexuses. These sympathetic fibers arise and enter the spinal cord at T11–12, and, as a result, uterine pain is often referred to the lower abdomen.[13] The uterus receives motor parasympathetic fibers originating in the S2–4 level via the pelvic splanchnic nerves. The cervix receives innervation through the paracervical ganglia. Cervical cancer pain is commonly felt over the lower back. The vagina, vulva, and distal urethra receive innervation via S2–4.

The prostate receives innervation through the prostatic plexus via the inferior hypogastric plexus. The prostate capsule is densely innervated and is very easily damaged by surgical resection or locally invasive cancer. Pain from the prostate is commonly referred to the scrotum. The scrotum receives innervations from the inferior hypogastric and pudendal nerves, whereas the testes are innervated by the renal plexus. The penis receives autonomic innervation from the cavernous nerves, which receives nerve fibers from inferior hypogastric plexus via the prostatic plexus.

EVALUATION OF PELVIC CANCER PAIN

The differential diagnosis for pelvic pain is extremely diverse and involves many systems. Common causes of pelvic pain include pelvic inflammatory disease, urinary tract infection, dysmenorrhea, diverticulitis, nephrolithiasis, ovarian or testicular torsion, ovarian cyst, appendicitis, endometriosis, ectopic pregnancy, and prostatitis. Lastly, although organic disease should be ruled out first, functional disorders should always be taken seriously and be considered on the differential.

All work-up should start with a thorough and detailed history and physical.[14] An essential part of the history is to begin to differentiate between the types of pain: somatic, visceral, or neuropathic. The patient should always be asked to describe his or her pain using his or her own words. Like the evaluation of all symptoms, it is important to elucidate the basics of onset, location, duration, characteristics, alleviating or aggravating factors, radiation, treatments attempted, and overall severity of symptoms. When taking a history, it is crucial to obtain a complete review of systems—particularly, questions concerning any gynecological, obstetrical, urological, gastrointestinal, neurological, musculoskeletal, and psychological symptoms. For example, back pain or pathological fractures may be signs of metastatic prostate cancer. Painless hematuria may indicate bladder cancer. Psychological evaluation of the patient is indispensable, especially addressing concerns of anxiety, emotional distress, and depression. Past medical history and family history are also essential, given the greater prevalence of ovarian cancer in patients with hereditary genetic disorders such as BRCA.[15] A proper social history is important because of the relationship between certain habits and cancer; for example, smoking is a risk factor for bladder cancer.[16] Additionally, smoking status may affect types of treatment modalities and complications of those treatments. Active smokers with cervical cancer were found to have much higher complication rates (hazard ratio of 2.3) after radiation therapy than non-smokers.[17]

The physical exam should cover many systems, including the neurological, orthopedic, gynecological, urological, and gastrointestinal. Patients with stage II endometrial cancer had significantly more abnormal physical exam findings on cervical palpation and rectal parametrial examination than patients with stage I cancer.[18] Additionally, Pap smear and colposcopy continue to play a crucial role in the diagnosis of cervical cancer.[18] Signs of pathological fracture may indicate metastatic prostate cancer.[19] Digital rectal exam continues to play a role in the initial screening for prostate cancer.[20]

In many cases, it is necessary to obtain complimentary laboratory tests, diagnostic imaging, and ultimately, more invasive diagnostic procedures to support or confirm one's differential diagnosis. As with all diagnostic work-ups, it is important to be judicious and goal-directed when ordering tests. Moreover, it is critical to have an organized, stepwise approach that is centered on the patient to avoid unnecessary invasive procedures.

When evaluating pain, given its inherent subjectivity, it is important to use reproducible assessment tools. The patient's pain should be evaluated on the initial visit and used on subsequent visits to monitor for the effectiveness and progression of therapy. There are various validated self-report assessment tools for pain, including the Numerical Rating Scale (NRS), Visual Analog Scale (VAS), Verbal Rating Scale (VRS), and Adjective Rating Scale (ARS). VRS and NRS were shown to have similar sensitivity in detecting a change in symptoms.[21] In a study comparing the use of VAS to NRS in lung cancer patients, a strong concordance between the two assessment tools was found.[22]

In children, many of the standard pain assessment modalities are inappropriate secondary to cognitive limitations. Validated pain assessment tools in children include the Face, Legs, Activity, Consolability scale, poker chip tool, Revised Faces Pain Scale, and the Body Outline Pain Scale.[23,24] In addition to monitoring pain, the evaluator needs to gain an understanding of how the pain is affecting the patient's activities of daily living (ADL). Each tool has its own advantages and disadvantages, and it is the physician's job to use both the patient's preferences and abilities to find the most effective scale.

MANAGEMENT OF PELVIC CANCER PAIN

Pharmacological Therapy

Goals in pain management are to maximize patient functionality and to improve quality of life. Medications should be given orally in preference to other routes, when possible. Simple daily or twice-daily dosing of medications is preferred. The regimen also must fulfill the patient's needs, based on the type of pain they are experiencing.

Medications can be given in both short-acting and sustained-released formularies.

Managing a cancer patient's pain requires a stepwise approach. The World Health Organization's (WHO) three-step ladder is the preferred approach to treatment of cancer pain. Using numerical rating, patients describe their pain on a scale of 0–10. At Step 1, for patients with mild pain (1–3), the individual should be started on a non-opioid analgesic. When choosing the appropriate initial therapy, taking a thorough history is necessary to avoid inappropriate drug administration. Additionally, a complete list of currently prescribed medications is required to avoid any overdoses or drug–drug interactions. There is a variety of choices of non-opioid analgesics, including aspirin, acetaminophen, and NSAIDS. Acetaminophen is an antipyretic and analgesic without anti-inflammatory properties. The exact mechanism of acetaminophen is unknown. When prescribing acetaminophen, it is extremely important to make sure patients are not taking other medications containing acetaminophen, which would cause the patient to exceed 4 g in 24 hours. NSAIDs provide analgesia by blocking the production of prostaglandins, which are involved in both the peripheral and central pain pathways. NSAIDs should be avoided or prescribed judiciously in patients with peptic ulcer disease, renal disease, cerebrovascular disease, coronary artery disease, or coagulopathy.

Step 2, for moderate pain (4–6), or if the individual continues to have poorly controlled symptoms on the initial therapy, a "weak" opioid (Tramadol or meperidine), or a combination of a non-opioid and opioid analgesic should be started. Tramadol is both a weak opioid agonist and a norepinephrine and serotonin reuptake inhibitor, which both play a role in its analgesic properties. As a result, tramadol should be avoided in patients already on antidepressants. Meperidine is a synthetic pure opioid agonist, which is of limited use because of its short duration of action and side-effect profile. Meperidine is broken down in the liver to normeperidine, which, if not cleared, can cause severe neurotoxicity and ultimately lead to seizures. The combination therapies include an opioid and a non-opioid medication. For example: acetaminophen/hydrocodone, acetaminophen/oxycodone, ibuprofen/hydrocodone, or acetaminophen/codeine. The combination medications provide superior analgesia by affecting nociceptive pathways at different sites. Moreover, by decreasing the opioid requirement, one curtails the risk of side effects. These medications rely on first-order kinetics for elimination, and as a result have a ceiling effect largely determined by the maximum safe dose of the non-opioid medication.

Step 3, if the patient continues to have pain or is having severe pain (on the order of 7–10), the patient should be started on a pure opioid agonist; i.e., morphine, hydromorphone, fentanyl, methadone, etc. Unlike the prior two steps, step 3 medications have no ceiling effect or maximum dose. Opioids may be administered orally, intranasally, rectally, buccally, transdermal, subcutaneously, or intravenously. Again, oral administration is always the preferred route when possible. Rectal administration may be preferred when the patient is unable to take PO or the patient is unable to absorb medications enterally. Intravenous administration may be preferred when there is a desire to avoid first past metabolism or need for quicker onset. Transdermal patches are ideal for providing long-acting analgesia for patients with severe chronic pain. Intraspinal administration is appropriate when the patient is unable to tolerate the side effects of systemic opioids or is having poor pain control with escalating doses. Titrating opioids requires close attention to details in order to avoid potentially life-threatening side effects. When starting a new opioid, it takes approximately five half-lives to reach steady state. As a result, it is important to always be mindful of the time course of any changes in one's regimen in order to avoid an overdose.

In addition to the medications used in steps 1–3, adjuvant therapies can be added at any step to enhance the effects of the opioid, reduce the dose of opioids needed, and address pain pathways that opioids may not be effectively covering.[25] Adjuvant medications in general have other primary indications, but they also possess some analgesic properties. Different adjuvant therapies have diverse mechanisms of action, and as result, are indicated for treating specific types of pain. Adjuvant medications include anticonvulsants, tricyclic antidepressants (TCA), corticosteroids, bisphosphonates, alpha2-adrenergic agonists, neuroleptics, and N-methyl-D-aspartate receptor (NMDA) antagonists. Anticonvulsants—specifically gabapentin and pregabalin—are effective for treating neuropathic pain in cancer patients.[26] TCAs, like anticonvulsants, are particularly effective for treating neuropathic pain.[27] When prescribing TCAs, it is important to be aware of their side-effect profile, specifically their anticholinergic effects. If the patient is not tolerating the tertiary amines, a change to a secondary amine may provide a more favorable side-effect profile. Unlike TCAs, selective serotonin reuptake inhibitors do not appear to be as useful in the treatment of neuropathic pain.[27] Corticosteroids are effective for neuropathic, somatic, and visceral pain. Corticosteroids are specifically useful for metastatic bone pain.[28] Additionally, corticosteroids are both orexigenic and an anti-emetic, which is of particular importance in cancer patients. Consequences of long-term steroid therapy include weight gain, hyperglycemia, adrenal suppression, fluid retention, increased intraocular pressure, and increased risk of infections in patients who may already be immunosuppressed.

Bisphosphonates and calcitonin, like corticosteroids, are effective adjuvant therapies for metastatic bone pain.[29] The mechanism is believed to be secondary to anti-osteoclast activity. Bisphosphonates help delay and prevent skeletal events in patients with metastatic disease.[29] This utility is of particular importance for prostate cancer patients who are on treatments like androgen-deprivation therapy and other antineoplastic agents that place them at increased risk of fracture.[30] Neuroleptics in cancer pain patients who are also experiencing some cognitive dysfunction have been shown to both decrease opioid usage and improve pain scores.[31] The mechanism of action may be secondary to a decrease in patient anxiety or by direct analgesic effects of the antipsychotic. Additionally, neuroleptics as a class have antiemetic properties. NMDA receptors have been shown to play a role in central sensitization and hyperalgesia.[32] NMDA antagonists have been shown to decrease pain and opioid dosage.[33] Additionally, they have been shown to inhibit the development of opioid tolerance.[32]

Non-pharmacological Management

Cancer pain therapy should not be limited to pharmacological therapy, but rather requires a multidisciplinary approach. When appropriate, it is crucial to utilize non-pharmacological treatments in addition to pharmacological and interventional therapies. Non-pharmacological therapies should be used early and often in a patient's treatment regimen. These therapies include, but are not limited to, physical therapy, exercise, heat, cold, education, acupuncture, and spiritual and psychiatric counseling. These psychological and behavioral therapies have be shown to reduce pain scores.[34,35] Clinicians and other healthcare workers should help patients gain access to and coordinate a more complete treatment plan. Of note, these therapies should never replace the use of appropriate pharmacological or interventional therapies.

Interventional Modalities

When conservative measures, such as pharmacological therapy, fail to control a patient's pain, more invasive procedures may be needed. There are two main categories of interventional treatment modalities used by anesthesiologists for cancer pain. One is intrathecal/epidural medications, and the other is targeted peripheral nerve blocks. Historically, interventional procedures have been considered the "fourth step" in the WHO pain ladder. They are mainly utilized when medical therapy is either insufficient or the side-effects of medications are too significant. But there is growing support and evidence for earlier interventional therapy, which shows that it provides better pain control and reduction in the use of systemic opioids.[36,37] When choosing an interventional procedure, it is important to consider life expectancy, quality of life, surgical risks, side effects, and cost in order to select the most appropriate modality.

Epidural and intrathecal medications are extremely effective for providing analgesia. Unlike systemic opioids, neuraxial analgesia is administered with greater proximity to its site of action—the central nervous system. As a result, dosages are greatly reduced, and the side-effect profile is considerably more favorable. Neuraxial analgesia is usually administered as continuous therapy. A plethora of different medications can be given, ranging from opioids alone, to combinations of opioid and local anesthetics, opioids and other adjuvant therapies, and ultimately, neurolytic therapies.

In a randomized control trial comparing the use of comprehensive medical management versus comprehensive medical management plus continuous intrathecal morphine for intractable cancer pain, there was a clinically significant reduction in pain and side effects in the group with intrathecal morphine.[38] Additionally, equivalent opioid administration was significantly reduced in the morphine group.[38]

In addition to opioid therapy, combination therapy of intrathecal opioids with a local anesthetic is an effective option for improving cancer pain and reducing opioid requirements.[39] In a prospective study of 55 opioid-tolerant patients with intractable cancer pain (including 13 patients with pelvic cancer), the combination of continuous intrathecal morphine and levobupivacaine showed significant improvement in pain scores from initiation of therapy until time of death, compared to their prior oral regimen.[40] Furthermore, oral use of opioids and their concurrent side effects decreased with intrathecal therapy.[40]

In addition to local anesthetics, other adjuvant therapies, including clonidine, ziconotide, ketamine, neostigmine, and steroids, can be used to enhance opioid therapy. Clonidine has been shown to act synergistically with intrathecal opioids and local anesthetics to improve pain control in patients with severe cancer-related pain.[41,42] Ziconotide, a N-type voltage-gated calcium blocker, is FDA-approved for intrathecal use to treat severe, refractory, chronic pain. In a double-blinded, placebo-controlled, randomized trial comparing intrathecal ziconotide to placebo, there was a statistically and clinically significant reduction in both pain scores and opioid usage among the ziconotide group.[43] Ziconotide's side-effect profile, especially its central nervous system effects, greatly limit its clinical use.[43] A systematic review of patients with cancer pain found that both intrathecal ketamine and epidural ketamine in combination with opioids improves pain control and reduces opioid requirements.[44] Additionally, the review suggests that neostigmine may also lower pain scores and reduce opioid needs.[44] In a case series of three patients with intractable pelvic cancer pain, intrathecal betamethasone was given, with significant pain relief beginning in about 10 minutes and lasting for at least 5 days.[45] In a case series of four terminally ill patients with prior bladder diversions suffering from intractable pelvic cancer pain, they were given intrathecal phenol, and all four had improvement in their pain symptoms and a >60% decline in their opioid usage.[46] The relief persisted from days to weeks, without any block-specific adverse effects.[46] Contraindications for use of epidural/intrathecal anesthesia include patient refusal, infection at the site of the procedure, coagulopathy, increased intracranial pressure, allergy, preexisting neurological deficits, demyelinating disease, valvular disease, sepsis, and uncooperative patients.

Nerve blocks are a targeted approach aimed at inhibiting the specific nerves involved in the pelvic cancer pain pathway. There are three main plexi that can be blocked for pelvic cancer pain relief: superior hypogastric plexus, inferior hypogastric plexus, and ganglion impar. There is a variety of other blocks that may be used separately or in combination with these blocks to provide pain relief. The two most commonly used neurolytic substances are alcohol (50–100%) and phenol (6–12%). Phenol provides the benefit of also being a local anesthetic and, unlike alcohol, is not painful on injection. Alcohol may be preferred given its ease of injection through a smaller needle. Problems with neurolysis arise when neuronal regeneration occurs, which can cause return of the original pain or creation of new pain. Given the uncertainty of the exact cause and innervations of the pain, a diagnostic block with a temporary local anesthetic is preferred prior to the actual neurolytic block.

The superior hypogastric plexus, found in the retroperitoneum just inferior to the aortic bifurcation and anterior to L4–S1, is crucial in the nociceptive pathway of the pelvic viscera. As a result, the superior hypogastric plexus block (SHPB) is a clear target for relief of pelvic cancer pain. Plancarte first introduced the SHPB in a small study of 28 patients with pelvic cancer pain, finding a 70% reduction in VAS scores.[47] The procedure is performed in the prone position. Once positioned, the L4–5 interspace is identified by both exam and fluoroscopy. After local anesthetic skin infiltration, bilateral 7-inch 22-G short beveled needles are inserted 5–7 cm lateral to midline. The needles are directed medially toward the anterolateral aspect of the L5 vertebral body. The needle is advanced approximately 1 cm past the vertebral body. After negative aspiration, appropriate placement is confirmed by fluoroscopy with contrast in both the anteroposterior (AP) and lateral view. Appropriate placement shows confinement of contrast in the midline region on AP view, and a smooth posterior contour corresponding to the anterior psoas fascia in the lateral view. Once placement is confirmed, local anesthetic is injected for diagnostic blocks and phenol or alcohol for neurolytic blocks.

The classic prone procedure has limitations secondary to the difficulty of needle placement. The iliac crest and transverse process act as obstacles to proper needle insertion. In a randomized study of 30 patients, the classic prone SHPB was compared to a novel transdiscal approach for treatment of pelvic cancer pain.[48] In both the classic prone approach and transdiscal approach, the VAS scores and the daily morphine consumption significantly decreased from baseline values at 24 hours, one week, one month, and two months.[48] Of note, there were no significant differences in VAS scores or morphine usage between the two groups.[48] Interestingly, the transdiscal approach took an average of 32 minutes' less time. In the classic prone approach group, two patients had ineffective blocks. Additionally, in the classic approach group, two patients had a vascular puncture, and four patients had aspiration of urine during the procedure. There were no failures of the block, no urinary injury nor vascular puncture in the transdiscal approach group. Importantly, follow-up CT showed no signs of discitis, rupture, or herniation in the transdiscal group.

In contrast to fluoroscopy-guided SHPB, an anterior ultrasound-guided approach may be performed when the patient cannot lie in the prone position. Additionally, unlike the fluoroscopy or CT-guided approach, the ultrasound-guided SHPB can be performed at bedside and involves no radiation exposure. In a blinded, randomized study of fifty patients with pelvic pain secondary to advanced gynecological cancers, anterior ultrasound-guided SHPB was compared to standard WHO therapy.[49] The procedure is performed in the supine position. A 22-G Chiba needle is advanced in an out-of-plane technique and aimed towards the fifth lumbar vertebral body. Once 1–2 mm from the vertebral body, 50% ethanol and .25% bupivacaine is injected, and spread is confirmed under real-time sonography.[49] In both groups, there was a statistically significant ($p < 0.05$) decrease in the VAS scores compared to baseline, although the ultrasound group provided greater relief at one week, one month, two months, and three months.[49] Additionally, the daily morphine consumption at all time points was less in the ultrasound-guided SHPB group.[49] Interestingly, the side-effect profile was better in SHPB compared to the morphine-only group, and no significant permanent adverse effects occurred in the anterior ultrasound-guided group.

Although the SHPB is an effective block for visceral pelvic pain, it does not always cover the lower pelvic organs, perineum, or genitalia. A block of the inferior hypogastric plexus, which runs along the ventral surface of the sacrum medial to the sacral foramen bilaterally, is a viable option for more complete coverage of the lower pelvic viscera. Additionally, the risk of injuring the intestines and common iliac arteries that exists with a SHPB is eliminated with an inferior hypogastric plexus block (IHPB). Neurolysis of the inferior hypogastric plexus was performed in 20 patients with poorly controlled pelvic cancer pain on opioid and adjuvant therapies.[50] The block is performed with the patient in the prone position under fluoroscopic guidance. Once S1–S4 foramina are identified, a 25-G spinal needle is advanced through the medial bony edge of ventral sacral foramen. Optimal position is achieved when cephalad and caudad spread is seen along the presacral plane. After confirmation of position, 6–8 cc of 10% phenol is injected bilaterally. Prior to the procedure, VAS scores were 7.21 ± 1.31. Following the procedure, the patients had a significant decrease in their VAS scores ($p < 0.05$) at 24 hours, one week, two weeks, one month, and two months.[50] The most significant results occurred at one week, with a 43.8% reduction from baseline pain scores.[50] Interestingly, patients with lower pelvic or perineal pain had the most significant pain relief.[50] Mean consumption of morphine prior to the procedure was 106.67 ± 32.9 and was significantly reduced ($p < 0.05$) at all time points except two months.[50] Similarly, the maximum decrease in morphine occurred at one week, with a 40.3% reduction from baseline usage.[50] Although larger controlled studies are needed, IHPB is a good alternative for lower pelvic or perineal cancer pain.

Similar to the IHPB, a block of the ganglion impar, located in the retroperitoneum at the sacrococcygeal junction, is a viable option for perineal pain secondary to pelvic cancer. In study of 16 patients with chronic perineal pain (CPP) mostly secondary to pelvic cancer, a ganglion impar block or neurolysis was performed.[51] Using a transsacrococcygeal approach under fluoroscopic guidance, a 22-G needle was advanced just anterior to the sacrococcygeal ligament. Position was confirmed with contrast. The neurolytic block was performed using 4–6 ml of 8% phenol. The average time of the procedure for the neurolytic block was 5.7 ± 1.11 minutes.[51] Approximately 12 minutes after the procedure, all patients had >50% reduction in their VAS scores from baseline.[51] Additionally, all patients maintained a clinically and statistically significant decrease in their pain scores throughout the two months' study.[51] There were no clinically significant complications of the procedure. In similar case series of three patients with refractory perineal pain secondary to pelvic cancer pain, a transsacrococcygeal ganglion impar block was performed. All three patients had VAS scores >8 prior to procedure and maintained VAS scores <3 for the entire six-month follow-up after the procedure.[52] Transsacrococcygeal is a safe, quick, and effective procedure for perineal pain secondary to pelvic cancer, but larger randomized control studies are still needed.

In a subset of pelvic cancer patients who are not candidates for surgery, radiofrequency ablation of the tumor (RFA), a minimally invasive procedure causing protein coagulation and ultimately cell death, may be a promising alternative. RFA may be practically useful in patients with short life expectancy when more invasive therapies are less desirable. In a study of 12 patients with severe pelvic pain secondary to recurrent rectal cancer, RFA was attempted to improve pain control. The patients had a mean reduction of their pain by 86% at one week.[53] Furthermore, the patients maintained lower pain scores throughout the duration of the study at 22 months.[53] RFA has significant morbidity, with complications including fistulas, ureteric obstruction, and abscess formation.

Surgical Management

Neurosurgical interventions include dorsal rhizotomy, myelotomy, and cordotomy. Given their invasive nature and inherent neurological sequelae, they are generally reserved for severely resistant pain in terminally ill patients. In a group of six individuals with advanced pelvic cancer and lumbosacral plexopathies, dorsal rhizotomy was utilized to treat their refractory neuropathic pain.[54] The patients were all on maximum tolerable opioid therapy and multiple other adjuvant therapies, including antiepileptics and antidepressants.[54] Furthermore, all patients had failed neuraxial therapy with morphine combined with a local anesthestic.[54] When compared to their prior symptoms, all patients had significant reductions in pain scores and opioid use.[54]

Myelotomy is another modality that may be an effective palliative option for intractable cancer pain.[55] The importance of the midline of the dorsal column compared to the classic spinothalamic tract in the visceral nociception pathway is unclear and currently under debate.[56] In a case series of six patients with intractable visceral pain secondary to cancer, a punctate midline myelotomy at the thoracic level was performed with significant reduction in visceral pain and medication usage.[57] In the study, none of the patients experienced persistent motor, autonomic, or sensory dysfunction from the procedure.[57]

In contrast to myelotomy, cordotomy involves creation of a lesion in the anterolateral region of the spinal cord containing the spinothalamic tract. The spinothalamic pathway decussates within the spinal cord one to two levels above the axons' point of entry. As a result, cordotomy at a specific level will produce anesthesia one to two levels below the site of the lesion. Cordotomy may be performed percutaneously or via open surgery. The procedure is classically reserved for patients who have failed all other modalities and have a life expectancy of less than 1–2 years. The procedure has significant side effects, including respiratory failure.[58] A retrospective case review of nine patients with pelvic cancer including rectal, gynecological, and sarcoma of the ischium were treated with a cordotomy for their intractable pain. Many of the patients had motor weakness and incontinence prior to the procedure. The individuals had tried a variety of other therapies, such as opioids, NSAIDs, steroids, ketamine, transcutaneous electrical nerve stimulation, neuraxial infusions, pudendal and caudal nerve blocks, lumbar sympathectomy, and palliative radiation/chemotherapy, without adequate response. In the study, eight of the nine patients had a reduction in their median daily morphine use from 580 mg to 160 mg.[58] There were no major complications, including respiratory dysfunction, following the procedure.[58]

SUMMARY

The majority of patients with pelvic cancer will experience pain; however, many of these patients can achieve adequate relief with pharmacological therapy using the standard WHO ladder approach. In the remaining patients, neurolysis of both sympathetic and parasympathetic nervous systems provides a safe and efficacious option for relief. Furthermore, these modalities have been shown to lower opioid usage, and as a result, reduce associated side effects. Currently, there is growing evidence that interventional modalities should be considered as adjuvant therapies and not reserved for refractory pain for the terminally ill.[37] It is crucial for pain practitioners to be familiar with the many available options, in order to maximally reduce the suffering of patients with cancer.

REFERENCES

1. Jemal A, Siegel R, Ward E, Hao Y, Xu J, Thun MJ. Cancer statistics, 2009. *CA Cancer J Clin.* 2009;59:225–249.
2. Siegel R, Naishadham D, Jemal A. Cancer statistics, 2012. *CA Cancer J Clin.* 2012;62:10–29.
3. Hausheer FH, Schilsky RL, Bain S, Berghorn EJ, Lieberman F. Diagnosis, management, and evaluation of chemotherapy-induced peripheral neuropathy. *Semin Oncol.* 2006;33:15–49.
4. Lema MJ, Foley KM, Hausheer FH. Types and epidemiology of cancer-related neuropathic pain: the intersection of cancer pain and neuropathic pain. *Oncologist.* 2010;15(Suppl 2):3–8.
5. Shaheen PE, Legrand SB, Walsh D, et al. Errors in opioid prescribing: a prospective survey in cancer pain. *J Pain Symptom Manag.* 2010;39:702–711.
6. van den Beuken-van Everdingen MH, de Rijke JM, Kessels AG, Schouten HC, van Kleef M, Patijn J. Prevalence of pain in patients with cancer: a systematic review of the past 40 years. *Ann Oncol ESMO.* 2007;18:1437–1449.
7. Aukst-Margetic B, Jakovljevic M, Margetic B, Biscan M, Samija M. Religiosity, depression and pain in patients with breast cancer. *Gen Hosp Psychiatry.* 2005;27:250–255.
8. Ko HJ, Seo SJ, Youn CH, Kim HM, Chung SE. The association between pain and depression, anxiety, and cognitive function among advanced cancer patients in the hospice ward. *Kor J Fam Med.* 2013;34:347–356.
9. O'Mahony S, Goulet JL, Payne R. Psychosocial distress in patients treated for cancer pain: a prospective observational study. *J Opiod Manag.* 2010;6:211–222.
10. Kroenke K, Theobald D, Wu J, Loza JK, Carpenter JS, Tu W. The association of depression and pain with health-related quality of life, disability, and health care use in cancer patients. *J Pain Symptom Manag.* 2010;40:327–341.
11. Brown LF, Kroenke K, Theobald DE, Wu J, Tu W. The association of depression and anxiety with health-related quality of life in cancer patients with depression and/or pain. *Psycho-oncology.* 2010;19:734–741.
12. Temel JS, Greer JA, Muzikansky A, et al. Early palliative care for patients with metastatic non-small-cell lung cancer. *N Engl J Med.* 2010;363: 733–742.
13. Marcus DA. Epidemiology of cancer pain. *Curr Pain Headache Rep.* 2011;15:231–234.
14. Jacox A, Carr DB, Payne R. New clinical-practice guidelines for the management of pain in patients with cancer. *N Engl J Med.* 1994;330:651–655.
15. Garcia C, Wendt J, Lyon L, et al. Risk management options elected by women after testing positive for a BRCA mutation. *Gynecol Oncol.* 2014;132: 428–433.
16. Sasco AJ, Secretan MB, Straif K. Tobacco smoking and cancer: a brief review of recent epidemiological evidence. *Lung Cancer.* 2004;45 Suppl 2:S3–S9.
17. Eifel PJ, Jhingran A, Bodurka DC, Levenback C, Thames H. Correlation of smoking history and other patient characteristics with major complications of pelvic radiation therapy for cervical cancer. *J Clin Oncol.* 2002;20:3651–3657.
18. Pristauz G, Winter R, Fischerauer E, et al. Can routine gynecologic examination contribute to the diagnosis of cervical involvement by primary endometrial cancer? *Eur J Gynaecol Oncol.* 2009;30:497–499.
19. Oster G, Lamerato L, Glass AG, et al. Natural history of skeletal-related events in patients with breast, lung, or prostate cancer and metastases to bone: a 15-year study in two large US health systems. *Support Care Cancer.* 2013;21:3279–3286.
20. Bunker CH, Patrick AL, Konety BR, et al. High prevalence of screening-detected prostate cancer among Afro-Caribbeans: the Tobago Prostate Cancer Survey. *Cancer Epidemiol Biomark Prev.* 2002;11:726–729.
21. Ripamonti CI, Brunelli C. Comparison between numerical rating scale and six-level verbal rating scale in cancer patients with pain: a preliminary report. *Support Care Cancer.* 2009;17:1433–1434.
22. Hollen PJ, Gralla RJ, Kris MG, McCoy S, Donaldson GW, Moinpour CM. A comparison of visual analogue and numerical rating scale formats for the Lung Cancer Symptom Scale (LCSS): does format affect patient ratings of symptoms and quality of life? *Qual Life Res.* 2005;14:837–847.
23. Bossert EA, Van Cleve L, Savedra MC. Children with cancer: the pain experience away from the health care setting. *J Pediatr Oncol Nursing.* 1996;13:109–120.
24. da Silva FC, Santos Thuler LC, de Leon-Casasola OA. Validity and reliability of two pain assessment tools in Brazilian children and adolescents. *J Clin Nursing.* 2011;20:1842–1848.
25. Lussier D, Huskey AG, Portenoy RK. Adjuvant analgesics in cancer pain management. *Oncologist.* 2004;9:571–591.
26. Jongen JL, Huijsman ML, Jessurun J, et al. The evidence for pharmacologic treatment of neuropathic cancer pain: beneficial and adverse effects. *J Pain Symptom Manag.* 2013;46:581–590 e1.
27. Saarto T, Wiffen PJ. Antidepressants for neuropathic pain. *Cochrane Database Syst Rev.* 2007:CD005454.
28. Auchus RJ, Yu MK, Nguyen S, Mundlec SD. Second-line treatment of metastatic prostate cancer. Prednisone and radiotherapy for symptom relief. *Prescrire Int.* 2013;22:74–78.

29. Lluch A, Cueva J, Ruiz-Borrego M, Ponce J, Perez-Fidalgo JA. Zoledronic acid in the treatment of metastatic breast cancer. *Anti-Cancer Drugs*. 2014; 25:1–7.

30. Tolia M, Zygogianni A, Kouvaris JR, et al. The key role of bisphosphonates in the supportive care of cancer patients. *Anticancer Res*. 2014;34:23–37.

31. Khojainova N, Santiago-Palma J, Kornick C, Breitbart W, Gonzales GR. Olanzapine in the management of cancer pain. *J Pain Symptom Manag*. 2002;23:346–350.

32. Parsons CG. NMDA receptors as targets for drug action in neuropathic pain. *Eur J Pharmacol*. 2001; 429:71–78.

33. Grande LA, O'Donnell BR, Fitzgibbon DR, Terman GW. Ultra-low dose ketamine and memantine treatment for pain in an opioid-tolerant oncology patient. *Anesth Analg*. 2008;107:1380–1383.

34. Sheinfeld Gorin S, Krebs P, Badr H, et al. Meta-analysis of psychosocial interventions to reduce pain in patients with cancer. *J Clin Oncol*. 2012;30:539–547.

35. Syrjala KL, Jensen MP, Mendoza ME, Yi JC, Fisher HM, Keefe FJ. Psychological and behavioral approaches to cancer pain management. *J Clin Oncol*. 2014;32:1703–1711.

36. Birthi P, Sloan P. Interventional treatment of refractory cancer pain. *Cancer J*. 2013;19:390–396.

37. Bhatnagar S, Khanna S, Roshni S, et al. Early ultrasound-guided neurolysis for pain management in gastrointestinal and pelvic malignancies: an observational study in a tertiary care center of urban India. *Pain Pract*. 2012;12:23–32.

38. Smith TJ, Staats PS, Deer T, et al. Randomized clinical trial of an implantable drug delivery system compared with comprehensive medical management for refractory cancer pain: impact on pain, drug-related toxicity, and survival. *J Clin Oncol*. 2002;20:4040–4049.

39. van Dongen RT, Crul BJ, van Egmond J. Intrathecal coadministration of bupivacaine diminishes morphine dose progression during long-term intrathecal infusion in cancer patients. *Clin J Pain*. 1999;15: 166–172.

40. Mercadante S, Intravaia G, Villari P, et al. Intrathecal treatment in cancer patients unresponsive to multiple trials of systemic opioids. *Clin J Pain*. 2007;23:793–798.

41. Tay W, Ho KY. The role of interventional therapies in cancer pain management. *Ann Acad Med Singapore*. 2009;38:989–997.

42. Newsome S, Frawley BK, Argoff CE. Intrathecal analgesia for refractory cancer pain. *Curr Pain Headache Rep*. 2008;12:249–256.

43. Staats PS, Yearwood T, Charapata SG, et al. Intrathecal ziconotide in the treatment of refractory pain in patients with cancer or AIDS: a randomized controlled trial. *JAMA*. 2004;291: 63–70.

44. Walker SM, Goudas LC, Cousins MJ, Carr DB. Combination spinal analgesic chemotherapy: a systematic review. *Anesth Analg*. 2002;95: 674–715.

45. Taguchi H, Shingu K, Okuda H, Matsumoto H. Analgesia for pelvic and perineal cancer pain by intrathecal steroid injection. *Acta Anaesthesiol Scandinav*. 2002;46:190–193.

46. Slatkin NE, Rhiner M. Phenol saddle blocks for intractable pain at end of life: report of four cases and literature review. *Am J Hospice Palliat Care*. 2003;20:62–66.

47. Plancarte R, Amescua C, Patt RB, Aldrete JA. Superior hypogastric plexus block for pelvic cancer pain. *Anesthesiology*. 1990;73:236–239.

48. Gamal G, Helaly M, Labib YM. Superior hypogastric block: transdiscal versus classic posterior approach in pelvic cancer pain. *Clin J Pain*. 2006;22:544–547.

49. Mishra S, Bhatnagar S, Rana SP, Khurana D, Thulkar S. Efficacy of the anterior ultrasound-guided superior hypogastric plexus neurolysis in pelvic cancer pain in advanced gynecological cancer patients. *Pain Med*. 2013;14:837–842.

50. Mohamed SA, Ahmed DG, Mohamad MF. Chemical neurolysis of the inferior hypogastric plexus for the treatment of cancer-related pelvic and perineal pain. *Pain Res Manag Canada*. 2013;18:249–252.

51. Toshniwal GR, Dureja GP, Prashanth SM. Transsacrococcygeal approach to ganglion impar block for management of chronic perineal pain: a prospective observational study. *Pain Physician*. 2007;10:661–666.

52. Eker HE, Cok OY, Kocum A, Acil M, Turkoz A. Transsacrococcygeal approach to ganglion impar for pelvic cancer pain: a report of 3 cases. *Region Anesth Pain Med*. 2008;33:381–382.

53. Pusceddu C, Sotgia B, Melis L, Fele RM, Meloni GB. Painful pelvic recurrence of rectal cancer: percutaneous radiofrequency ablation treatment. *Abdomin Imag*. 2013;38:1225–1233.

54. Son BC, Yoon JH, Kim DR, Lee SW. Dorsal rhizotomy for pain from neoplastic lumbosacral plexopathy in advanced pelvic cancer. *Stereotact Funct Neurosurg*. 2014;92:109–116.

55. Viswanathan A, Burton AW, Rekito A, McCutcheon IE. Commissural myelotomy in the treatment of intractable visceral pain: technique and outcomes. *Stereotact Funct Neurosurg*. 2010;88:374–382.

56. Hong D, Andren-Sandberg A. Punctate midline myelotomy: a minimally invasive procedure for the treatment of pain in inextirpable abdominal and pelvic cancer. *J Pain Symptom Manag*. 2007;33: 99–109.

57. Nauta HJ, Soukup VM, Fabian RH, et al. Punctate midline myelotomy for the relief of visceral cancer pain. *J Neurosurg*. 2000;92:125–130.

58. Jones B, Finlay I, Ray A, Simpson B. Is there still a role for open cordotomy in cancer pain management? *J Pain Symptom Manag*. 2003;25:179–184.

15

Surgical Treatment of Pelvic Pain

ADAM R. DUKE AND KAREN WANG

Chronic pelvic pain (CPP) is defined as non-menstrual pelvic pain of at least six months' duration that is severe enough to cause functional disability or require treatment (Howard, 1993). In the United States, CPP is a commonly encountered problem and may affect up to one in seven women (Mathias, Kuppermann, Liberman, Lipschutz, & Steege, 1996). In primary care offices, 39% of women complain of pelvic pain (Jamieson, Steege, 1996) and CPP accounts for 10% of all referrals to a gynecologist (Mathias et al., 1996). Direct healthcare expenditure related to CPP is estimated at $880 million annually, while direct and indirect costs are estimated at more than $2 billion annually (Mathias et al., 1996).

A multitude of causes have been implicated in the development of CPP, and many—including irritable bowel syndrome, interstitial cystitis/painful bladder syndrome, and physical and/or sexual abuse—have little or nothing to do with the "gynecological organs." Indeed, one such study found that gynecological conditions may account for only 20% of chronic pelvic pain (Zondervan et al., 1999). Studies have demonstrated that there is also significant cross-over of causes, with multiple etiologies often present in the same patient (Zondervan et al., 2001). This can complicate both diagnosis and treatment options.

Despite the multitude of non-gynecological symptoms that can contribute to CPP, the gynecologist often feels compelled to intervene, and both evaluation and treatment of pelvic pain account for a significant number of surgeries. A 2006 study revealed that in the United States, approximately 130,000 women annually undergo outpatient laparoscopy for work-up of their pelvic pain (Tu & Beaumont, 2006), and other studies estimate that CPP may account for 40% of all gynecological laparoscopies performed in the

United States (Howard, 1993). Of the 600,000 hysterectomies performed annually in America, approximately 12% cite pelvic pain as the primary indication for surgery (Howard, 1993). It is thus imperative to understand the role of surgery in the treatment of chronic pelvic pain.

PRE-SURGICAL EVALUATION

As many non-gynecological causes can contribute to the development of CPP, it is critical that a thorough history and physical be performed. The history is especially important because, in addition to helping identify the source of pain, it can help establish rapport and trust between patient and provider (Howard, 2003). The history should also identify the location of pain, its onset and duration, timing of symptoms, and pain severity and quality. The practitioner should also not hesitate to inquire about any history of emotional, physical, and sexual abuse, as these types of trauma can manifest in CPP. A pelvic pain intake questionnaire, available free of charge from the International Pelvic Pain Society, can aid in the history-taking. Additional useful resources include the McGill Present Pain Index and a pain Visual Analog Score.

A thorough physical exam is also essential in the pre-operative evaluation. A systematic approach should be used to attempt to duplicate the patient's symptoms, both in location and in severity. This may involve examining the patient in multiple positions: standing, supine, sitting, etc. Surgical scars should be noted and palpated. A vaginal exam should include palpation of the pelvic floor muscles to note any tenderness or muscle spasm. The external genitalia should also be examined with a Q-tip and pin to note the presence of allodynia or hyperalgesia. During the examination, the surgeon should be speaking with the patient and asking frequent questions about the location and severity of pain. Non-visual clues such as "guarding" are also important to note during the examination (Howard, 2003).

Pelvic pain specialists have long advocated a multidisciplinary "team" approach to the diagnosis and treatment of CPP, and studies confirm the utility of this approach (Hooker et al., 2013; Peters et al., 1991). This team of providers includes pelvic floor physical therapists, psychiatrists, and counsellors. Despite these recommendations, however, it is estimated that 90% of women with chronic pelvic pain have already had some type of unsuccessful surgery for their pain prior to the utilization of a multidisciplinary approach (Lamvu et al., 2006). It is essential that, prior to performing surgery for pelvic pain, the surgeon ask two questions: (1) "Am I truly qualified to provide the most effective surgery my patient needs?" and (2) "Will surgery benefit the patient?" If the answer to either of these questions is no, then surgery should be postponed, as it is likely to do more harm than good. At that time, the patient should be reevaluated with a multidisciplinary approach in mind, and most probably referred to a physician with expertise in chronic pelvic pain.

APPROACH TO TREATMENT

Controversy remains as to whether pelvic pain is a symptom or a disease. Some experts even propose that, after six months, pain itself becomes the disease, not just a symptom, though the pathogenesis of this transformation remains unclear (Howard, 2003). Therefore, treatment can focus on either the symptom or the disease, though these two treatment pathways need not be mutually exclusive. It is also important that both the practitioner and the patient understand that, unlike acute pain, a "cure" for chronic pelvic pain is often not achieved; rather, the focus should be on minimizing symptoms and allowing the patient to lead as close to a "normal" life as possible.

Prior to performing surgery, all attempts should be made to maximize medical therapy for at least 6–12 months. Mainstays of medical therapy include analgesics and antidepressants, but therapy should also target specific conditions such as interstitial cystitis, irritable bowel syndrome, or endometriosis, if such conditions can be identified. If medical treatment is not effective or the practitioner believes surgery will aid medical therapy, then procedures such as hysterectomy, lysis of adhesions, and neuroablative and neural release/decompression procedures can be performed.

Hysterectomy

Hysterectomy remains one of the mainstays of surgical treatment for CPP, despite controversy about its effectiveness. Certainly, if an identifiable uterine pathology such as fibroids or adenomyosis can be confidently diagnosed pre-operatively, then hysterectomy can provide relief. However, as discussed, the etiologies of CPP are often complex and rarely act alone, so it must again be stressed that, prior to proceeding with hysterectomy, a thorough evaluation should be performed to rule out concomitant causes of pain.

In patients without an identifiable uterine pathology contributing to pain, the role of hysterectomy is controversial, and only relatively recently an area of study. The first major study to assess outcomes of hysterectomy on CPP was performed in 1990 by Stovall and colleagues. Ninety-nine women underwent hysterectomy for pain that was presumed to be related to the uterus; the assumption was that the majority of women would improve with uterine removal. Long-term follow-up (15–64 months; mean, 21.6 months) demonstrated that, although the vast majority of patients experienced relief, 22% still complained of pelvic pain. This was a larger-than-expected number, especially when compared to pain improvement rates in other studies examining hysterectomy outcomes in the general population (as opposed to just those patients with pelvic pain) (Stovall, Ling, & Crawford, 1990). A 1995 study by Hillis and colleagues mirrored Stovall's findings. A total of 308 women with pelvic pain for at least six months underwent hysterectomy. At the one-year follow-up, the majority experienced relief of pain, but 21% reported continued but decreased pain, and 5% reported unchanged or *increased* pain. Alarmingly, in unadjusted analyses, women under the age of 30 were at increased risk for continued pain, while in adjusted analyses, an increased probability of persistent pain was observed in women who had no identified pelvic pathology (Hillis, Marchbanks, & Peterson, 1995).

These two studies demonstrated that a majority—about 75%—of patients would experience relief of pain with hysterectomy. A large number of patients, however, would continue to suffer. It has also been pointed out that both studies have major limitations, probably because they were performed before an understanding of the multidisciplinary approach to treatment of pelvic pain had been established. Lamvu comments that both studies suffered from a small cohort of patients, and neither had a pain-free comparison group (Lamvu, 2011). More important is that these studies did not take into account confounding variables that may contribute to pain after surgery—notably, depression, anxiety, and history of abuse. The influence of these confounders cannot be underestimated; indeed, a 2004 study of 1,249 women with pain and/or depression demonstrated that, 24 months after hysterectomy for CPP, only 9.3% of women with pain only had continued symptoms, while 19.4% of women with pain and depression continued to be symptomatic. When compared to the women who had neither pain nor depression, women with pain and depression were three to five times more likely to continue to suffer from dyspareunia, pain, and impaired quality of life (Hartmann et al., 2004).

Hillis and colleagues' finding that 5% of women experienced an unchanged or increased amount of pain is an area of concern. It is well known that certain surgeries such as thoracotomy, amputation, and mastectomy with axillary lymph node dissection are associated with a risk of developing chronic post-surgical pain (Schnabel & Pogatzki-Zahn, 2010). Despite the vast number of hysterectomies performed annually, research is still ongoing as to whether surgery itself can lead to the development of pain. A questionnaire based study of 1,135 women examined pain characteristics both before and one year after hysterectomy and found that 32% of women had chronic postoperative pain (Brandsborg, 2012). Risk factors for post-operative pain were identified, including pre-operative pelvic pain, prior cesarean delivery, pain as main indication for surgery, and a history of pain problems elsewhere in the body. Worryingly, of the women reporting chronic post-operative pain, 14.9% had no pain pre-operatively, indicating that hysterectomy itself may play a role in the development of chronic pelvic pain (Brandsborg, 2012). Based on these findings, the same authors performed a prospective study of 90 women undergoing hysterectomy for benign reasons. They noted that, at four months, 15 (16.7%) continued to

have CPP. In 11 women, the pain mimicked their pre-operative pain, and in the other four, pain was probably related to post-surgical discomfort. Their conclusion was that persistent pain after hysterectomy is most often related to pre-operative factors, and that the relative contribution of surgery to the development of pain is probably small (Brandsborg, Dueholm, Nikolajsen, Kehlet, & Jensen, 2009). However, given the staggering 14.9% of women who developed pelvic pain after hysterectomy (as reported in an earlier paper by the same authors), more investigation is needed. Stovall and colleagues' conclusion to their 1990 paper thus seemed prophetic: "Physicians must be vigilant in monitoring long-term outcomes in patients undergoing hysterectomy for chronic pelvic pain so that the appropriate role for this operation can be found" (Stovall et al., 1990).

Bilateral oophorectomy for treatment of pelvic pain is even more controversial. Certain experts advocate the removal of ovaries at time of surgery for pelvic pain, especially if there is a strong family history of breast and ovarian cancer or if endometriosis is present, as it is well established that endometriosis is hormonally responsive (Martin & Ling, 1999). However, in the case of deep infiltrating endometriosis, especially that affecting the uterosacral ligaments or the rectovaginal septum, patients may continue to experience pain and dyspareunia despite estrogen reduction (Redwine, 1994; Te Linde & Scott, 1950). Moreover, increasing evidence is demonstrating an increased risk of death in women who have undergone bilateral oophorectomy (Grover, Kuppermann, Kahn, & Washington, 1996; Rocca, Grossardt, de Andrade, Malkasian, & Melton, 2006). As there is no clear evidence that bilateral oophorectomy improves pelvic pain, and the risks may outweigh the benefits, the decision to remove the ovaries should be left up to the surgeon after discussion with the patient.

Presacral Neurectomy

Presacral neurectomy is indicated in the treatment of severe and disabling midline pain secondary to endometriosis, or pain associated with chronic pelvic inflammatory disease (Polan & DeCherney, 1980). First performed in 1899, the procedure has been well studied, and multiple trials have shown relatively good pain improvement rates—up to 85% in some cases (Black, 1955; Ingersoll & Meigs, 1948; Tjaden, Schlaff,

Kimball, & Rock, 1990). Additionally, there is a relatively low complication rate to the procedure.

The term "presacral nerve" is a misnomer; what is being removed is actually a plexus of nerves known as the "superior hypogastric plexus." Moreover, it is actually pre-lumbar, not pre-sacral. The superior hypogastric plexus is a direct extension of the aortic plexus and courses out beneath the bifurcation of the aorta. From here, it runs over the sacral promontory to become the middle and lower hypogastric plexus, before eventually anastomosing with the pelvic plexus. Afferent fibers accompanying the sympathetic nerves transmit pain from the cervix, uterine corpus, and proximal fallopian tubes. A successful—and complication-free—procedure requires intimate understanding of the anatomy of the interiliac triangle. The interiliac triangle is bordered laterally by the common iliac artery and ureter on the right and the common iliac vein on the left. The triangle is defined cephalad by the bifurcation of the aorta. Running through the center of the pre lumbar space are the inferior mesenteric, superior hemorrhoidal, and midsacral arteries. Further complicating the procedure is that the rectosigmoid and mesocolon often lie over the area of dissection. These structures typically cover the left ureter and can impair general visualization. It is often necessary to suture the mesocolon to the sidewall to deviate it away from the area of dissection.

Once visualization has been established and major arteries are identified, the peritoneum over the pre-lumbar space is incised vertically. The opening is extended to the aortic bifurcation superiorly and the sacral promontory inferiorly. The retroperitoneal fatty tissue is removed, and the nerve plexus is visualized. The plexus is grasped with atraumatic forceps, and blunt and sharp dissection are used to coagulate and excise the nerves. It is important that all nerves within the interiliac triangle are removed; in some patients, this may be an 8–10-cm-long plexus of nerves. Bleeding is not usually brisk, but it is important to meticulously coagulate any oozing in this area. The peritoneum is then closed with a running absorbable suture.

Presacral neurectomy may be performed open but has been performed recently laparoscopically with excellent results. One of the earliest randomized trials of patients with endometriosis and midline pelvic pain found 15/17 patients undergoing open presacral neurectomy to be pain-free

at 42 months, compared to none of the nine patients undergoing surgical excision of endometriosis only (Tjaden et al., 1990). A 25-year retrospective study of nearly 10,000 patients estimated a nearly 80% success rate of open presacral neurectomy. In 1992, one of the earliest papers addressing laparoscopic presacral neurectomy was published by Nezhat and colleagues. Fifty-two patients had laparoscopic presacral neurectomy, and of these, 49 (94%) reported improvement in pain, with 27 (51.2%) reporting complete resolution of pain. Notably, all patients were discharged home within 24 hours, and there were no major complications (Nezhat, 1992). Subsequent papers have found similar results with the laparoscopic technique (Chen, Chang, Chu, & Soong, 1996; Zullo et al., 2003)

Major complications with presacral neurectomy are fortunately rare (Cotte, 1949). The most important to consider are major vascular injuries, as the interiliac triangle is bordered by the aorta and common iliac arteries and veins. If the procedure is performed laparoscopically and one of the structures is damaged, immediate laparotomy is necessary. Troublesome bleeding can be encountered if the middle sacral vessels are damaged, as they lie under the hypogastric plexus and just above the periosteum of the sacral promontory. These can usually be coagulated or ligated to provide hemostasis.

Additional complications include ureteral injury, urinary difficulties, and defecatory dysfunction. Cotte noted only one ureteral injury in a review of 1,500 patients (Cotte, 1949). Constipation has been observed in 3–4% of patients and in most cases can be successfully treated with medical therapy (Lee, Stone, Magelssen, Belts, & Benson, 1986; Zullo et al., 2003). Urinary retention with need for catheterization was reported in 50% of patients in one study, though this had resolved in all patients by post-op day 7 (Ingersoll & Meigs, 1948). In a review of 50 patients, one patient had a long-term complication of urinary urgency and had lost the sensation of a full bladder (Lee et al., 1986). Other studies demonstrate a very low rate of urinary urgency. It is unclear whether this urgency is responsive to anticholinergic medications.

Uterosacral Nerve Transection and Ablation

Relief of pelvic pain and dysmenorrhea by uterosacral nerve transection was first described by Doyle in 1963. Performed transvaginally, the technique treated dysmenorrhea with 85–90% efficacy (Doyle, 1955). However, due to technical aspects, it was not a particularly popular procedure until the more recent advent of laparoscopy. Laparoscopic uterosacral nerve ablation—or LUNA as it's popularly called—involves the destruction of afferent pain fibers exiting the uterus and coursing through the uterosacral ligaments. Typically a 2–3 cm portion of nerve is destroyed. LUNA is technically less difficult than presacral neurectomy, and complication rates are extremely low, though there have been reports of ureteral transection and prolapse (Check, 2011).

Anecdotal evidence from experienced surgeons demonstrated potential for the technique, and, indeed, an early review of two small randomized studies concluded that there was "some evidence" of the effectiveness of LUNA when compared to controls (Proctor, Latthe, Farquhar, Khan, & Johnson, 2005). However, it has been demonstrated that the effect of LUNA is short-lived, with the relief of symptoms rapidly diminishing over a few years, possibly due to regrowth of uterine nerves (Chen et al., 1996). Two large, randomized prospective studies comparing LUNA to laparoscopy alone have unfortunately failed to demonstrate a benefit to the procedure. In both trials, LUNA failed to decrease either the severity or the frequency of dysmenorrhea and pelvic pain, and quality of life was not improved. In addition, time to recurrence of pain was similar in both groups (Daniels et al., 2009; Vercellini et al., 2003). Thus, LUNA should not be used as an adjunct treatment in the management of pelvic pain.

Adhesiolysis

Meta-analysis demonstrates the clear role of adhesions in intestinal obstruction and infertility (ten Broek et al., 2013). However, their role in the development of chronic pelvic pain is unknown. Thus lysis of adhesions—like hysterectomy—remains a controversial part of the surgical treatment plan for chronic pelvic pain. The notion of adhesions as a causative factor in CPP stems from an early study demonstrating a higher incidence of adhesions at time of laparoscopy in women with pelvic pain compared to those without pain (25% vs. 17%, respectively) (Howard, 1993). Additional observational studies as well as conscious pain-mapping also suggested an association between

adhesions and pain (Howard, El-Minawi, & Sanchez, 2000; Steege & Stout, 1991; Sutton & MacDonald, 1990).

Unfortunately, at this writing, only two randomized prospective studies exist that explore the role of adhesiolysis in the management of pelvic pain. In the first, 48 women with pelvic pain were randomized to adhesiolysis or expectant management. At nine months to one year, there was no difference between the groups with regard to pain—both groups reported about a 50% improvement (Peters, Trimbos-Kemper, Admiraal, Trimbos, & Hermans, 1992). An additional study randomized 100 patients to laparoscopic adhesiolysis vs. diagnostic laparoscopy alone. Both groups reported improvement in pain and quality of life but there was no significant difference in improvement rates between the two cohorts (Swank et al., 2003). Both of these studies recommended abandoning adhesiolysis in the treatment of pelvic pain. However, criticism of the second paper noted that there was insufficient statistical power to reject the null hypothesis that adhesiolysis was beneficial and that an "erroneous conclusion" had been reached (Roman, Hulsey, Marpeau, & Hulsey, 2009).

A very recent double-blind RCT compared laparoscopic adhesiolysis to laparoscopy alone. At six months, an improvement in Visual Analogue Scale (VAS) scores was noted in the adhesiolysis group compared to control. However, this study was abandoned before recruitment had reached the statistically powered sample size, due to difficulty with enrollment and lack of continued funding (Cheong et al., 2014). Though most experts agree that adhesiolysis probably does not add a surgical benefit to the patient with CPP, there may be insufficient data to justify abandoning the procedure all together. In the hands of the experienced surgeon, it may be of some benefit. Clearly, additional study of the topic is needed.

Pudendal Nerve Decompression

Recent controversy surrounding the use of synthetic mesh in pelvic organ prolapse surgery has brought much attention to the role of pudendal neuralgia in the development of chronic pelvic pain. Other than surgery, multiple causes have been implicated in the etiology of pudendal neuralgia, including viral infection, autoimmune disease, and mechanical trauma (such as long-distance cycling) (Campbell & Meyer, 2006). "Entrapment" of the nerve may also occur as a result of pelvic floor muscle spasm, and pressure from surrounding sacrospinous and sacrotu-berous ligaments (Hibner, Desai, Robertson, & Nour, 2010).

In general, the incidence of nerve injury following pelvic surgery is about 2%, though most of these injuries are due to retractors or patient positioning, not actual surgical trauma (Cardosi, Cox, & Hoffman, 2002). One study, of 183 patients who had uterosacral suspension—often the most utilized surgery for apical prolapse—estimated the development of neu-ropathic pain in the S2–S4 distribution at 3.8% (Flynn, Weidner, & Amundsen, 2006). The best treatment is often prevention, and, indeed, any patient complaining of new-onset neuropathic pain—burning, itching, stabbing—in the vulva, buttocks, or posterior leg after prolapse sur-gery should be immediately taken back to the operating room for release of the compressing suture or mesh. In patients in whom symptoms of pudendal nerve compression are not imme-diately recognized or the patient's initial com-plaints are minimized or ignored by the surgeon as being part of normal post-operative pain, there is risk of permanent damage.

Criteria have been proposed (Nantes criteria) to identify true pudendal neuralgia by pudendal nerve entrapment. The five essential diagnostic criteria are:

1. Pain in the anatomical territory of the pudendal nerve
2. Worsened by sitting
3. The patient is not woken at night by the pain
4. No objective sensory loss on clinical examination
5. Positive anesthetic pudendal nerve block (Labat et al., 2008)

Patients meeting these requirements are gener-ally first treated conservatively with pelvic floor physical therapy, gabapentin, narcotics, and pudendal nerve blocks. Conservative treatment is preferred because the technical aspects of pudendal nerve decompression can be beyond the surgical skill level of most gynecologists, and also because there is less chance of complication with conservative therapy. Most experts agree a reasonable timeframe should be given to see improvements with conservative therapy, typi-cally 12–16 weeks.

In the event that conservative therapy is unsuc-cessful, surgical decompression of the pudendal nerve becomes necessary. This involves a keen understanding of the anatomy of the pudendal nerve distribution. The pudendal nerve arises from the second, third, and fourth sacral nerve roots, then exits the pelvis through the greater sciatic foramen. The nerve then reenters the pelvis via the lesser sciatic foramen and enters Alcock's canal, which is a fascial sheath on the medial aspect of the obturator internus muscle. From here, the nerve passes behind the lateral part of the sacro-spinous ligament and posterior to the ischial spine. As the ischial spine is also the attachment for the arcus tendineus fascia pelvis, it is here that the nerve is at risk of injury or entrapment during pel-vic reconstructive procedures such as sacrospinous fixation.

The first of the two decompression meth-ods is a transgluteal approach first described by Robert (Robert, Labat, Riant, Khalfallah, & Hamel, 2007). An incision is made across the gluteal region over the area of the sacrotuberous ligament. The gluteal muscle is then separated with gentle dissection until the sacrotuberous ligament is encountered. The ligament is tran-sected, and the pudendal nerve is then identi-fied underneath. The pudendal nerve is then decompressed along its entire length, from the piriformis muscle to Alcock's canal. In the event that mesh from a previous surgery is dis-covered in this area, then this is also resected. Dr. Michael Hibner and colleagues advocate placing a segment of Neuragen (Origin Biomed, Inc.; Halifax, Nova Scotia, Canada), a nerve-protecting tubing made of a collagen matrix, to prevent re-scarring of the nerve and help in the healing process (Hibner et al., 2010).

The second type of decompression method involves a laparoscopic approach described by Nieves. The space of Retzius is entered by mak-ing a trans-peritoneal incision 2–3 cm above the bladder reflection; identification of loose areolar tissue confirms the correct entry point. Once the space of Retzius is entered, the loose areolar tissue is dissected away bluntly, allow-ing development of the retropubic space. Here, Cooper's ligament is identified; great care must be taken to identify a possible aberrant obtu-rator vein, which may be present in as many as 70% of patients. Dissection continues later-ally until the obturator neurovascular bundle is identified. This complex must be completely identified and respected, as injury here can be life-threatening. Posterior dissection is con-tinued until the arcus tendineus fascia pelvis and its attachment to the ischial spine are identified. Here, the pudendal nerve may be visualized, and any surrounding scar tissue is resected. If mesh is present, it is grasped at its insertion into the sacrospinous ligament and resected to free the attachment. If a significant amount of fibrotic tissue is present that may be contributing to entrapment of the pudendal nerve, then portions of the sacrospinous ligament can be resected here until the pudendal nerve is completely free of scarring.

Additional approaches such as the perianal and trans-ischiorectal (Bautrant et al., 2003) have been described, but the aforementioned techniques are those most commonly used. Advocates for both techniques insist their approach is the best, and there is unfortunately a paucity of data regarding outcomes. The first RCT of its kind was performed by Robert using the trans-gluteal approach. Thirty-two patients were assigned to surgical decompression vs. conservative therapy (16 in each arm). At three months, a significantly higher proportion of the surgical group was improved (50% of the surgery group reported improvement in pain at 3 months versus 6.2% of the non-surgery group). Additionally, no complications were reported in the surgical group. At 12 months, 71.4% of the surgery group, compared with 13.3% of the non-surgery group, were improved (Robert et al., 2005). A retrospective Turkish study analyzed 27 patients who underwent pudendal nerve decompression using the laparoscopic approach. In patients followed for more than six months, reduction in VAS score of >80% was achieved in 13 of the 16 patients (81.2%). Additionally, no complications were encountered (Erdogru, Avci, & Akand, 2014).

Surgical decompression of the pudendal nerve requires an intimate understanding of the anatomy as well as a high level of surgical skill. Because of this, there are very few centers worldwide that can offer this modality, and these tend to be highly specialized pelvic pain centers. Until the technique becomes more common and more outcomes-based prospective trials are performed, this technique should only be attempted by specially trained surgeons. Referral to these surgeons is appropriate for the patient requiring pudendal nerve decompression.

CONCLUSION

The more that is discovered about the complex etiology of pelvic pain, the more complicated the treatment becomes; the convoluted nature of the disease makes for convoluted data regarding outcomes. In the novel *Love in the Time of Cholera*, Gabriel García Márquez's protagonist remarks, "The scalpel is the greatest proof of the failure of medicine." I would suggest instead that surgery is an integral part of the armamentarium of available treatments and can be a highly effective one in the right hands. However, it must be stressed to patient and physician alike that are no clear-cut recommendations regarding the role of surgery in the treatment of pelvic pain. Ultimately, the practitioner must be an advocate for the patient, presenting different options, utilizing or being part of a multidisciplinary approach, and never pushing any particular treatment—especially surgery—on a patient. Beneficence—that fundamental tenet of medicine—still applies, and it is especially important when approaching pelvic pain.

REFERENCES

Bautrant E, de Bisschop E, Vaini-Elies V, et al. (2003). [Modern algorithm for treating pudendal neuralgia: 212 cases and 104 decompressions]. *J Gynecol Obstet Biol Reprod (Paris)*. 32(8 Pt 1):705–712.

Black WT, Jr. (1955). Presacral neurectomy: report of 70 cases. *South Med J*. 48(2):120–126.

Brandsborg B. (2012). Pain following hysterectomy: epidemiological and clinical aspects. *Dan Med J*. 59(1), B4374.

Brandsborg B, Dueholm M, Nikolajsen L, Kehlet H, Jensen TS. (2009). A prospective study of risk factors for pain persisting 4 months after hysterectomy. *Clin J Pain*. 25(4):263–268. doi: 10.1097/AJP.0b013e31819655ca

Campbell JN, Meyer RA. (2006). Mechanisms of neuropathic pain. *Neuron*. 52(1):77–92. doi: 10.1016/j.neuron.2006.09.021

Cardosi RJ, Cox CS, Hoffman MS. (2002). Postoperative neuropathies after major pelvic surgery. *Obstet Gynecol*. 100(2):240–244.

Check JH. (2011). Chronic pelvic pain syndromes—traditional and novel therapies: part I, surgical therapy. *Clin Exp Obstet Gynecol*. 38(1):10–13.

Chen FP, Chang SD, Chu KK, Soong YK. (1996). Comparison of laparoscopic presacral neurectomy and laparoscopic uterine nerve ablation for primary dysmenorrhea. *J Reprod Med*. 41(7):463–466.

Cheong YC, Reading I, Bailey S, Sadek K, Ledger W, Li TC. (2014). Should women with chronic pelvic pain have adhesiolysis? *BMC Women's Health*. 14(1):36. doi: 10.1186/1472-6874-14-36

Cotte G. (1949). Technique of presacral neurectomy. *Am J Surg*. 78(1):50–53.

Daniels J, Gray R, Hills RK, et al.; Collaboration LT. (2009). Laparoscopic uterosacral nerve ablation for alleviating chronic pelvic pain: a randomized controlled trial. *JAMA*. 302(9):955–961. doi: 10.1001/jama.2009.1268

Doyle JB. (1955). Paracervical uterine denervation by transection of the cervical plexus for the relief of dysmenorrhea. *Am J Obstet Gynecol*. 70(1):1–16.

Erdogru T, Avci E, Akand M. (2014). Laparoscopic pudendal nerve decompression and transposition combined with omental flap protection of the nerve (Istanbul technique): technical description and feasibility analysis. *Surg Endosc*. 28(3):925–932. doi: 10.1007/s00464-013-3248-1

Flynn MK, Weidner AC, Amundsen CL. (2006). Sensory nerve injury after uterosacral ligament suspension. *Am J Obstet Gynecol*. 195(6):1869–1872. doi: 10.1016/j.ajog.2006.06.059

Grover CM, Kuppermann M, Kahn JG, Washington AE. (1996). Concurrent hysterectomy at bilateral salpingo-oophorectomy: benefits, risks, and costs. *Obstet Gynecol*. 88(6):907–913.

Hartmann KE, Ma C, Lamvu GM, Langenberg PW, Steege JF, Kjerulff KH. (2004). Quality of life and sexual function after hysterectomy in women with preoperative pain and depression. *Obstet Gynecol*. 104(4):701–709. doi: 10.1097/01.AOG.000014068 4.37428.48

Hibner M, Desai N, Robertson LJ, Nour M. (2010). Pudendal neuralgia. *J Minim Invasive Gynecol*. 17(2):148–153. doi: 10.1016/j.jmig.2009.11.003

Hillis SD, Marchbanks PA, Peterson HB. (1995). The effectiveness of hysterectomy for chronic pelvic pain. *Obstet Gynecol*. 86(6):941–945.

Hooker AB, van Moorst BR, van Haarst EP, van Ootegehem NA, van Dijken DK, Heres MH. (2013). Chronic pelvic pain: evaluation of the epidemiology, baseline demographics, and clinical variables via a prospective and multidisciplinary approach. *Clin Exp Obstet Gynecol*. 40(4):492–498.

Howard FM. (1993). The role of laparoscopy in chronic pelvic pain: promise and pitfalls. *Obstet Gynecol Surv*. 48(6):357–387.

Howard FM. (2003). Chronic pelvic pain. *Obstet Gynecol*. 101(3):594–611.

Howard FM, El-Minawi AM, Sanchez RA. (2000). Conscious pain mapping by laparoscopy in women with chronic pelvic pain. *Obstet Gynecol*. 96(6):934–939.

Ingersoll FM, Meigs JV. (1948). Presacral neurectomy for dysmenorrhea. *N Engl J Med*. 238(11):357–360. doi: 10.1056/NEJM194803112381103

Jamieson DJ, Steege JF. (1996). The prevalence of dysmenorrhea, dyspareunia, pelvic pain, and irritable bowel syndrome in primary care practices. *Obstet Gynecol*. 87(1):55–58.

Labat JJ, Riant T, Robert R, Amarenco G, Lefaucheur JP, Rigaud J. (2008). Diagnostic criteria for pudendal neuralgia by pudendal nerve entrapment (Nantes criteria). *Neurourol Urodyn*. 27(4):306–310. doi: 10.1002/nau.20505

Lamvu G. (2011). Role of hysterectomy in the treatment of chronic pelvic pain. *Obstet Gynecol*. 117(5):1175–1178. doi: 10.1097/AOG.0b013e31821646e1

Lamvu G, Williams R, Zolnoun D, et al. (2006). Long-term outcomes after surgical and nonsurgical management of chronic pelvic pain: one year after evaluation in a pelvic pain specialty clinic. *Am J Obstet Gynecol*. 195(2):591–598; discussion 598–600. doi: 10.1016/j.ajog.2006.03.081

Lee RB, Stone K, Magelssen D, Belts RP, Benson WL. (1986). Presacral neurectomy for chronic pelvic pain. *Obstet Gynecol*. 68(4):517–521.

Martin DC, Ling FW. (1999). Endometriosis and pain. *Clin Obstet Gynecol*. 42(3):664–686.

Mathias SD, Kuppermann M, Liberman RF, Lipschutz RC, Steege JF. (1996). Chronic pelvic pain: prevalence, health-related quality of life, and economic correlates. *Obstet Gynecol*. 87(3):321–327.

Nezhat C, Nezhat F. (1992). A simplified method of laparoscopic presacral neurectomy for the treatment of central pelvic pain due to endometriosis. *Br J Obstet Gynaecol*. 99(8):659–663.

Peters AA, Trimbos-Kemper GC, Admiraal C, Trimbos JB, Hermans J. (1992). A randomized clinical trial on the benefit of adhesiolysis in patients with intraperitoneal adhesions and chronic pelvic pain. *Br J Obstet Gynaecol*. 99(1):59–62.

Peters AA, van Dorst E, Jellis B, van Zuuren E, Hermans J, Trimbos JB. (1991). A randomized clinical trial to compare two different approaches in women with chronic pelvic pain. *Obstet Gynecol*. 77(5): 740–744.

Polan ML, DeCherney A. (1980). Presacral neurectomy for pelvic pain in infertility. *Fertil Steril*. 34(6):557–560.

Proctor ML, Latthe PM, Farquhar CM, Khan KS, Johnson NP. (2005). Surgical interruption of pelvic nerve pathways for primary and secondary dysmenorrhea. *Cochrane Database Syst Rev* (4), CD001896. doi: 10.1002/14651858.CD001896.pub2

Redwine DB. (1994). Endometriosis persisting after castration: clinical characteristics and results of surgical management. *Obstet Gynecol*. 83(3):405–413.

Robert R, Labat JJ, Bensignor M, et al. (2005). Decompression and transposition of the pudendal nerve in pudendal neuralgia: a randomized controlled trial and long-term evaluation. *Eur Urol*. 47(3):403–408. doi: 10.1016/j.eururo.2004.09.003

Robert R, Labat JJ, Riant T, Khalfallah M, Hamel O. (2007). Neurosurgical treatment of perineal neuralgias. *Adv Tech Stand Neurosurg*, 32, 41–59.

Rocca WA, Grossardt BR, de Andrade M, Malkasian GD, Melton LJ 3rd. (2006). Survival patterns after oophorectomy in premenopausal women:

a population-based cohort study. *Lancet Oncol.* 7(10):821–828. doi: 10.1016/S1470-2045(06)70869-5

Roman H, Hulsey TF, Marpeau L, Hulsey TC. (2009). Why laparoscopic adhesiolysis should not be the victim of a single randomized clinical trial. *Am J Obstet Gynecol.* 200(2):136, e131–134. doi: 10.1016/j.ajog.2008.04.011

Schnabel A, Pogatzki-Zahn E. (2010). [Predictors of chronic pain following surgery. What do we know?]. *Schmerz.* 24(5):517–531; quiz 532–513. doi: 10.1007/s00482-010-0932-0

Scott RB, Te LR. (1950). External endometriosis—the scourge of the private patient. *Ann Surg.* 131(5): 697–720.

Steege JF, Stout AL. (1991). Resolution of chronic pelvic pain after laparoscopic lysis of adhesions. *Am J Obstet Gynecol.* 165(2):278–281; discussion, 281–273.

Stovall TG, Ling FW, Crawford DA. (1990). Hysterectomy for chronic pelvic pain of presumed uterine etiology. *Obstet Gynecol.* 75(4): 676–679.

Sutton C, MacDonald R. (1990). Laser laparoscopic adhesiolysis. *J Gynecol Surg.* 6(3):155–159.

Swank DJ, Swank-Bordewijk SC, Hop WC, et al. (2003). Laparoscopic adhesiolysis in patients with chronic abdominal pain: a blinded randomised controlled multi-centre trial. *Lancet.* 361(9365): 1247–1251.

ten Broek RP, Issa Y, van Santbrink EJ, et al. (2013). Burden of adhesions in abdominal and pelvic surgery: systematic review and meta-analysis. *BMJ.* 347:f5588. doi: 10.1136/bmj.f5588

Tjaden B, Schlaff WD, Kimball A, Rock JA. (1990). The efficacy of presacral neurectomy for the relief of midline dysmenorrhea. *Obstet Gynecol.* 76(1):89–91.

Tu FF, Beaumont JL. (2006). Outpatient laparoscopy for abdominal and pelvic pain in the United States, 1994 through 1996. *Am J Obstet Gynecol.* 194(3): 699–703. doi: 10.1016/j.ajog.2005.09.001

Vercellini P, Aimi G, Busacca M, Apolone G, Uglietti A, Crosignani PG. (2003). Laparoscopic uterosacral ligament resection for dysmenorrhea associated with endometriosis: results of a randomized, controlled trial. *Fertil Steril.* 80(2):310–319.

Zondervan KT, Yudkin PL, Vessey MP, Dawes MG, Barlow DH, Kennedy SH. (1999). Patterns of diagnosis and referral in women consulting for chronic pelvic pain in UK primary care. *Br J Obstet Gynaecol.* 106(11):1156–1161.

Zondervan KT, Yudkin PL, Vessey MP, et al. (2001). Chronic pelvic pain in the community—symptoms, investigations, and diagnoses. *Am J Obstet Gynecol.* 184(6):1149–1155. doi: 10.1067/mob.2001.112904

Zullo F, Palomba S, Zupi E, et al. (2003). Effectiveness of presacral neurectomy in women with severe dysmenorrhea caused by endometriosis who were treated with laparoscopic conservative surgery: a 1-year prospective randomized double-blind controlled trial. *Am J Obstet Gynecol.* 189(1):5–10.

16

Chronic Pelvic Pain and Psychological Disorders

MOHAMMED ISSA AND RAHEEL BENGALI

Chronic pelvic pain (CPP) is a prevalent, costly condition for which diagnosis and management are often difficult because of the complexities of causative factors and the multitude of involved structures. The evaluation and treatment of chronic pelvic pain have been both a clinical challenge and a source of controversy in medical literature. There continues to be little consensus in the literature about whether organic or psychological factors are primarily implicated in the etiology of chronic pelvic pain. The majority of investigators have suggested that psychological factors are primary, while a small number of studies point to organic causes. Childhood sexual abuse and adult sexual adjustment disorders have been repeatedly reported in patients with chronic pelvic pain. Other common psychosocial conditions seen in patients with chronic pelvic pain have included major depression, anxiety, somatization disorders, and chaotic family backgrounds.

The first contributions of psychological and biological factors in chronic pelvic pain were discussed in the literature by Duncan and Taylor.[1] They investigated the psychological background of 36 women with chronic pelvic pain without apparent physical cause, and reported a prominence of emotional disturbance in them. This led the investigators to suggest a psycho-pathological etiology to chronic pelvic pain.

Chronic pelvic pain has an important impact on the quality of life. Society and the scientific community, in spite of the available abundant research, still have difficulty valuing the significant role of psychological disorders in chronic pelvic pain, whether they precede, or occur as a result of, the pain. Successful intervention for one and not the other will be difficult; therefore, the pain physicians must be adept in recognizing, evaluating, and treating concurrent psychological disorders.

UNDERSTANDING THE PSYCHOLOGICAL COMPONENTS OF PELVIC PAIN

More and more models integrate psychological factors found in persistent pelvic pain with our current neurobiological understanding of pain. Symptom-related anxiety and central pain amplification have been repeatedly linked in several disorders, including endometriosis. The various mechanisms of facilitation, amplification, failure of inhibition, and difficulty disengaging from painful stimuli can influence an individual's experience of pain and result in increased distress and restriction of activities. Chronic emotional disturbances early in life might be associated with the development of chronic pelvic pain.[2] Conflicts with parents, lower interest of a father figure in the daughter's life, conflicts with regard to sexuality, and negative perceptions of menarche or puberty are greater in chronic pelvic pain patients.[3] Low self-esteem and body perceptions with poor body awareness are also commonly seen.[4]

Fear-Avoidance Model (FAM) of Chronic Pelvic Pain

Although treatment approaches directed at improving physical impairments are fundamental, increasing evidence suggests that women with chronic pelvic pain may fare better with a treatment approach that incorporates cognitive-behavioral interventions directed at decreasing certain pain-related cognitions, including pain-related fear, pain-related anxiety, and catastrophizing. These variables are the cornerstone of the fear-avoidance model (FAM), a conceptual model that theorizes how particular psychological variables may contribute to the maintenance of musculoskeletal pain.

FAM was first introduced by Lethem et al.[5] as a theoretical model to explain why some people recover from a painful injury, whereas others who exhibit certain pain-related behaviors and cognitions develop chronic pain. The initial model was based on the central idea of fear of pain and was developed to provide an understanding of how exaggerated pain perception contributes to the maintenance of chronic pain problems. FAM includes three central components that contribute to the cycle of fear and avoidance behaviors: pain-related fear, pain-related anxiety, and pain-catastrophizing. These variables are believed to lead to avoidance/escape behaviors, disuse, and disability, placing an individual at risk for reinjury, perpetuation of negative-related cognitions and behaviors, or both.

"Pain-related fear" refers to fear of the sensation of pain, fear of movement or reinjury, and fear of physical activities that are assumed to cause pain.[6] People with pain-related fear are likely to avoid activities or movements that they believe will cause pain, further exacerbating negative pain-related cognitions about these activities, disuse, and deconditioning. This results in the development of chronic pain and disability.

"Pain catastrophizing" describes how an individual responds to an actual or impending pain experience, and its presence is thought to be a risk factor for the development of chronic pain.[7] It involves the tendency to focus on the pain sensation (rumination), to exaggerate the threat of pain (magnification), and to negatively self-evaluate the ability to deal with pain (helplessness).[8] There is considerable evidence of the association between catastrophizing and pain intensity in pain conditions and disabilities; evidence has shown that overall pain sensitivity was enhanced in patients who had catastrophizing thoughts about their pain.[9]

Pain-related anxiety is the third key component in the FAM of pain. It leads to preventive behaviors, including avoidance of and hypervigilance for perceived impending pain.[10] This may result in patients' directing their attention toward the potential threat of a painful stimulus while they disengage from neutral stimuli.

PAIN-RELATED PSYCHOLOGICAL VARIABLES ASSOCIATED WITH CHRONIC PELVIC PAIN

Several recent studies have shifted the focus from the biomedical mechanisms to the psychological variables associated with chronic pelvic pain, especially how these variable may contribute to the maintenance of different types of pelvic pain. Previous studies have documented significantly high levels of affective disorders in patients with chronic pelvic pain, which also correlated significantly with hypochondriacal beliefs.[11] Other studies have examined the relationship of psychological variables to intercourse and sexual arousal. Women with vulvodynia reported more hypervigilance for pain during intercourse (dyspareunia), suggesting that increased attention to a potentially painful stimulus during intercourse may interfere with sexual arousal and diminish the experience of intercourse. Women with vulvodynia also reported increased catastrophizing thoughts regarding intercourse-related pain.[12] A recent study revealed that catastrophizing was the only variable that contributed a substantial variance to intercourse-related pain.[13] Women with vulvodynia were found to have significantly lower heat pain thresholds compared to healthy women, while pain ratings and anxiety scores were significantly higher.[14] These results suggest that women with vulvodynia may have enhanced pain sensitivity, perhaps due in part to changes in central nervous system (CNS)-mediated pain processing.

In general, women with chronic pelvic pain are more likely to have histories of depression, somatization, sexual and physical abuse, and chronic psychological distress compared with controls.[15] Studies have shown an association of 30–80% between psychological comorbidities and chronic pelvic pain.[16,17] Childhood sexual and physical abuse have also been shown to subsequently lead to somatization, anxiety, and depression. The intensity of these psychosocial sequelae appears to be correlated with the duration and severity of the abuse.[18] These patients often have a characteristic psychological pattern: a sad childhood, and lack of parental interest and affection. The patient's marital and/or sexual relationships have often been unsuccessful, with various psychosexual dysfunctions such as loss of libido, lack of orgasm, and dyspareunia. Russo et al.[19] have shown that the number of non-organic causes of pelvic pain is linearly correlated with both the number of lifetime anxiety disorders, agoraphobia, and the degree of neuroticism. Walker et al.[20] highlighted the importance of recognizing that medically unexplained physical symptoms may be a proxy for psychiatric distress.

Depression

Pain and depression can be closely linked. Both may be mediated by the same neurotransmitters, such as noradrenaline (norepinephrine), serotonin, and endorphin. They also give rise to similar behaviors, such as behavioral and social withdrawal with limited interaction. Depression was found to predate the symptom of pain in 75% of cases.[21] Nolan et al.[22] found that 72% of patients with pelvic pain reported sleep disorders, and 51% were clinically depressed. Slocumb et al.[23] found gynecological patients with pelvic pain to be more anxious, depressed, hostile, and have more somatic symptoms than controls. Although there appears to be an association between chronic pelvic pain and depression, in many cases it is still unclear whether the depressive symptoms precede the development of pain or result from it.

Anxiety

Pain intensity positively correlates with anxiety severity. Up to 87.5% of patients with chronic pelvic pain have associated anxiety.[24] "Anxiety" may refer to fears of missed pathology as the cause of pain (like cancer) and/or to uncertainties about treatment options and prognosis. Asking about what the patient believes or fears is the cause of their pain may be more suitable in assessing their anxiety in the context of chronic pelvic pain than using a general anxiety questionnaire.[25]

Somatization Disorders

Patients with multiple physical complaints that are out of proportion to an organic cause of pain and cannot be fully explained by a known general medical condition may be given the diagnosis of "somatization disorder." Up to 70% of women with chronic pelvic pain may have a coexisting somatization disorder. Patients with chronic pelvic pain have an increased incidence of upper abdominal pain, diarrhea, constipation, low back pain, dyspareunia, dysmenorrhea, nausea, bloating, breathlessness, dizziness, weakness, and menstrual irregularity.[26] There is also an association between somatization and a history of sexual trauma in women with non-somatic pelvic pain.[27] Chronic somatic complaints, including gynecological problems, have also been linked to a personal and/or family history of alcohol abuse.

Physical and Sexual Abuse

Childhood physical and sexual abuse has been noted to be more prevalent in women with chronic pelvic pain compared with those with other types of pain and with control groups (52% and 12%, respectively).[28] There is a specific association between major sexual abuse and chronic pelvic pain, and a more general association between physical abuse and chronic pain. Women with pelvic pain who had a previous history of sexual abuse had a significantly higher risk of having a current diagnosis of major depression and somatoform pain disorder compared with those with no abuse or less severe abuse.[15] Toomey et al.[29] found that 53% of patients with chronic pelvic pain reported previous abuse, and that sexual abuse was reported more frequently than physical abuse. Rapkin et al.[15] reported that 39% of patients with chronic pelvic pain had been physically abused during childhood, and in this study, physical abuse was more common than sexual abuse in the majority of these cases. However, many studies have failed to adopt comparative groups of patients with pain of equal chronicity. It is, therefore, difficult to exclude the possibility that psychological disturbances may have arisen from long term experiences of pain.

Sexual Desire and Arousal

Evidence suggests that women with chronic pelvic pain exhibit lower levels of sexual desire and arousal than healthy women.[30] Payne et al.[31] reported that women with vulvodynia experienced more difficulty with sexual arousal, lubrication, and sexual desire than women without pain, and that they had more catastrophizing thoughts and hypervigilance related to pain with intercourse. Brauer et al.[32] assessed how fear of a painful stimulus may affect sexual arousal by using the threat of pain at a distal location (the ankle). Interestingly, there was no difference in the extent of decreased sexual arousal between women with dyspareunia and women without sexual dysfunction; both groups exhibited less arousal with the threat of a painful stimulus, suggesting that the threat of pain may decrease arousal even in the absence of reported sexual dysfunction. In another study, Brauer et al.[33] demonstrated that negative appraisals were also associated with diminished arousal in women both with and without dyspareunia. These results suggest that the negative emotional appraisal of an experience associated with pain, such as intercourse, may affect arousal in women despite their level of sexual dysfunction. Accordingly, it is important to ask patients about their levels of sexual desire and arousal when screening for psychological variables, even when they do not report pain with intercourse.

PSYCHOLOGICAL APPROACH TO CHRONIC PELVIC PAIN

Available evidence suggests that psychological factors play an important role in the perception of pain, behaviors, and attitudes toward experimental and sexual stimuli in women with chronic pelvic pain. Physicians should be able to identify such variables with proper screening tools, and the presence of these variables should influence how treatment interventions are delivered. Psychological interventions, including cognitive-behavioral therapy, should be integrated into the comprehensive treatment of women with sexual pain disorders. Despite these recommendations, interventions that target psychological factors and pain-related cognitions, such as fear of pain, catastrophizing, or anxiety about pain, do not yet appear to be widely used by physicians to complement traditional interventions.[34]

Screening questionnaires for pain-related psychological variables, such as the Pain Catastrophizing Scale,[35] the Fear of Pain Questionnaire,[36] and the State-Trait Anxiety Inventory,[37] should be included in routine practice during evaluation and assessment of patients with chronic pelvic pain. These scales are likely to provide important information about the presence of psychological variables, including catastrophizing, fear, and anxiety, in patients with chronic pelvic pain, which can alter the treatment approach used. In addition, their continued use over the course of treatment can help assess whether changes in pain-related psychological variables have occurred and may signal the need for referral to another healthcare provider, such as a clinical psychologist or sex therapist.

Cognitive-behavioral therapy has been repeatedly demonstrated to be an effective treatment intervention for women with chronic pelvic pain.[38,39] Cognitive coping strategies should include education about how certain psychological factors and attentional bias to pain during intercourse may affect sexual functioning and other activities for which patients may report pain. These strategies also should include specific instructions about decreasing hypervigilance and expectations of painful stimuli during activities reported to cause pain; self-coping skills, such as relaxation training, during periods of pain; and gradual exposure to activities reported to cause pain.

Another psychological intervention that has been studied extensively in patients with chronic low back pain is graded exposure to activities associated with pain-related fear, with the goal of encouraging patients to engage more in such activities. For women with chronic pelvic pain and resultant dyspareunia, one of these activities is often intercourse. However, there have not yet been trials comparing the efficacy of a graded-exposure protocol with cognitive-behavioral therapy or other interventions for pain and sexual function in patients with chronic pelvic pain. For women with chronic pelvic pain, these protocols should be designed to include interventions that actually simulate intercourse rather than just simple vaginal dilation exercises.

In addition to rehabilitative interventions, collaborative psychosexual treatment of women with chronic pelvic pain is essential. Referral to a sex counselor or therapist is recommended for women who have pelvic pain complaints and report sexual dysfunction or intimacy problems secondary to pelvic pain complaints. Sex therapists may be helpful in addressing low libido or arousal problems, in addition to the effects of sexual dysfunction on intimate relationships.[40] Psychological assessment and psychotherapy should be initiated first if any signs of psychopathology are present.[41]

In summary, the approach to patients with chronic pelvic pain must be therapeutic, supportive, and sympathetic. Follow-up appointments should be given, because requesting patients to return "only if pain persists" can reinforce pain behavior. Different psychotherapeutic approaches such as depth psychotherapy, systemic psychotherapy, psychodynamic-interpersonal therapy, biofeedback therapy, and hypnosis have been shown to be effective in achieving symptomatic relief from pain, as well as palliative reduction in pain intensity. Hypnosis has been suggested to help in breaking up the harmful and well-established pain reflexes through "synaptic ablation." Anxiety and depression can also be reduced when psychosocial functioning improves, including return to work, increased social activities, and improved sexual activity.

REFERENCES

1. Duncan CH, Taylor HC. A psychosomatic study of pelvic congestion. *Am J Obstet Gynecol.* 1952;64:1–12.

2. Collins ML. Personality correlates of endometriosis. Doctoral thesis. Michigan: Western Michigan University. 1979.

3. Roth H. *Psychosomatische Aspekte der Endometriose*. Kiel, Germany: Universität Kiel, 1996.

4. Haugstad GK, Haugstad TS, Kirste UM, Leganger S, Klemmetsen I, Malt UF. Mensendieck somatocognitive therapy as treatment approach to chronic pelvic pain: results of a randomized controlled intervention study. *Am J Obstet Gynecol*. 2006;194(5):1303–1310.

5. Lethem J, Slade PD, Troup JD, Bentley G. Outline of a Fear-Avoidance Model of exaggerated pain perception. *Behav Res Ther*. 1983;21(4):401–408.

6. Vlaeyen JW, Kole-Snijders AM, Boeren RG, van Eek H. Fear of movement/(re)injury in chronic low back pain and its relation to behavioral performance. *Pain*. 1995 Sep;62(3):363–372.

7. Keefe FJ, Rumble ME, Scipio CD, Giordano LA, Perri LM. Psychological aspects of persistent pain: current state of the science. *J Pain*. 2004 May;5(4):195–121.

8. Sullivan MJ, Thorn B, Haythornthwaite JA, et al. Theoretical perspectives on the relation between catastrophizing and pain. *Clin J Pain*. 2001 Mar;17(1):52–64.

9. George SZ, Wittmer VT, Fillingim RB, Robinson ME. Sex and pain-related psychological variables are associated with thermal pain sensitivity for patients with chronic low back pain. *J Pain*. 2007 Jan;8(1):2–10.

10. Leeuw M, Goossens ME, Linton SJ. The fear-avoidance model of musculoskeletal pain: current state of scientific evidence. *J Behav Med*. 2007;30: 77–94.

11. Kellner R, Slocumb JC, Rosenfeld RC, Pathak D. Fears and beliefs in patients with the pelvic pain syndrome. *J Psychosom Res*. 1988;32:303–310.

12. Pukall CF, Binik YM, Khalife S, et al. Vestibular tactile and pain thresholds in women with vulvar vestibulitis syndrome. *Pain*. 2002;96:163–175.

13. Desrochers G, Bergeron S, Khalife S, et al. Fear, avoidance and self-efficacy in relation to pain and sexual impairment in women with provoked vestibulodynia. *Clin J Pain*. 2009;25:520–527.

14. Granot M, Friedman M, Yarnitsky D, Zimmer EZ. Enhancement of the perception of systemic pain in women with vulvar vestibulitis. *BJOG*. 2002;109:863–866.

15. Rapkin AJ, Kames LD, Darke LL, et al. History of physical and sexual abuse in women with chronic pelvic pain. *Obstet Gynecol*. 1990;76:92–96.

16. Peveler R, Edwards J, Daddow J, Thomas E. Psychosocial factors and chronic pelvic pain: a comparison of women with endometriosis and with unexplained pain. *J Psychosom Res*. 1996;40(3):305–315.

17. Paras ML, Murad MH, Chen LP et al. Sexual abuse and lifetime diagnosis of somatic disorders: a systematic review and meta-analysis. *JAMA*. 2009:302(5):550–561.

18. Reiter RC, Shakerin LR, Gambone JC, et al. Correlation between sexual abuse and somatization in women with somatic and non-somatic chronic pelvic pain. *Am J Obstet Gynecol*. 1991;165: 104–109.

19. Russo J, Katon WJ, Sullivan H, et al. Severity of somatization and its relationship to psychiatric disorders and personality. *Psychosomatics*. 1994;35:546–556.

20. Walker EA, Gelfand AN, Gelfand MD, et al. Chronic pelvic pain and gynecological symptoms in women with irritable bowel syndrome. *J Psychosom Obstet Gynaecol*.1996:17:39–46.

21. Walker EA, Katon WJ, Harrop-Griffiths J, et al. Relationship of chronic pelvic pain to psychiatric diagnosis as childhood sexual abuse. *Am J Psychiatry*. 1980;145:75–80.

22. Nolan TE, Metheny WP, Smith RP. Unrecognized association of sleep disorder and depression with chronic pelvic pain. *South Med J*. 1992;85:1181–1183.

23. Slocumb JC, Kellner R, Rosenfield RC, et al. Anxiety and depression inpatients with abdominal pelvic pain syndrome. *Gen Hosp Psychiatry*. 1989;11:48–53.

24. Sepulcri RP, do Amaral VF. Depressive symptoms, anxiety, and quality of life in women with pelvic endometriosis. *Eur J Obstet Gynecol Reprod Biol*. 2009;142(1):53–56.

25. Howard FM. Chronic pelvic pain. *Obstet Gynecol*. 2003 Mar;101(3):594–611.

26. Reiter RC, Gambone JC. Nongynecologic somatic pathology in women with chronic pelvic pain and negative laparoscopy. *J Reprod Med*. 1991;36: 253–259.

27. Walling MK, Reiter RC, O'Hara MW, et al. Abuse history and chronic pelvic pain in women: I. Prevalences of sexual abuse and physical abuse. *Obstet Gynecol*. 1994;84:193–199.

28. Walker EA, Stenchever MA. Sexual victimization and chronic pelvic pain. *Obstet Gynecol Clin North Am*. 1993;20:795–807.

29. Toomey TC, Hernandez JT, Gittelman DF, et al. Relationship of sexual and physical abuse to pain and psychological assessment variables in chronic pelvic pain patients. *Pain*. 1993;53:105–109.

30. Desrochers G, Bergeron S, Landry T, Jodoin M. Do psychosexual factors play a role in the etiology of provoked vestibulodynia? A critical review. *J Sex Marital Ther*. 2008;34(3):198–226.

31. Payne KA, Binik YM, Pukall CF, et al. Effects of sexual arousal on genital and non-genital

sensation: a comparison of women with vulvar vestibulitis syndrome and healthy controls. *Arch Sex Behav.* 2007;36:289–300.

32. Brauer M, ter Kuile MM, Janssen SA, Laan E. The effect of pain-related fear on sexual arousal in women with superficial dyspareunia. *Eur J Pain.* 2007;11:788–798.

33. Brauer M, ter Kuile MM, Laan E. Effects of appraisal of sexual stimuli on sexual arousal in women with and without superficial dyspareunia. *Arch Sex Behav.* 2009;38:476–485.

34. Hartmann D, Strauhal MJ, Nelson CA. Treatment of women in the United States with localized, provoked vulvodynia: practice survey of women's health physical therapists. *J Women Health Phys Ther.* 2007;31(3):5.

35. Sullivan MJ, Bishop SR, Pivik J. The Pain Catastrophizing Scale: development and validation. *Psychol Assess.* 1995;7:9.

36. McNeil DW, Rainwater AJ., III Development of the Fear of Pain Questionnaire—III. *J Behav Med.* 1998;21:389–410.

37. Barnes LLB, Harp D, Jung WS. Reliability generalization of scores on the Spielberger State-Trait Anxiety Inventory. *Educ Psychol Meas.* 2002;62:603–618.

38. Bergeron S, Binik YM, Khalife S, et al. A randomized comparison of group cognitive-behavioral therapy, surface electromyographic biofeedback, and vestibulectomy in the treatment of dyspareunia resulting from vulvar vestibulitis. *Pain.* 2001;91:297–306.

39. Masheb RM, Kerns RD, Lozano C, et al. A randomized clinical trial for women with vulvodynia: cognitive-behavioral therapy vs. supportive psychotherapy. *Pain.* 2009;141:31–40.

40. Rosenbaum TY. Physiotherapy treatment of sexual pain disorders. *J Sex Marital Ther.* 2005;31: 329–340.

41. Weijmar Schultz W, Basson R, Binik Y, et al. Women's sexual pain and its management. *J Sex Med.* 2005;2:301–316.

17

The Physical Therapy Approach to Pelvic Pain

Evaluation

LILA BARTKOWSKI-ABBATE AND AMY STEIN

Chronic pelvic pain is estimated to affect one in four women—particularly reproductive women, among whom some 14.7–25.4% experience it—while chronic prostatitis and male pelvic pain affect 9% of the male population.[1] Since the complex actions of normal pelvic floor muscle function—tightening, lifting, squeezing, and relaxing—"support all organs within the pelvis, maintain continence, allow for bladder and bowel emptying, and contribute to sexual arousal and orgasmic function" as well as assisting with childbirth, any dysfunction giving rise to such pain can have a wide-ranging impact, affecting bladder, bowel, and sexual functions as well as causing pain in the pelvic, abdominal, back, and lower-extremity regions of the body. It is why patients with such pain or dysfunction tend to consult doctors representing such overlapping specialties as urology, gynecology, urogynecology, gastroenterology, and colorectal disorders.

While the dysfunction affects many systems (Table 17.1), its potential causes are many and are often difficult to determine. It can arise from abnormalities occurring throughout the neuromuscular and musculoskeletal systems within and surrounding the pelvis—for example, from muscular weakness, increased tone, or skeletal impairments.

The dysfunction may begin as early as in childhood and continue throughout the life cycle. It is not uncommon for a teenaged patient to consult a gynecologist for her inability to wear a tampon, later see a colorectal specialist for chronic constipation and defecation pain, then in college turn to a urologist for urinary urgency and frequency, head back to the gynecologist for dyspareunia as an adult, and seek help from an orthopedist for tailbone pain due to sitting in later maturity. Multiple systems appear to be involved, yet a single cause—a pelvic floor muscle problem—may be the source of all these symptoms.

Because pelvic floor physical therapy is capable of treating all the musculoskeletal impairments that contribute to pelvic pain, it has proven to be an invaluable part of treatment for musculoskeletal causes of functional pelvic pain.[2,3,4,5,6] This chapter is on evaluation and Chapter 18 is on physical therapy treatment approach to pelvic floor muscle dysfunction. We discuss first what the pelvic floor physical therapy evaluation should consist of and how it should be executed, then define and describe the various forms of treatment. Both evaluation and treatment of pelvic floor disorders require postgraduate training. We begin, however, with the context within which the physical therapy approach is applied—that is, in the anatomy of the pelvic floor and its dysfunction.

PELVIC ANATOMY, PELVIC DYSFUNCTIONS

The skeletal structure of the pelvis comprises four distinct bony segments—the two paired innominate bones (ilia), the sacrum, and the coccyx. The four are joined at four joint surfaces—the anterior pubic symphysis, the paired posterior sacroiliac joints, and the sacrococcygeal joint. The endopelvic portion of the pelvis cradles the pelvic organs—bladder and urethra, reproductive organs in women, prostate in men, and rectum—and includes the perineum, which serves to support the viscera as well as give structure to the triad of pelvic orifices—the urethra, vagina, and anus.[7] The abdominal peritoneum extends down to cover the reproductive organs, bladder, and rectum from above.

Dynamically, the pelvis functions to assist with the mobility and stability of the trunk; to

TABLE 17.1 MEDICAL SYSTEM BASED MUSCLE OVERACTIVITY SYMPTOMS

System	Female	Male
Urology	Urinary urgency	Urinary urgency
	Urinary frequency	Urinary frequency
	Pain with urination	Pain with urination
	Burning with urination	Burning with urination
	Chronic UTIs—feeling	Erection pain
	Post-coital UTI—feeling	Post-ejaculatory pain
		Penile-shaft pain or numbness
Gastroenterology	Abdominal pain	Abdominal pain
	Abdominal bloating	Abdominal bloating
	Inability to pass gas	Inability to pass gas
	Flatulence	Flatulence
Colorectal	Pain before, during, or after a bowel movement	Pain before, during, or after a bowel movement
	Tenesmus	Tenesmus
	Chronic constipation	Chronic constipation
	Incomplete bowel emptying	Incomplete bowel emptying
	Rectal burning	Rectal burning
Gynecology	Dyspareunia: initial penetration pain, deep thrusting pain	
	Post-sex pain with or without urinary urgency/frequency	
	Vaginal burning	
	Reproductive pain without an organic diagnosis	
Urogynecology	Pelvic organ prolapse	
	Urinary urgency	
	Urinary frequency	
	Pain with urination	
	Burning with urination	
	Chronic UTIs	
	Post-sex UTI—feeling	
	Dyspareunia: initial penetration pain, deep thrusting pain	
	Post-sex pain with or without urinary urgency/frequency	
	Vaginal burning	
	Reproductive pain without an organic diagnosis	
Orthopedic	Unexplained back, Sacroiliac, hip pain	Unexplained back, Sacroiliac, hip pain
	Referred Sacroiliac Joint Pain/Dysfunction	Referred Sacroiliac Joint pain/Dysfunction
	Tailbone pain	Tailbone pain
	Piriformis pain	Piriformis pain

provide for the transfer of weight-bearing forces between the trunk and the upper and lower limbs; to protect the pelvic organs and the attachments for muscle, fascia, and ligaments in and around the midsection; and to assist in childbirth. The ability of the pelvis to function is greatly influenced by the soft tissues that attach to it, including the pelvic floor muscles, both superficial and deep; the diaphragm and the abdominal muscles; the hip muscles; and the thoracolumbosacral muscles. Equally influential are the pelvic viscera and their fascial attachments within the pelvic confines, including the support system of the bladder and urethra, the bowel, reproductive organs, and the rectum.[8] Some authors suggest that the soft tissue of the pelvic floor is divided into layers.[9] The topmost layer comprises the pelvic viscera and its supportive endopelvic fascia.[9] These fascial structures are complex, composed of loose connective tissue, smooth muscle, elastic fibers, blood vessels, and nerves, more closely resembling a mesentery than skeletal ligaments. The endopelvic fascia serves to suspend the pelvic viscera from the pelvic sidewalls.[10] Distal to that are the levator ani muscles, which support the viscera and are part of the urethral, vaginal, and anal openings. More superficial is the urogenital diaphragm, or perineal membrane, which crosses the anterior pelvic outlet, connecting the perineal body to the ischiopubic rami and securing the distal urethra. Most superficial are the bulbocavernosus, ischiocavernosus, and superficial transverse perineal muscles of the anterior urogenital triangle and the anal sphincter of the posterior anal triangle (see Figures 17.1 and 17.2).

As a whole, the pelvic floor muscles function to support the pelvic organs, to assist in both fecal and urinary continence, to provide support for the rectum and inhibition to the bladder, to assist in "uploading" the spine and pelvic-spinal stability, and to contribute to sexual arousal and performance (see Figures 17.3 and 17.4).[11]

Support within the pelvis is multifaceted. Articular and fibrous cartilage support and bind the bony pelvis,[12] while the viscerofascia[9,10] suspends the organs. The organs themselves have an affinity for one another due to the serous fluids in and around them, even as they occupy all the physical space available within the bony confines.[8] Though the pelvic viscera are supported most inferiorly by the pelvic floor muscles, the pressure within the abdominal cavity also greatly influences their positioning, with the pressure being greatest just inferior to the respiratory diaphragm and decreasing distally.[8] When these support systems shorten and/or weaken due to such causes as surgery, multiple pregnancies, or age, the result can be pelvic organ prolapse; bladder, bowel, and sexual dysfunction; and pelvic, abdominal, and back pain.

A range of abnormalities—muscular weakness, increased tone, or skeletal impairments—occurring throughout the neuromuscular and musculoskeletal systems within and surrounding the pelvis can cause pelvic floor dysfunction,

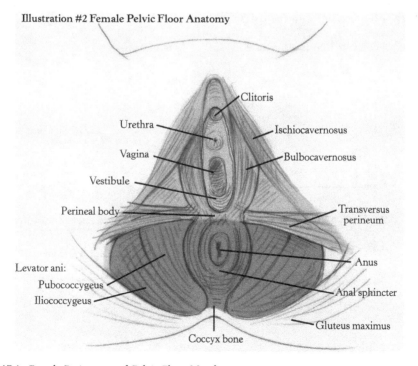

Illustration #2 Female Pelvic Floor Anatomy

Clitoris
Urethra
Ischiocavernosus
Vagina
Bulbocavernosus
Vestibule
Perineal body
Transversus perineum
Levator ani:
Pubococcygeus
Iliococcygeus
Anus
Anal sphincter
Gluteus maximus
Coccyx bone

FIGURE 17.1: Female Perineum and Pelvic Floor Muscles.

Heal Pelvic Pain by Amy Stein, DPT

Illustration #4 Male Pelvic Floor Anatomy

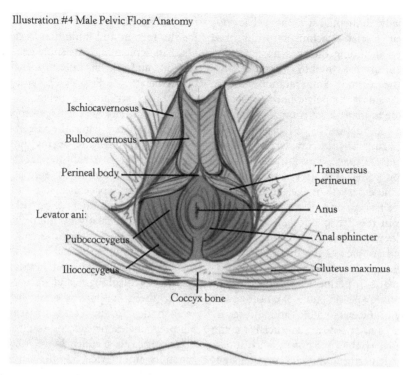

FIGURE 17.2: Male Perineum and Pelvic Floor Muscles.

Heal Pelvic Pain by Amy Stein, DPT

and the underlying cause of pelvic pain and related symptoms is therefore often difficult to determine. Singular events can cause changes in the physiology or biomechanics in the region of the pelvis. Events such as abdominal or pelvic surgery, an acute infection, a fall, or childbirth often leave the pelvic floor with lasting abnormalities that require effective care.

Illustration #1-Female Urogenital System (midsagittal section)

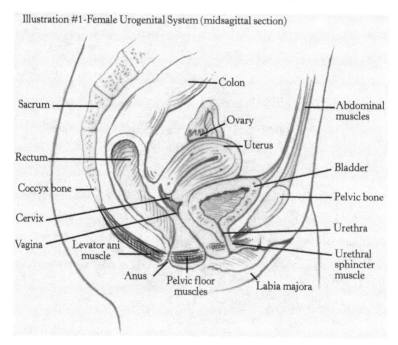

FIGURE 17.3: Female Pelvic Floor Muscles-Midsaggital.

Heal Pelvic Pain by Amy Stein, DPT

Illustration #3 Male Urogenital System (midsagittal section)

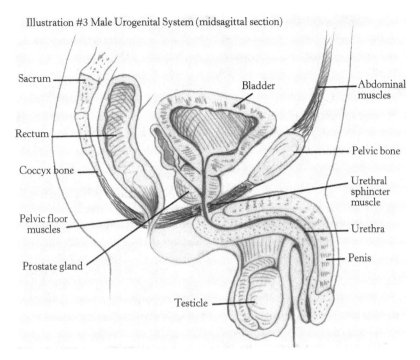

FIGURE 17.4: Male Pelvic Floor Muscles-Midsaggital.

Heal Pelvic Pain by Amy Stein, DPT

Moreover, a range of other pelvic pain disorders can cause either itching, burning, or a combination of the two in and around the genital region, creating increased tension in the pelvic floor. Examples of this include bladder infections, yeast infections, and such dermatological conditions or sexually transmitted diseases as lichen sclerosus, condyloma acuminatum (genital warts), squamous cell hyperplasia, and vulvar interepithelial neoplasia.[4] Typically, once these disorders are properly diagnosed and managed and the musculoskeletal dysfunction is addressed, normal pelvic floor tone is restored.

But pelvic floor dysfunction can be insidious and can range from childhood dysfunctional voiding to such inflammatory conditions as endometriosis,[13,14] interstitial cystitis,[6,15] and inflammatory bowel disorders,[16,17] to neuropathic pain.[18] Chemotherapy and radiation often have a lasting impact on pelvic floor function as well as on bowel, bladder, and sexual function. Hormonal imbalance, especially low estrogen causing vaginal atrophy, can play a part as well. We also know that the torments of psychological, physical, and/or sexual abuse[19] can leave lifelong abnormalities in and around the pelvis. Muscular changes occurring with poor posture, skeletal misalignment (especially in

the lumbo-sacral region), and prolonged and improper sitting postures can also commonly leave the pelvic floor structures compromised[20].

All of these conditions and eventualities may result in ongoing discomfort that causes pelvic floor muscle guarding and overactivity of the muscles.[21] Scarring and adhesions can occur, as can shortening of the pelvic floor muscles. Such biomechanical abnormalities as foramenal narrowing or scarring of a fascial nerve canal, myofascial trigger points, or connective tissue restrictions around the vaginal introitus[22] or genital region, or around nerves can also leave the pelvic floor muscles dysfunctional.

A noxious stimulus can trigger pelvic floor dysfunction—and vice versa: pelvic floor dysfunction can trigger a noxious stimulus. For example, in response to the chronic pain of hemorrhoids, patients may habituate a pelvic floor holding pattern that, over time, leaves the pelvic floor muscles hypertonic, with a shortening of sarcomeres and with subsequent and additional muscular pain. Or, a young man with a lifelong phobia about public toilets may develop an overactive pelvic floor from delaying the urge to empty his bowel and bladder. Over time, bowel and bladder retention disorders become a much bigger problem, increasing the possibility of recurrent urinary tract infections, chronic constipation, and hemorrhoids. The cycle of noxious stimuli, improper behavioral patterns, and pelvic floor dysfunction must be addressed, both physically and psychologically, before normal function can be regained.

A large portion of the literature dealing with pelvic floor issues is in the realm of urogynecology and deals with pelvic prolapse and incontinence.[23,24,25] When reviewing the literature on physical therapy and pelvic floor dysfunction, a fair number of studies can be found; most, however, lack stringent study protocols, with a limited number of randomized controlled studies (RTCs). Bo and her colleagues have published an excellent and highly recommended book describing evidence-based physical therapy care.[2] They, too, recognize that "good clinical practice always should be individualized and should be based on a combination of clinical experience, knowledge from high-quality RCTs and patient preferences ... [as well as] respect, empathy, and strong ethical grounding."[2] Many other studies do exist, however, dealing with the specifics of pelvic floor dysfunction as it relates to chronic pelvic pain syndromes,[3,26,27,21,28,29] sexual dysfunction,[30,31,32] painful bladder syndromes,[33,6,34,35] and incontinence.[36,37,38] (The references provided here are for example only and by no means represent all published data.)

THE
NEURALGIA FACTOR

Thanks to the constellation of nerves of the pelvic floor region, adverse neural tension due to physiological abnormalities can also be a major factor in pelvic pain.[6,39] One of the chief actors in that constellation in terms of the problems it may cause is the pudendal nerve. It originates from the sacral plexus (S2–S4) and contains 80% sensory and 20% motor fibers. The sensory pudendal nerve branches into three smaller nerves: the inferior rectal nerve, which innervates part of the rectum and the surrounding skin; the perineal nerve, innervating the perineum, vagina, male scrotum, labia, and urethra; and the dorsal nerve of the clitoris or penis. The motor branch of the nerve supplies the external anal sphincter, sphincter muscles of the bladder, and the levator ani muscles. The visceral referral pattern for the pudendal nerve is to the lower uterine segment, distal ureter, bladder, cervix, upper vagina, and rectum. A common site for adverse pudendal nerve tension may be at the sacrotuberous or sacrospinous ligaments

of the sacroiliac joint, the Alcock's canal, and/or at the obturator internus muscle.

Patients thus affected may complain of an increase in symptoms with tight clothing and with sitting, and of improvement upon standing or sitting on a toilet seat. They may present with bladder and bowel symptoms of frequency, urgency, retention, pain, and constipation. They may complain of pain in the genital or anal region. Dyspareunia is a common complaint, as is pain during or after orgasm. Patients may or may not present with an abnormal pudendal nerve motor latency test.

The pudendal nerve is also the only peripheral nerve that has both somatic and autonomic fibers. A person can therefore experience increased heart rate and blood pressure, decreased motility of the colon, decreased blood flow, and perspiration with pudendal nerve stimulation.

There are other nerves in the thoracolumbosacral region that can cause abdomino-pelvic pain. The *genitofemoral* nerve originates from the upper part of the lumbar plexus, L1 and L2, and divides into two branches. The femoral branch supplies the anterior portion of the upper thigh. The genital branch supplies the scrotal skin in males and the mons pubis and labia majora in females. Its motor innervation is the lateral portion of the bulbocavernosus. The visceral referral pattern is to the proximal tube and uterine fundus.

The *ilioinguinal* nerve originates from L1 and refers to the upper and medial portions of the thigh and to the lateral part of the scrotum and testicles in males and the lateral part of the labia majora and mons pubis in females. Its motor distribution is to portions of the abdominal muscles. Its visceral innervation is to the proximal tube and uterine fundus.

The *iliohypogastric* nerve emerges from T12 and L1, with sensory distribution to the lower abdomen and the superior gluteal region, and with motor innervation to portions of the abdominal muscles. The visceral referred pattern is to the ovaries and the distal fallopian tubes in women, and to the testicles in men.

The *lateral femoral cutaneous* nerve arises from L2–L3 and refers to the lateral and anterior portion of the thigh, with the visceral referred pattern to the fundus and lower uterine region.

The *posterior femoral cutaneous* nerve originates from the dorsal portion of S1–S2 and the ventral portion of S2–S3. It refers to the perineum, gluteal region, the posterior thigh, popliteal fossa, and the superior posterior portion of the lower leg.

The *femoral nerve* arises from the dorsal portion of L2–L4 and has a sensory innervation with the anterior and medial thigh and a motor innervation of the quadriceps and hip flexor muscles.

The *obturator nerve* emerges from the ventral portion of L2–L4 and refers from the groin area down the inner thigh area; its motor innervations are the adductor and hip flexor muscles.

The *sciatic nerve* originates from L4–S2 with sensory innervation to the posterior thigh, leg, and foot, and with motor innervation to the hamstring muscles.

The *superior hypogastric*, the *inferior hypogastric* plexus, and the *ganglion of impar* are bundles of nerves that all contain fibers of the sympathetic nervous system. The superior hypogastric nerve's origin is at T10–L2, and it ends as the inferior hypogastric plexus. The inferior hypogastric nerves contain both sympathetic and parasympathetic fibers from S2–S4, and they supply a portion of the viscera of the pelvic cavity. The ganglion of impar originates as four or five small sacral ganglia anterior to the sacrum and terminates at the coccyx. All connect the spinal cord to portions of the pelvic floor, perineum, and pelvic organs in some manner. Other important nerve bundles that innervate portions of the pelvic viscera are the lumbar splanchnic nerves, the sacral and pelvic splanchnic nerves, and the sacral sympathetic trunk.

Adverse neural tension anywhere in the pelvic region may result in nerve irritation and subsequent neuralgia in any or all areas that the nerve supplies, and it may manifest itself as sensations of itching, burning, tingling, cold, sharp and shooting pain, or as overactivity of the innervated muscles. The tension may derive from adhesions, from overactive or shortened pelvic floor muscles, from such biomechanical abnormalities as narrowing of a foramen or canal where the nerve travels, from myofascial trigger points, or from connective tissue restrictions surrounding the nerve. In turn, these physiological or biomechanical changes could be the result of a traumatic fall or injury; of abdominal, pelvic, or thigh surgery; of traumatic childbirth; emotional or physical abuse; hormonal imbalances; skeletal malalignment; and of other related first causes.[6,39]

Whatever the root origin of the tension, the peripheral nervous system of the pelvic floor can refer the pain to the somatic innervation or to the visceral innervation. The afferents of these nerves can converge on the dorsal horn of the spinal cord, both affecting the organs and giving rise to a pain pattern and to possible central sensitization. There are two possible results of this convergence. Either a dysfunction in the viscera will express itself somatically—a viscerosomatic reflex—or a dysfunction at the body's surface will be expressed to the viscera as a somatovisceral reflex.[40] The spinal cord in turn helps transmit the symptoms of the visceral and somatic systems.

VISCEROSOMATIC AND SOMATOVISCERAL REFLEXES

Viscerosomatic reflexes at the spinal cord level can result in somatic dysfunctions that develop in response to visceral pathology, and vice versa, with somatovisceral reflexes; they therefore constitute a possible explanation for pelvic floor nerve abnormalities and can be used as diagnostic tools for exploring such normalities.

Although the evidence is thus far incomplete, it is believed that these reflexes to and from the abdomino-pelvic region become much more sensitized with the increased sensitivity of the nerves. A viscerosomatic reflex might begin with an inflammation associated with visceral pathology and then result in activation of nociceptive, visceral afferent neurons. These afferent neurons return to the spinal cord, and the ongoing afferent stimulation results in irritability of the internuncial neurons of that spinal segment. When the afferent activity from the offending organ is sufficiently stimulated, it will result in a referred pain pattern from the ongoing internuncial firing. The afferent stimulation proceeds across synapses to the dorsal horn at the spinal cord segment; this activates the internuncial neurons, which then diffuse to the ventral horn motor neurons. The result is myospasticity and palpable tissue texture changes. The location of the reflex between the visceral pathology and the paravertebral soft tissue is consistent from one individual to another, which is why both viscerosomatic and somatovisceral reflexes are of diagnostic use.[41]

EVALUATING PELVIC FLOOR DYSFUNCTION FOR PHYSICAL THERAPY TREATMENT

To begin with, it is a given that any such evaluation requires complex interpretations of information to determine a proper diagnosis and plan of care. As the *Guide to Physical*

Therapist Practice puts it, "The physical therapist integrates the five elements of patient/client management—examination, evaluation, diagnosis, prognosis, and intervention—in a manner designed to optimize outcomes."[42] The initial aim, after collecting the patient's history and performing a detailed objective examination, is to determine how the physical findings cause and/or affect a patient's physical complaints and to classify the systems pattern at work in the patient's case—a cardiovascular/pulmonary, integumentary, or neuromuscular pattern, or a musculoskeletal pattern.

In patients who present with the complexity of pelvic pain, the musculoskeletal category is usually dominant, regardless of the other system patterns that are present. For example, a pelvic pain patient may present with such symptoms as vulvar skin inflammation (integumentary pattern) or burning symptoms from nerve compression (neurovascular) along with complaints of dull or achy abdominal and pelvic pain (musculoskeletal). Musculoskeletal dysfunctions can actually cause all of the symptoms that seem to come from other patterns. Most typically, pelvic pain patients fall into the Musculoskeletal Pattern 4D: impaired joint mobility, motor function, muscle performance, and range of motion (ROM) associated with connective tissue dysfunction.[42] Assessment of a musculoskeletal dysfunction typically follows the completion of basic medial diagnostic tests addressing the pelvic pain patient's complaints and ruling out any serious pathology or disease.

At a minimum, the evaluation should include, but will not be limited to:

- Posture and gait assessment
- Biomechanical and joint mobility assessment
- Myofascial restriction and trigger point assessment
- Connective tissue assessment
- Scar tissue assessment
- Spinosacral and peripheral nerve assessment
- Pelvic floor muscle evaluation
- Visceral mobilization assessment
- Core assessment
- Biofeedback and real-time ultrasound assessment

A plan of potential treatment options will then be directed toward the physical cause of the dysfunction, including pelvic floor muscle over-activity, visceral abnormalities, and the associated musculoskeletal issues that accompany the dysfunction. Treatment may consist of rehabilitation of the pelvic floor, abdominal, gluteal, spino-sacral, hip, and lower-extremity muscles; lumbosacral and peripheral nerve mobilization; connective tissue mobilization, and myofascial trigger point release of the surrounding muscles and tissues. Pelvic floor physical therapists may also perform range-of-motion and strengthening exercises of certain muscles to improve core and lower extremity mobility and stability. Depending on their symptoms, patients are educated in appropriate sitting postures and may be given bladder and bowel retraining, including toileting posture. They may be educated in the basics of water intake and of eating healthy, fiber-filled foods, as well as dietary changes for bladder and bowel health. Restoration of sexual activity is a key goal that may require education in the use of self-massage techniques, dilators, and sexual positions that can avoid pain. Central sensitization and reprocessing may also be part of the treatment paradigm, but specialized training in neurodynamic treatment, guided imagery, dynamic movement, and treatment of cognitive-behavioral approaches will be discussed in other chapters and does not form part of this chapter.

THE EVALUATION

First Impressions: Visual Assessment of Posture and Gait

A practitioner's evaluation begins at the moment of greeting the patient in the waiting room. This is when the therapist can observe the moment-in-time information embodied in the patient's sitting position, alignment, and holding pattern. Is the individual slumped, sitting extra tall, leaning to one side? How quickly and easily does the patient rise from the chair? Is the patient holding his or her abdomen in pain? If so, how severe does the pain seem to be? What is the strength of the patient's handshake? In addition, as the patient walks to the treatment room, the practitioner can observe and assess his or her gait-pattern, stride length, heel-to-toe foot strike, and the weight-bearing patterns through the lower extremity.[43] All these observations can enrich the practitioner's understanding of the patient's condition and level of pain—even before a single question has been asked.

The Intake

The aim of the intake process is to determine how the patient's symptoms started and how they progressed to the point that the patient sought or was referred to physical therapy as a remedy. This requires cataloguing the patient's past medical history, past surgical history, prior medical testing and outcomes, medications, current and past complaints, and whether the injury was traumatic, insidious, or unknown in nature. Ask the patient to describe his/her complaints within the 24-hour pain cycle, articulating the current pain level, what worsens or improves the symptoms, and any positions or actions that exacerbate or relieve symptoms; for example, some patients feel their symptoms worsen at the end of their day, others when they awake in the morning. The intake should also explore other musculoskeletal injuries thought to be benign and seemingly unrelated to the symptoms of pelvic pain. A female who is four months postpartum and presents with sexual dysfunction may not see the relationship of her current pain to falling off a slide and sustaining a coccyx fracture at the age of eight, but it may indeed be related to the presenting symptoms. That is why it is essential to press the patient about old musculoskeletal injuries: a severe ankle sprain from years ago, for example, can have taken years to manifest itself in pelvic pain symptoms.[44]

Examination

Biomechanical and Joint Mobility Assessment

Postural assessment of the patient is an important and effective clinical tool. The central nervous system's neuromuscular reaction to pain varies widely, so noting the compensatory posture of a patient in pain signals the nature of his/her neuromuscular response—for example, the "back-gripper" overactivation of the erector spinae, "the chest-gripper" overactivation of the external and internal obliques, or the "co-contraction brace—the trunk-gripper," a neutral posture in which there is co-activation of the trunk flexors and extensors.[12] In assessing the patient from cranium to foot and noting these gripping postures, the physical therapist must explore how the postures may be affecting the patient's pain and, taking into consideration the patient's history as well, whether there is a longstanding compensation that has been driving the pain. Further inspection of the pelvis to assess the bony relationships as well as neuromuscular control must also be taken into account as potential sources of symptoms.

While pelvic pain may arise from the structures themselves, it may also be the result of abdominal and levator ani trigger points; intrapelvic muscle strain (obturator internus, coccygeus, piriformis, pelvic floor myalgia/spasm); weakness in the levator, coccygeus, piriformis, abdominal, and gluteus maximus; anterior pelvic tilt; leg length/pelvic postural asymmetry; loss of hip range of motion; lumbar joint dysfunction; and iliopsoas adaptive shortening.[20] According to King Baker, posture plays a major role in all of chronic pelvic pain syndromes, and because of common innervations, it's not uncommon to find abnormalities in the thoracolumbar vertebrae, joint capsules, ligaments, discs, hip joints, and ligaments that also contribute to chronic pelvic pain.

As noted above, the bony pelvis is made up of a complex relationship of articulating structures—the two innominates that make up the pubic symphysis at the anterior portion of the pelvis with two posterior portions of the bone that articulate with the sacrum. The sacrum articulates with the coccyx on its inferior pole and with the lumbar spine on the superior pole. All pelvic articulations are weight-bearing in all positions—sitting, lying, and standing—as the lumbar spine loads and as femurs compress through the acetabula during weight-bearing tasks.[45] By comparing specific bony landmarks on the pelvis, the physical therapy practitioner can check for pelvic bony symmetry across all planes. Even a millimeter of excess movement in any plane of motion can cause severe pain due to abnormal muscle and nerve tension, and these minor movements may not appear in radiographic images. Moreover, as sacroiliac joints vary from person to person and between genders in terms of morphology and mobility, determining if those millimeters of movement are a limiting factor or affect patients' pain patterns can be a clinical challenge to the treating physical therapist or other practitioners.[46]

Palpation is the methodology for making this determination. With palpation, the examining practitioner checks via touch for symmetry in bony landmarks, looks for torsions within the pelvis or spine, checks muscle tone, and screens for the range of motion of specific joints. The aim is to note any areas of dysfunction—in particular, those that stand out as needing to be addressed early on in the treatment plan.

By instructing the patient to sit tall, then move to a slumped position, or to shift weight in standing or to shift weight by standing on one leg, the practitioner can perform a biomechanical assessment of the external pelvis. Asking the patient to execute a functional task like stepping forward to simulate walking, or stepping up on a step, lets the physical therapist check pelvic position and movement and thus identify such areas of dysfunction as pelvic obliquity and asymmetrical mobility of the pelvic bones.[12] Poor alignment or scoliosis may also be noted; each plays a role above and below the pelvis. If a pelvic bone is out of alignment, the internal and external muscles could be stretched or shortened, and nerves may be compressed, a less than optimal condition that can create pain.

Deficits in normal muscle length and full joint range of motion are a possible cause of or at minimum a contributing factor in pelvic pain. Restrictions within any joint or decreased muscle length or muscle glide can create areas of connective tissue restriction, a form of nerve compression that can lead to compensations above and below the area of pain. The physical therapist performing an evaluation of a patient's pelvic pain symptoms must therefore assess joint ROM and muscle length of the lower extremities, the lumbar spine, and the thorax.

Assessment of hip ROM is also clinically relevant, as hip pathology can refer pain into the posterior pelvis and thigh, the groin, or the anterior thigh and leg.[47] Symptomatology of hip dysfunction can mimic pelvic floor muscle overactivity, and vice versa, to produce such symptoms as urinary urgency/frequency, pain with sitting, and groin pain. Current research shows there is a relationship between hip labral tears and the concurrence of pelvic pain. It is therefore important that the practitioner conduct a full assessment of hip ROM in all planes of motion, along with checking the integrity of the hip capsule, of the wearing surfaces of the femoral head, and of the acetabulum. Hip pain of a non-arthritic origin in post-partum women has gained recent attention.[48] Women can develop "hip pain during pregnancy and/or after delivery that is caused by a labral tear." The position of the femur and inability of the hip to externally rotate may cause this tear and could be a causative factor in pelvic pain.

Myofascial Restriction and Trigger Point Assessments

Myofascial trigger points are found in skeletal muscle or muscle fascia and are an extremely prevalent cause of persistent pain disorders within the abdomino-pelvic region— exacerbated even further by poor posture, poor body mechanics, psychological stress or depression, and poor sleep or nutrition.

Trigger points are characterized by deep aching pain referred to any structure from focal tender points in taut bands of skeletal muscle; those taut bands are the actual trigger points. Trigger points resulting in or from pelvic pain have been well documented and can be found in the following muscles: levator ani muscles, obturator internus, coccygeus, abdominal, gluteals, adductors, piriformis, quadratus lumborum, paraspinals, iliotibial band and tensor fascia lata, quadriceps, and hamstrings.[49]

Pelvic floor myofascial trigger points typically occur when the muscles are overloaded from trauma, repetitive overuse, pelvic organ disease, inflammation in the area, or from sympathetically mediated tension resulting in a holding or guarding pattern.[50] Precisely because the pelvic floor muscles support the pelvic and abdominal organs; assist with functions of the bladder, bowel, and sexual activity; and provide stability and mobility of the trunk with the lower extremities, they are easily susceptible to developing myofascial trigger points. In the posterior pelvic region, trigger points typically result in symptoms in the rectum, anus, coccyx, and sacrum. Trigger points in the anterior portion may result in more urogenital pain. Dyspareunia, as well as bladder and bowel dysfunction, can be the result of pelvic floor trigger points and can cause sharp, dull, aching, deep, or superficial pain.[51,6,5,52]

Diagnosis of a trigger point depends on accurate palpation with 2–4 kg/cm2 of pressure for 10–20 seconds over the suspected trigger point to allow the referred-pain pattern to develop. In addition, to ensure that all trigger points and myofascial restrictions are noted, it is advisable to conduct both an internal muscle assessment and an external biomechanical assessment of muscle function of the patient performing a functional task.[49]

Connective Tissue Assessment

Connective tissue needs to be assessed in the physical therapy evaluation because it envelops everything within the body and because its extensibility can become restricted or can be misused by something as basic as prolonged sitting. We have seen fascial restrictions as cranial as the rib cage and as caudal as the knee joints in patients who present with pelvic pain.[44] It is thus essential for the practitioner to examine connective tissue extensibility in areas prone to being restricted—for example, around bony prominences or in areas of complex neurovascular bundles. This assessment will form the basis of a treatment plan of connective tissue massage aimed at improving circulation, restoring tissue integrity, decreasing ischemia, and eliminating adverse reactions in viscera, and decreasing adverse neural tension in peripheral nerve branches.[44]

Scar Tissue Assessment

Scar tissue formation is a necessary healing function after any skin or soft-tissue injury or following surgical incision. Scars range from simple—a pimple, for example—to severe keloid scarring, and while they are essential for healing, they can interfere with the normal mobility of organs, muscles, nerves, and fascia. These tissue restrictions can progress into a source of abdomino-pelvic pain. For example, when superficial nerves that traverse the anterior portion of the pelvis become entrapped in the scar tissue of cesarean section scars from traditional Pfannenstiel incisions, this can create genital and pelvic pain.[53] Moreover, these C-section scars can run deep and tend to compress near the bladder, which thereby limits bladder extensibility, prevents normal filling, and creates symptoms of urinary urgency and frequency.

Abdominal scar tissue can constrict portions of the colon, thereby slowing colon transit time. Superficial episiotomy scars and the internal vaginal scars from normal childbirth that create any grade of vaginal and rectal tearing can create vaginal and/or rectal pain. Rectal scarring from hemorrhoidectomies can create pain and tissue immobility in both men and women. Scar tissue within muscle can create muscle weakness or its opposite—i.e., muscle shortening and overactivity in tissue surrounding the scar.

The practitioner can assess these dysfunctions using connective tissue and myofascial release mobilization (MFR), skin rolling, and some deep-tissue manual assessment. These actions can establish the amount of decreased mobility and shortening of the tissue under and around the scar tissue.

Spinosacral and Peripheral Nerve Assessment

A nerve should traverse through a foramen, around bony prominences, and through fascia like dental floss through clean teeth. If it does not, if the nerve is entrapped or compressed within a nerve tunnel, neurological symptoms may result. Entrapment or compression within the abdomino-pelvic area's external and internal nerve systems as well as in the nerves of the lower extremities can cause symptoms of itching, swelling, burning, and numbness.[44,43] For these reasons, an assessment of the spinosacral and peripheral nerves is essential.

As noted above, one of the innervations of the pelvic floor is supplied by the sacral nerves of S2, S3, and S4 that make up the pudendal nerve. Patient symptoms can direct the physical therapist performing the evaluation to the appropriate branch of the pudendal nerve—the inferior rectal branch, the perineal branch, or the dorsal branch. For example, a patient with a unilateral pelvic fracture presents to the clinic as being continent with regard to stool but not to urine; through palpation, the practitioner can determine through light touch or deep pressure which branches of the nerve are still supplying sensation.

While the pudendal nerve and the other sacral nerves are the first to come to mind when considering pelvic and genital nerves, the other nerve branches must also be evaluated—specifically, the lumbar, genitofemoral (L1), ilioinguinal (L1), iliohypogastric (T12 and L1), and lateral and posterior femoral cutaneous nerves (L2, L3, and sacral plexus). These all supply sensation to the lower abdomen, upper thigh, genitalia, gluteus regions, and lateral, anterior, and posterior portions of the thighs, and can thus also cause pelvic pain. During a physical therapy evaluation, therefore, it is important to assess T10 through L5 vertebrae to note rotations, increased muscle tension in the paraspinals, and ring shifts (rib placement) throughout the thorax[54,12] that might irritate or compress those specific nerve roots and thereby create symptoms in the above-mentioned areas.

Within the pelvis, the obturator internus is the only muscle interior to the pelvic walls that is innervated with slips of L5, S1, and S2.[43,54]

Pelvic Floor Muscle Evaluation

For the pelvic floor muscle evaluation, the practitioner's aim is to assess muscle tone (overactive or underactive), bony landmarks, and muscle length from origin to insertion, and to evaluate tissue integrity, fascial restriction, nerve assessment, and muscle strength. Muscle coordination can be assessed externally (partially) and internally (which can be more uncomfortable) and can be assessed vaginally in women and rectally in both women and men.

To assess pelvic floor muscle coordination, patients are typically directed to perform an excursion test that can measure their ability to relax.[43] This test enables the practitioner to assess muscle activity, normal muscle firing, and coordination. Are the muscles completing the task at hand? If there is no muscle lengthening, nor a bulge at the completion of the excursion test, it could be an indication of pelvic floor muscle overactivity and a signal that the patient is having difficulty with some or all of the functions of the pelvic floor—sphincteric, sexual, or bowel- and bladder-related.

Both the vaginal and rectal evaluations include visual and palpable external and internal assessments. The rectal evaluation is required in both male and female patients: in the female, the rectal side of the deep transverse perineal, puborectalis, and iliococcygeus muscles need to be fully examined in order to assess the full muscle length and tone of the vaginal pelvic floor muscles. A rectal examination gives access to the anterior surface of the coccyx and its position as well as the coccygeus and the internal and external anal sphincter muscles, thus ensuring a comprehensive evaluation of all the pelvic floor muscles.

The External Pelvic Floor Assessment: Visual

The external visual examination in both male and female should make a general muscle assessment of the urogenital triangle. The practitioner should direct the patient to perform an excursion test in which the patient contracts the pelvic floor muscles, relaxes, performs a Valsalva maneuver, then relaxes the muscles again.[55] Asking the patient to repeat this test once or twice should provide the practitioner with sufficient information to make a quick muscle assessment. (*Note*: Performed by male patients in the hook-lying position, this excursion test enables a practitioner to assess the male perineal area.)

For the female patient, on external visual examination of the vagina, the labia minora should sit somewhat closed. If the labia sit open, it can be surmised that there is some prolapse from an anterior or posterior compartment beyond the opening. If the labia sit somewhat open with no prolapse noted, there may be vaginal estrogenization.[56] The visual examination should assess tissue integrity to determine if the tissue is moist or atrophic and to note any dermatological changes. In observing the vaginal external tissue, practitioners must also look at the skin as a potential source of pain.

The External Pelvic Floor Assessment: Palpation

Through external palpation using a cotton swab, the practitioner can detect areas of pain and assess tissue tenderness; in women, palpation also lets the practitioner note any hypersensitivity of the vestibular area and the surrounding vaginal tissue. Cotton-swab palpation can also tell the physical therapist performing the palpation if the problem is right-sided vs. left-sided and whether it is located in the upper urogenital diaphragm area or the anal triangle area. When pain is present on palpation, it should be documented as mild, moderate, or severe. By stroking each side of the rectal meatus in turn, the practitioner can assess reflex in the perineal area and/or anal area.[43] The reflex may be absent in patients with muscle overactivity and spasm[43] or with neurological involvement.

After assessing the patient using the cotton swab, the practitioner digitally palpates the external tissue to assess the tone of the underlying muscle. External palpation of the urogenital diaphragm and the superficial fibers of the deep pelvic floor muscles with the second digit provides the ability to assess tone of the muscle and restriction of the external fascia.

The Vaginal Assessment: Palpation

In proceeding to internal vaginal palpation in female patients, a systematic approach is essential. Caution must be exercised upon entering the vagina to ensure against eliciting pain prematurely. Even gentle pressure can cause the patient to wince in pain. Unlike a physician's examination that looks for space-occupying lesions or pathologies, this internal vaginal palpation uses no speculum and applies no corkscrewing motion of the palpating finger. The use of both hands—not just the dominant hand for palpation—ensures that each side of the internal pelvis is examined in turn, and the two evaluations are then compared one to the other.

The feel of a normal, healthy, lubricated, reproductive vaginal vault can be likened to that of smooth velvet. It should feel a little slippery, plump, and firm. Upon entering the vaginal vault, separate the labia with the thumb and index finger,[57] and enter with the index finger of the *other* gloved hand, with the lubricated finger pad down, taking note of the position of the urethra to avoid it. Gently lay the pad of your second digit as deep as the first knuckle (distal phalangeal joint) onto the perineal body; this should feel moderately firm. Four muscles are originating here: two superficial transverse perineal muscles at the outer layer, one from each side, and the deep transverse perineal muscle, also one from each side, adjacent and a layer deeper. These muscles will insert on the ischial tuberosity on either side.

Enter the vaginal vault either to the right or left side of the perineal body. If using the right hand, you are examining the right side of the patient's vaginal vault. It should feel like dropping down a bit into the vaginal vault, but it should not feel like a significant step down; if it does, that may indicate muscle overactivity.

For accurate muscle assessment, think of the internal pelvis as divided into right side and left side with the urethra at the top of midline—the 12 o'clock position—and the perineal body at the bottom portion of midline (6 o'clock). The examination should proceed muscle by muscle in order to determine trigger point areas, areas of tightness and shortening, and areas of provoked pain.[43] Starting at the crus of the clitoris are two muscles—the bulbocavernosus, located within the lower portion of the labia minora, and the ischiocavernosus, hugging the pubic rami. Within the pelvis, the obturator internus is on the lateral wall of the ilium. Where the obturator internus ends at the fascial layer of the archis tendonius levator ani (ATLA), the iliococcygeus begins and travels down the midline into the coccyx. The very prominent coccygeus runs toward the ischial spine parallel with the sacrospinous ligament. At the edge of the bowel, closer to the vaginal opening, the physical therapist assesses the puborectalis and the integrity of the vaginal-rectal septum. The tissue should have equal side-glide mobility when comparing sides within the pelvis. If the pelvic floor muscles are overactive and have been shortened over a prolonged period of time, the muscles will have no give when pressed upon, and the fibers may feel like guitar or banjo strings. This may result in symptoms of bladder, bowel, or sexual dysfunction, and/or abdomino-pelvic pain.

Returning to the perineal body and turning the finger pad side up cranially, the practitioner can palpate the structures and muscles of the urogenital diaphragm. The urethra is very sensitive and must be palpated gently. This palpation enables assessment of the peri-urethral space on either side of the urethra, addressing the compressor urethra and surrounding tissue. The practitioner can note areas of muscle overactivity, trigger point areas, decreased fascial movement, and areas of tenderness and pain that can cause patients symptoms of urinary retention or a burning sensation during urination.

The Rectal Assessment: Visual

For the visual assessment, the male or female is placed in either a prone, hook-lying, or side-lying position. The prone position makes it easier to spread apart the butt cheeks to observe the rectal opening and surrounding tissues. Skin tags, small fissures, or hemorrhoids may be noted; along with a notably thick or thin skin texture: these may indicate bowel movement straining. Normal muscle tone will show tight puckering of the outside skin. The external anal sphincter can be almost one inch deep. If no puckering is noted, this may be an area of de-innervation; this is called a "dovetail sign," where flaccidity of the muscle causes the skin to look smooth, not puckered. Such de-innervation may be anywhere within the 360-degree rectal opening. Women with a history of stage III or IV episiotomy tears may show dovetail signs years later, with subsequent symptoms of fecal incontinence.

The patient should be directed to execute an excursion test, during which the practitioner will observe contraction and coordination of the rectal pelvic floor muscles.

The Rectal Assessment: Palpation

The practitioner performing internal rectal palpation must be sure to allow the anal reflex to diminish before entering, and must take care, once within the rectal compartment, to use no cork-screwing motion of the palpating finger, as this can cause discomfort to the patient.

After applying a significant amount of gel to the tip of the examining finger, the physical therapist performing the evaluation should rest the gloved finger at the rectal opening for a moment before entering; the practitioner then cues the patient to bear down and bulge. As the patient bulges, the examiner enters, thereby curtailing the reflex so that the examination and treatment will be a bit more comfortable. On entering the rectal canal, the examiner palpates to the approximate depth of the first knuckle (distal phalangeal joint) to assess the external anal sphincter for tone and length. Ask the patient for a contraction at this point in order to assess both the strength of the external anal sphincter and its ability to relax. Again, ask the patient to bear down, and at this point increase the depth of insertion to the second knuckle; the examiner will feel the internal anal sphincter on the edges of the palpating finger and can assess its bogginess or firmness. At the distal tip of the finger, the examiner touches the edge of the puborectalis. Ask the patient to contract the muscles. If the contraction gently pulls the examiner's finger toward the pubic bone, that is an appropriate contraction. It provides information on muscle strength and on the firmness of the tissue that gives awareness of stool in the area. In addition, it should tell the examiner whether the muscles are acting appropriately or in an uncoordinated manner—known as "paradoxical pelvic floor function." If the muscles feel very overactive and firm, the patient may tend to experience a feeling of *tenesmus* or incomplete emptying. If particularly tight, the muscles themselves can occupy space, giving the patient the feeling that he or she is sitting on a golf or tennis ball.

To examine and assess the coccyx, a two-handed technique is required. The external digit finds the coccyx, while the internal palpating finger is turned pad side up to gently sink posterior to find the bony landmark.[43] The anterior face of the coccyx will be felt when the muscles and fascia have relaxed sufficiently. This may take longer in patients with muscle overactivity. Palpation of the coccyx enables the examiner to determine its level of flexion, whether it is midline or deviated to the right or left, and how much either or both coccygeus muscles are pulling. The examiner can also mobilize the coccyx in a posterior-anterior direction to assess the glide of the coccyx toward extension. Should the coccyx be positioned more posteriorly, the opposite—a posterior-anterior glide—will determine the coccyx's ability to move toward flexion.

Visceral Mobility Assessment

Because visceral restrictions have musculoskeletal connections, it is useful and advisable to assess visceral mobility in all pelvic pain patients. For example, a visceral mobility assessment of a patient with chronic constipation showed that full colon transit time had not been restored following scar tissue release therapy that was causing only a portion of the patient's pain; visceral restrictions were still present and were generating the pain.

Jean-Pierre Barral, a French osteopath and physical therapist, developed visceral manipulation as a form of manual therapy based on his theory of visceral mobility—i.e., the ability of each organ to display an inherent, normal tissue motion. According to the theory, each internal organ rotates on a physiological axis and has a relationship with its adjacent organ and, through fascial attachments, with the spine and other surrounding tissues. Like joints, organs must move to stay healthy.[58,59] When the mobility and motility of the viscera become dysfunctional, it can become apparent as a viscerosomatic reflex at a segmental level. For example, a facilitated segment (a vertebral body rotation), which creates spinal pain at the T10–L2 areas, when provoked can be a segmentally related visceral pathology. Organ dysfunction can present as provoked pain to corresponding segmental levels, which can be identified through palpation—and should be treated.[60]

Core Assessment

Weakness in the core muscles or an imbalance in the musculoskeletal system can create a slew of different dysfunctions in the back, pelvis, sacroiliac joint, ligaments, discs, and hip joints. These dysfunctions may eventually lead to such other disorders as osteoarthritis, degenerative disk disease, incontinence, and prolapsed pelvic organs. In relation to abdomino-pelvic pain syndromes, loss of core stabilization can cause the pelvic floor muscles to overcompensate, become overactive, and eventually cause pain.

It is important also to assess for diastasis recti. This separation of the right and left sides of the rectus abdominus can occur in men and women of all ages, although it is most common in women as a result of pregnancy. It can contribute to pelvic pain and weakness disorders due to the synergistic effect of the abdominal and pelvic floor muscles. The separation can occur at different points within the life cycle and may be caused by trauma—as with an abdominal surgery or an emergency infra-umbilical cesarean section—in pregnancy, and with advancing age. While men may complain of chronic constipation and low back pain, women add complaints of urinary incontinence, pelvic organ prolapse,[12,61] and pelvic pain. As Fitzgerald and Kotarinos assert, "optimal function of the pelvic floor muscles will not be achieved while any significant diastasis of the abdominal wall remains, i.e., closure of any diastasis is critically important in rehabilitation of this region."[62]

Digital palpation along the rectus where the two sides join is convenient and widely used in the clinic to determine if a patient has diastasis recti, but inter-rater reliability of results is poor. A more objective measurement is the use of calipers and real-time ultrasound, as used in medical research.[63]

Biofeedback and Real-Time Ultrasound Assessment

Biofeedback is a process that enables an individual to learn how to change her/his physiological activity in order to improve health and performance (The Association for Applied Psychophysiology and Biofeedback, Inc [AAPB]). For pelvic pain patients, it is most effectively used in conjunction with digital palpation that assesses muscle activity by helping to make patients aware of their breath, muscle activity, and muscle holding patterns; in so doing, it can also help them reduce voluntary muscle tension and change unwanted muscle activity through muscle downtraining.[64]

For use with a pelvic pain patient, internal sensors—an intra-vaginal sensor for women or intra-rectal sensor for men or women—or external sensors can be used, depending on symptoms and the severity of the internal pelvic floor muscle overactivity. The aim is to assess holding patterns or muscle overactivity. External sensors tend to be unreliable due to the "cross-talk" of external muscles.

Small, randomized research studies have demonstrated that patients who present with muscle overactivity can have either "heightened or decreased muscular electromyographic response to a stimulus,"[65] and this can be misleading if biofeedback is the sole methodology used to determine muscle overactivity. That is why surface electromyography (SEMG-assisted biofeedback) results should always be interpreted in conjunction with intra-vaginal or intra-rectal digital palpation to be certain that the finding of muscle shortening or overactivity holds. Biofeedback has certainly proven to be a useful clinical tool that gives patients a window into their bodies, providing a visual or audible sense of muscle events or holding patterns and showing patients how their actions can change long-standing habits. But palpation skills that can confirm the diagnostic findings of biofeedback, or suggest another line of inquiry, are an essential complement to the biofeedback findings[26] and an essential ingredient in the practitioner's toolkit.

Real-time ultrasound (RTUS) is another clinical tool that can provide both the clinician and the patient the "dynamic study (real-time images) of muscle groups as they contract."[66] By using an ultrasound unit that can capture a picture on a screen, the RTUS helps the patient reeducate and recoordinate his or her muscle-firing patterns using neuromuscular cueing techniques. Even small muscle injuries, not to mention large injuries, can cause edema that may shut muscles down, thus creating inappropriate firing patterns. It has become evident that, in patients who present with chronic low back and pelvic-girdle pain, the issue is one of "altered neuromuscular control as opposed to decreased strength or functional capacity."[66] One of the compensations for this loss of neuromuscular control can be pelvic floor muscle overactivity. RTUS can serve as an adjunct to "display the subtleties of muscle behavior so that they can be discussed and modified."[66]

RTUS uses assorted ultrasound technologies and varying external and internal sensors to provide a range of information. For example, an ultrasound probe held on a patient's lateral abdomen can demonstrate the recruitment of the transverse abdominus and of how the external and internal obliques function during an activity. If the supine patient is then directed to lift a leg so as to simulate walking—the Active Straight Leg Raise (ALSR) test—the examiner can see the firing pattern of the muscles of the trunk as it relates to the functional task of walking. With expert "translation" of the findings, this picture can identify which muscle is overactive or which may not be activated enough during the task. With appropriate cueing by the practitioner, the patient can work on recruiting the correct muscles, redirecting the muscle, and normalizing the pattern required.

Using an ultrasound transducer and placing the head supra-pubically enables the practitioner to view the bladder neck, bladder, and an outline of the pelvic floor muscles. Asking the patient to contract the pelvic floor muscles, the practitioner will view movement of the bladder, which demonstrates the symmetrical or asymmetrical firing patterns of the pelvic floor muscles. This can also be a useful tool for patients with urinary urgency and frequency, as the RTUS can actually demonstrate to a patient that his or her bladder is indeed empty or barely full. It thus provides a visual and scientific "contradiction" of a patient's belief that his or her bladder filled to capacity during the physical treatment session.

An internal sensor—a long circumferential wand—can assess vaginal and rectal pelvic floor function. The rectal sensor is inserted and shows layers of the external and internal anal sphincters and puborectalis muscles. It enables the examiner to detect thinness or lacerations in the layers that can lead to symptoms of involuntary flatulence or fecal soiling. This methodology also serves as a biofeedback tool for appropriate strengthening and deep fiber recruitment.

CONCLUSION

The physical therapy evaluation of patients presenting with pelvic pain requires a range of often highly complex observations and assessments. In a very complicated patient, multiple evaluation sessions may be needed to obtain all the objective information required and to measure the various sources of the patient's complaints.

REFERENCES

1. Hilton S, Vandyken C. The puzzle of pelvic pain—a rehabilitation framework for balancing tissue dysfunction and central sensitization, I: pain physiology and evaluation for the physical therapist. *J Women Health Phys Ther*. 2011; 35(3): 103–113.

2. Bo K, Berghmans B, Morkved S, Van Kampen M. *Evidence-Based Physical Therapy for the Pelvic Floor*. 1st ed. Philadelphia, PA: Churchill Livingstone Elsevier; 2007.

3. Bergeron S, Lord M-J. The integration of pelviperineal re-education and cognitive-behavioural therapy in the multidisciplinary treatment of the sexual pain disorders. *Sex Relation Ther*. 2003;18(2): 135–141.

4. Haefner HK, Collins ME, Davis GD, et al. The vulvodynia guideline. *J Low Genit Tract Dis*. 2005;9(1):40–51.

5. FitzGerald MP, Kotarinos R. Rehabilitation of the short pelvic floor. I: Background and patient evaluation. *Int Urogynecol J*. 2003;14(4):261–268.

6. Weiss JM. Pelvic floor myofascial trigger points: manual therapy for interstitial cystitis and the urgency-frequency syndrome. *J Urol*. 2001;166(6): 2226–2231.

7. Calais-Germain B. *The Female Pelvis: Anatomy and Exercises*. Seattle, WA: Eastland Press; 2003.

8. Barral JP, Mercier P. *Visceral Manipulation*. Seattle, WA: Eastland Press; 2005.

9. Ashton-Miller JA, DeLancey JO. Functional anatomy of the female pelvic floor. *Ann N Y Acad Sci*. 2007;1101(1):266–296.

10. Laycock J, Haslam J. *Therapeutic Management of Incontinence and Pelvic Pain: Pelvic Organ Disorders*. London: Springer; 2002.

11. Sapsford R, Bullock-Saxton J, Markwell S. *Women's Health: A Textbook for Physiotherapists*. London: WB Saunders; 1998.

12. Lee DG. *The Pelvic Girdle: An Integration of Clinical Expertise and Research*. 4th ed. Philadelphia, PA: Churchill Livingstone Elsevier; 2011.

13. Wesselmann U, Lai J. Mechanisms of referred visceral pain: uterine inflammation in the adult virgin rat results in neurogenic plasma extravasation in the skin. *Pain*. 1997;73(3):309–317.

14. Ferrero S, Esposito F, Abbamonte LH, Anserini P, Remorgida V, Ragni N. Quality of sex life in women with endometriosis and deep dyspareunia. *Fertil Steril*. 2005;83(3):573–579.

15. Whitmore K, Siegel JF, Kellogg-Spadt S. Interstitial cystitis/painful bladder syndrome as a cause of sexual pain in women: a diagnosis to consider. *J Sex Med*. 2007;4(3):720–727.

16. Porpora MG, Picarelli A, Prosperi Porta R, Di Tola M, D'Elia C, Cosmi EV. Celiac disease as a cause of chronic pelvic pain, dysmenorrhea, and deep dyspareunia. *Obstet Gynecol*. 2002;99(5):937–939.

17. Fass R, Fullerton S, Naliboff B, Hirsh T, Mayer EA. Sexual dysfunction in patients with irritable bowel syndrome and non-ulcer dyspepsia. *Digestion*. 1998; 59(1):79–85.

18. Vecchiet L, Giamberardino MA, Dragani L, Albe-Fessard D. Pain from renal/ureteral calculosis: evaluation of sensory thresholds in the lumbar area. *Pain*. 1989;36(3):289–295.

19. Lampe A, Solder E, Ennemoser A, Schubert C, Rumpold G, Sollner W. Chronic pelvic pain and previous sexual abuse. *Obstet Gynecol*. 2000;96(6): 929–933.

20. Baker PK. Musculoskeletal origins of chronic pelvic pain. Diagnosis and treatment. *Obstet Gynecol Clin North Am*. 1993;20(4):719–742.

21. Pukall CF, Smith KB, Chamberlain SM. Provoked vestibulodynia. *Women Health*. 2007;3(5):583–592.

22. Reissing ED, Brown C, Lord MJ, Binik YM, Khalife S. Pelvic floor muscle functioning in women with vulvar vestibulitis syndrome. *J Psychosom Obstet Gynaecol*. 2005;26(2):107–113.

23. Wall LL, DeLancey JO. The politics of prolapse: a revisionist approach to disorders of the pelvic floor in women. *Perspect Biol Med*. 1991;34(4):486–496.

24. Bump RC, Mattiasson A, Bo K, et al. The standardization of terminology of female pelvic organ prolapse and pelvic floor dysfunction. *Am J Obstet Gynecol*. Jul 1996;175(1):10–17.

25. Messelink B, Benson T, Berghmans B, et al. Standardization of terminology of pelvic floor muscle function and dysfunction: report from the Pelvic

Floor Clinical Assessment Group of the International Continence Society. *Neurourol Urodyn*. 2005; 24(4):374–380.

26. Bergeron S, Binik YM, Khalife S, Pagidas K. Vulvar vestibulitis syndrome: a critical review. *Clin J Pain*. 1997;13(1):27–42.

27. Hartmann EH, Nelson CA. The perceived effectiveness of physical therapy treatment on women complaining of chronic vulvar pain and diagnosed with either vulvar vestibulitis syndrome or dysesthetic vulvodynia. *J Women Health Phys Ther*. 2001;25:13–18.

28. Fenton BW. Limbic associated pelvic pain: a hypothesis to explain the diagnostic relationships and features of patients with chronic pelvic pain. *Med Hypotheses*. 2007;69(2):282–286.

29. Goetsch MF. Surgery combined with muscle therapy for dyspareunia from vulvar vestibulitis: an observational study. *J Reprod Med*. 2007; 52(7):597–603.

30. Rosenbaum TY. Pelvic floor involvement in male and female sexual dysfunction and the role of pelvic floor rehabilitation in treatment: a literature review. *J Sex Med*. 2007;4(1):4–13.

31. Verit FF, Verit A, Yeni E. The prevalence of sexual dysfunction and associated risk factors in women with chronic pelvic pain: a cross-sectional study. *Arch Gynecol Obstet*. 2006;274(5):297–302.

32. Bergeron S, Brown C, Lord MJ, Oala M, Binik YM, Khalife S. Physical therapy for vulvar vestibulitis syndrome: a retrospective study. *J Sex Marital Ther*. 2002;28(3):183–192.

33. Peters KM, Carrico DJ, Kalinowski SE, Ibrahim IA, Diokno AC. Prevalence of pelvic floor dysfunction in patients with interstitial cystitis. *Urology*. 2007;70(1):16–18.

34. Peters KM, Carrico DJ. Frequency, urgency, and pelvic pain: treating the pelvic floor versus the epithelium. *Curr Urol Rep*. 2006;7(6):450–455.

35. Rehman I, Oyama IA, Rejba A, Lukban JC, Fletcher E. Modified thiele massage as therapeutic intervention for female patients with interstitial cystitis and high-tone pelvic floor dysfunction. *Urology*. 2004;64(5):862–865.

36. Dumoulin C, Hay-Smith J. Pelvic floor muscle training versus no treatment for urinary incontinence in women: a Cochrane systematic review. *Eur J Phys Rehabil Med*. 2008;44(1):47–63.

37. Hay-Smith EJ, Bo K, Berghmans LC, Hendriks HJ, de Bie RA, van Waalwijk van Doorn ES. Pelvic floor muscle training for urinary incontinence in women. *Cochrane Database Syst Rev*. 2006(1):CD001407.

38. Dannecker C, Wolf V, Raab R, Hepp H, Anthuber C. EMG-biofeedback assisted pelvic floor muscle training is an effective therapy of stress urinary or mixed incontinence: a 7-year experience with 390 patients. *Arch Gynecol Obstet*. 2005;273(2):93–97.

39. Prendergast SA, Weiss JM. Screening for musculoskeletal causes of pelvic pain. *Clin Obstet Gynecol*. 2003;46(4):773–782.

40. Mein EA, Richards DD, McMillin DL, McPartland JM, Nelson CD. Physiological regulation through manual therapy. *Physical Medicine and Rehabilitation: State of the Art Reviews*. Vol. 14, no 1. Philadelphia, PA: Hanley & Belfus; 2000.

41. Van Buskirk RL. Nociceptive reflexes and the somatic dysfunction: a model. *J Am Osteopath Assoc*. 1990;90(9):792–794, 797–809

42. American Physical Therapy Association. *Guide to Physical Therapist Practice*. 2nd ed: American Physical Therapy Association; 2003.

43. Hull M, Corton MM. Evaluation of the levator ani and pelvic wall muscles in levator ani syndrome. *Urol Nurs*. 2009;29(4):225–231.

44. Prendergast S, Rummer E. *Demystifying Pudendal Neuralgia as a Source of Pain: A Physical Therapist's Approach*. Chicago, IL: International Pelvic Pain Society Annual Meeting, 2009.

45. Hesch J. *The Hesch Method of Treating Sacroiliac Joint Dysfunction: Integrating the SI, Symphysis Pubis, Pelvic, Hip and Lumbar Spine, Basic and Intermediate Workbook* Henderson; Self-publish; 2010.

46. Dalton E, Aston J, Gracovetsky S, et al. *Dynamic Body: Exploring Form, Expanding Function*. Oklahoma: Freedom From Pain Institute; 2011.

47. Prather H, Hunt D, Fournie A, Clohisy JC. Early intra-articular hip disease presenting with posterior pelvic and groin pain. *PM&R*. 2009;1(9): 809–815.

48. Brooks AG, Domb BG. Acetabular labral tear and postpartum hip pain. *Obstet Gynecol*. 2012; 120(5):1093–1098.

49. Travell JG, Simons DG. *Myofascial Pain and Dysfunction: The Trigger Point Manual. Vol. 2: The Lower Extremities*. Baltimore, MD: Williams & Wilkins; 1992.

50. Weiss JM. Chronic pelvic pain and myofascial trigger points. *Pain Clinic*. 2000;2(6):13–18.

51. Bernstein AM, Philips HC, Linden W, Fenster H. A psychophysiological evaluation of female urethral syndrome: evidence for a muscular abnormality. *J Behav Med*. 1992;15(3):299–312.

52. Schmidt RA, Vapnek JM. Pelvic floor behavior and interstitial cystitis. *Semin Urol*. 1991;9(2):154–159.

53. Loos MJ, Scheltinga MR, Mulders LG, Roumen RM. The Pfannenstiel incision as a source of chronic pain. *Obstet Gynecol*. 2008;111(4):839–846.

54. Hollinshead WH. *Textbook of Anatomy*. 4th ed. Philadelphia, PA: Harper & Row Publishers; 1985.

55. Castello K. Myofascial syndromes. In: *Chronic Pelvic Pain: An Integrated Approach*. Philadelphia, PA: Saunders; 1998:251–266.

56. Trutnovsky G, Guzman-Rojas R, Martin A, Dietz HP. Pelvic floor dysfunction—does menopause duration matter? *Maturitas.* 2013;76(2):134–138.

57. Haslam J. Pelvic floor muscle exercise in the treatment of urinary incontinence. In: *Therapeutic Management of Incontinence and Pelvic Pain: Pelvic Organ Disorders.* London: Springer 2007: 89–94.

58. Russell J. What is visceral manipulation? *Directions in Physiotherapy.* Autumn 2008.

59. Barral JP. *Urogenital Manipulation.* Seattle, WA: Eastland Press; 1993.

60. Nelson KE, Glonek T. *Somatic Dysfunction in Osteopathic Family Medicine.* Baltimore, MD: Lippincott Williams & Wilkins; 2007.

61. Spitznagle TM, Leong FC, Van Dillen LR. Prevalence of diastasis recti abdominis in a urogynecological patient population. *Int Urogynecol J Pelvic Floor Dysfunct.* 2007;18(3):321–328.

62. FitzGerald MP, Kotarinos R. Rehabilitation of the short pelvic floor. II: Treatment of the patient with the short pelvic floor. *Int Urogynecol J Pelvic Floor Dysfunct.* 2003;14(4):269–275.

63. Chiarello CM, McAuley JA. Concurrent validity of calipers and ultrasound imaging to measure interrecti distance. *J Orthop Sports Phys Ther.* 2013;43(7):495–503.

64. Wise D, Anderson R. *A Headache in the Pelvis: A New Understanding and Treatment for Chronic Pelvic Pain Syndromes.* 6th ed. Occidental, CA: National Center for Pelvic Pain; 2012.

65. Gentilcore-Saulnier E, McLean L, Goldfinger C, Pukall CF, Chamberlain S. Pelvic floor muscle assessment outcomes in women with and without provoked vestibulodynie and the impact of a physical therapy program. *J Sex Med.* 2010;7(2):1003–1022.

66. Whittaker JL. *Ultrasound Imaging for Rehabilitation of the Lumbopelvic Region: A Clinical Approach.* Philadelphia, PA: Churchill Livingstone Elsevier; 2007.

18

The Physical Therapy Approach to Pelvic Pain

Treatment

AMY STEIN, MPT, DPT, BCB-PMD, IF

As mentioned in the physical therapy evaluation chapter, pelvic floor physical therapy has proven to be an invaluable component of treatment* for the musculoskeletal causes of functional pelvic pain.[21,1,22,23,24,13,25] A conservative and extremely effective treatment option for men, women, and children, physical therapy offers a holistic approach to help address the biopsychosocial aspects of the patient's pain.

Treatment may consist of a range of such manual therapies as neural mobilization, connective tissue and joint mobilization, and myofascial trigger-point release to address the medical aspects of chronic pelvic pain; behavioral therapies for muscle retraining; treatments to address central sensitization; therapeutic exercises for range of motion (ROM) and for core strengthening; and an assortment of modalities like biofeedback, real-time ultrasound, low-level laser,

---

* While there are a range of studies dealing with pelvic floor dysfunction as it relates to chronic pelvic pain syndromes,[1,2,3,4,5,6] sexual dysfunction,[7,8,9,10] painful bladder syndromes,[11,12,13,14] and incontinence,[15,16,17] a large portion of the literature is in the realm of urogynecology and deals with pelvic prolapse and incontinence.[18,19,20] Many of these studies, however, lack stringent study protocols and offer only a limited number of randomized controlled studies (RTCs). In this review of the manual therapy techniques and modalities commonly used by physical therapists, references provided are for example only and by no means represent all published data. But we wholeheartedly endorse the work of Kari Bo and her colleagues, *Evidence-Based Physical Therapy for the Pelvic Floor,* and we applaud its affirmation that "good clinical practice always should be individualized and should be based on a combination of clinical experience, knowledge from high-quality RCTs and patient preferences ... [as well as] respect, empathy, and strong ethical grounding."

and other modalities that may be suggested by the treating physical therapist to complement these treatment approaches. Whatever the recommended treatment, the patient's symptoms should be repeatedly reassessed for improvement or progression. Such validated treatment tools as the Visual Analog Scale (VAS) pain scale[26] and a bladder, bowel, and/or sexual function scale should be used during and after each treatment session and home program In order to monitor the patient's symptoms and progression. The references provided throughout this chapter are for example only, and by no means represent all published data.

MANUAL THERAPIES

Through their increasing involvement in treating chronic pelvic pain (CPP), physical therapists have developed valuable tools of manual therapy that can provide both mobility and effective analgesic response throughout the body tissues to deal with the many physical abnormalities that generate the pain.[27,1,10,3] As one expert states,

> It is appropriate that the role of the short, painful and/or hypertonic pelvic floor in the development of chronic genitourinary conditions has now begun to inform physiotherapeutic interventions aimed at rehabilitation; whether the somatic abnormalities are primary or secondary. Research is now showing that specialized manual therapy is clinically beneficial.[31]

Myofascial Release and Myofascial Trigger Point Release

As noted in the evaluation chapter 17, myofascial pain is associated with myofascial trigger points found in skeletal muscle or in the fascia, the fine sheet of connective tissue that surrounds, separates, or connects muscles, organs, and other soft structures of the body—and studies have shown that these trigger points and tissue restrictions are key components of pain in as many as 93% of patients in a pain clinic.[28]

Travell and Simons define a "trigger point" as a highly irritable spot in a nodule occurring in a palpably taut band of the muscle or fascia, and biopsy tests have shown them to be hyperirritable and electrically active muscle spindles in general muscle tissue.[28] The nodule containing these trigger points feels like a knot or a small lump that can range from the size of a pinhead to the size of a pea.

Whatever their size, trigger points can give rise to characteristic referred pain in clear and consistent patterns, to tenderness, and to autonomic phenomena.[29] Muscles containing trigger points are characteristically short with limited ROM, are weak, and present with increased tone, loss of coordination, and substitution patterns.[23,24,30] As a result, the muscles have to work harder to produce the same effects, and the surrounding muscles may become altered, potentially disturbing the proprioceptive, nociceptive, and autonomic functions of the affected region.[28]

Trigger points can go unrecognized unless a skilled practitioner actively palpates and locates them in the muscle tissue. Once they are located, the application of sustained pressure to reduce fascial restrictions can reduce the pain, improve range of motion, relax the muscles, and assist in relieving any nerve irritation or compression. Techniques of strumming,

kneading, oscillations, vibrations, stripping of the muscle fibers, and myofascial shortening and lengthening may also be used. Stretching and such proprioceptive neuromuscular facilitation as contraction/relaxation, reciprocal inhibition, active release technique, and other muscle energy techniques will also help facilitate muscle relaxation and lengthening. In all these manual techniques, the therapist must address superficial tissues, bony contours, muscle play, and muscle tone while looking for restrictions at the depth, direction, and angle of maximal limitation. Trigger point injections and dry needling may also be recommended as an adjunct to the manual treatment.[23,24]

Manual therapies of myofascial and trigger point release, as demonstrated in Figure 18.1, have been found to be highly effective. In women with interstitial cystitis/painful bladder syndrome, Fitzgerald et al. found that a significantly higher proportion responded to treatment with myofascial physical therapy versus global therapeutic massage, achieving an overall improvement in symptoms.[31] Weiss reported an 83% reduction in symptoms, including a reduction in neurogenic bladder inflammation, a decrease in central nervous sensitization, and a reduction in pelvic floor hypertonicity through manual release of myofascial trigger points.[13] And Anderson et al. reported a 72% improvement—described as "moderate to marked"—in chronic pelvic pain and urinary symptoms in men, through a combination of myofascial trigger point release of the pelvic floor muscles and paradoxical relaxation.

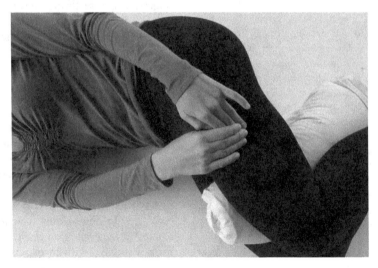

FIGURE 18.1: Myofascial trigger point release technique.

Heal Pelvic Pain by Amy Stein, DPT

Connective Tissue Manipulation

Connective tissue manipulation, as demonstrated in Figure 18.2, is the movement of one layer of skin over the other to release tension in the tissue and to increase ROM in the joint or the limb. It is effective for a range of subcutaneous connective tissue restrictions; these restrictions should be assessed, and manipulation should be performed as indicated throughout the course of pelvic floor physical therapy.

Pelvic pain patients typically present with connective tissue abnormalities in and around the abdomino-pelvic region, lower extremities, back, and buttocks. As an example, restrictions in the inferomedial buttocks and the ischiorectal fossa may also contribute to the patient's pain and cause sensitivity to tight clothing and underwear, and upon the assumption of certain seated positions.[23,24] Trigger points and any neural tension also commonly respond to connective tissue manipulation.[23,24]

The manipulation creates a sensation of a sharp scratch—the so-called "nails" sensation—and the tighter the tissue, the sharper the sensation. When the tension is released, the blood flow to the area increases, thereby removing toxins from that region, decreasing pain, and ultimately allowing more movement to occur. With each treatment, there is further reduction in connective tissue tension, and this reduction can be maintained.

Scar Tissue Mobilization

Scar tissue and *adhesions*, fibrous bands of scar tissue that form between surfaces within the body, may result from such pelvic pain conditions as endometriosis or any abdomino-pelvic surgery. They may be superficial or deep, and they can adhere to the internal anatomy, including the reproductive organs, genitals, bladder, and the bowels.[32] These areas must therefore be mobilized to allow proper movement and to help mitigate the pain. Such manipulative mobilizations as stroking and strumming between fingers and thumbs on and around the scar have been shown to loosen the surrounding tissue and the scar itself, thereby easing any pain the scar or surrounding tissue may be causing or to which it may be contributing.[23,24]

Visceral Manipulation

Adhesions, abnormal tone, or displacement may result in disharmonious movement between internal organs, which in turn may lead to chronic irritation and pain. Visceral manipulation uses gentle palpation and manual therapy to evaluate and correct the imbalances.

Developed by Jean-Pierre Barral, a French osteopath, along with several of his colleagues, visceral manipulation is based on the understanding that the health of any system in the body is measured by its ability to move. When that ability is lessened or restricted over an extended period of time, the system itself becomes damaged. Barral's techniques of visceral manipulation both identify and can correct the mobility dysfunctions. They are aimed at restoring the body's mobility and inherent

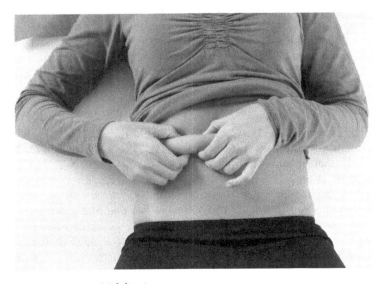

FIGURE 18.2: Connective Tissue Mobilization.

Heal Pelvic Pain by Amy Stein, DPT

motility—and thereby restoring also the health of the body's systems.[33]

Specifically, visceral manipulation is aimed at adhesions, fixations, organ ptosis, and viscerospasms throughout the visceral systems of the thorax, abdomen, and pelvis. Barral's reasoning is simple: Since it is rare that just a single organ system in the body is affected, the overall effect of treatment is to create a response in the tissues similar to the analgesic responses of acupuncture[34,35,36]—that is, to stimulate neurotransmitters (endorphins, serotonin, etc.) that in turn will stimulate the hypothalamus, pituitary, thyroid, and adrenal glands, producing hormones like. Thyroid-stimulating hormone and Follicle-stimulating hormone (TSH, FSH), and adrenaline. Barral's studies suggest that tissue metabolism is improved and the production of serotonin is increased by his manual techniques; this, in turn, stimulates greater cerebral activity and increased activity in the smooth muscles of the blood vessels, digestive tract, and respiratory tract.[33]

Visceral manipulation allows therapists to deal with the tension that occurs throughout the viscera, specifically within the abdominal and pelvic organs. It is suggested that the viscera and the musculoskeletal systems interact and that the visceral spasm therefore produces muscular pain and tension; the reverse will also be true. Effective treatment, therefore, includes releasing the tension in both systems simultaneously. Hartmann's research showed that when treating women with vulvodynia (either localized or generalized), visceral manipulation was included in a treatment regimen that led to a 71% improvement in overall symptoms, a 62% improvement in sexual function, and a 50% increase in quality-of-life issues.[3] Physical therapy, including visceral manipulation, is therefore now included in the multidisciplinary approach to treating women with vulvodynia.[22]

Neural Mobilization

The nervous system is a continuous structure throughout the body that should slide, glide, bend, stretch, and move as we move.[37] Anything that interrupts the normal movement of neural tissues—a sacroiliac dysfunction, a bulging disk, a muscle spasm, scar tissue or swollen compartments—will cause pain, will decrease blood supply to the nerve, and may displace the myelin sheath.

Neural mobilization helps restore mobility to the neural tissue through manual treatment.

The technique is a gentle, flossing-like technique with active or passive muscle release, aimed at freeing up a specific compromised nerve from its surrounding structures. In addition, myofascial trigger points, connective tissue restrictions, and any imbalance of joint mobility and stability need to be addressed if they are contributing to the adverse neural tension. As noted in the evaluation chapter, with chronic pelvic pain, it is commonly the pudendal nerve and other surrounding nerves that may be compromised; neural mobilization can free these nerves, which is essential to facilitate healing.

Joint Mobilization

Joints in and around the pelvis may be hypermobile or hypomobile, and both conditions can cause or contribute to pelvic pain. Also, because of networked innervation, it's not uncommon to find that abnormalities in the lumbar vertebrae, joint capsules, discs, hip joints, and ligaments also lead to chronic pelvic pain, according to King Baker's work.[38] Joint normalization is therefore often necessary—along with soft-tissue corrections. Indeed, its use is widespread, reportedly used by 78% of therapists treating women with localized provoked vulvodynia.[3]

Pelvic floor disorders must not be seen as purely isolated problems, it is important to note that skilled stretching and mobilization of associated joints may indeed be indicated when impairment is present, especially in the spine, hips, pubic symphysis, and sacroiliac and sacrococcygeal articulations.[39] Oscillations and vibrations may also be applied, while thrust techniques, which require advanced training, should only be performed by qualified physical therapists. Stability exercises may also be recommended, as demonstrated in Figure 18.3.

BEHAVIORAL THERAPIES FOR PELVIC FLOOR MUSCLE RETRAINING: MOTOR LEARNING AND MOTOR CONTROL

Pelvic floor muscle retraining helps develop or improve motor control for bladder, bowel, and sexual function and pelvic pain.[40,41] People suffering from chronic pelvic pain, dyspareunia, or any urgency-frequency dysfunction tend to present with overactive pelvic floor muscles.[42,12,30,43,44] This overactivity could be the result of the person developing holding patterns, which eventually

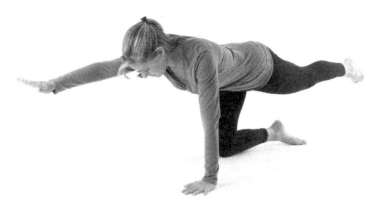

FIGURE 18.3: A Stability Exercise.

Heal Pelvic Pain by Amy Stein, DPT

result in shortened muscle fibers and connective tissues. This, in turn, perpetuates a continued cycle of dysfunction and pain.

Behavioral therapy is therefore a necessary adjunct to pelvic floor muscle rehabilitation, and such strategies as the operant learning model and cognitive behavioral therapy should be integrated into the treatment approach in order to help break this cycle of dysfunction and pain. Education and training should focus on proper motor control—e.g., relaxing the pelvic floor muscles with voiding and with intercourse rather than contracting or "tensing" the muscles out of fear of pain. This is learned by practice in discerning the difference between contracting, elongating, and relaxing the pelvic floor and is achieved through verbal cueing, biofeedback, and other techniques. Such behavioral modifications as scheduled voiding, urge control, posture retraining, and pelvic floor muscle relaxation and self-massage prior to or following sexual activity are also key to pelvic floor rehabilitation.

Patients can also apply helpful techniques at home—for example, stretching (i.e., Pelvic floor stretch shown in Figure 18.4), external massage, or use of a dilator or internal massage device—to help eliminate myofascial trigger points and to further elongate the shortened pelvic floor and surrounding muscles and tissues. A female with pain at the vaginal introitus can also passively stretch the tissues at the introitus.[45] Stress management, relaxation breathing, pelvic floor muscle relaxation, relaxing by taking a walk, soaking in a hot bath, and practicing yoga and meditation are all examples of behavioral modifications that can help with physiological quieting.

Pelvic muscle exercises (Kegels) are not indicated in the case of overactive or shortened pelvic floor muscles. These exercises help strengthen the pelvic floor muscles in the case of incontinence; if the patient is experiencing only pain and not leaking, however, it is likely that the pelvic floor muscles are not weak, but rather are shortened or tight, and pelvic floor muscle exercises may further exacerbate the shortening and tightening. If there is urinary or fecal leakage, lengthening these painful muscles through manual therapy will in many cases allow for proper ROM, and the leakage may subside. If the leaking does not subside, once trigger points are eliminated and muscles are restored to functional length, then pelvic floor muscles exercises can be administered under the guidance of an experienced pelvic floor physical therapist.

Bladder and Bowel Retraining

Regulation of bladder and bowel function is an essential part of the treatment of abdomino-pelvic pain. The pelvic floor muscles need to be relaxed during bladder and bowel emptying, and if the patient presents with a paradoxical contraction, muscle reeducation may be required.

Patients need to be in a comfortable and supportive position for voiding—commonly, with a stool under their feet for certain toilets. Toileting should not be rushed, a partial squat should be avoided, and straining should be avoided because of the pressure and stress it places on the pelvic floor muscle.[46]

Muscle reeducation can be a slow process for patients with a long history of overactive pelvic floor muscles. Distraction, breathing with voiding, imagery, and biofeedback are some of the tools that will help the process, helping

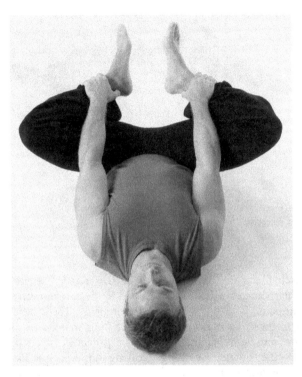

FIGURE 18.4: Pelvic Floor Stretch.

Heal Pelvic Pain by Amy Stein, DPT

the muscles relax so as to eliminate post-void dribble, bladder and bowel frequency, urgency, retention, hesitancy, and pain.

Bladder Reeducation

In addition, bladder reeducation should include reminders against pushing, training in the elimination of dietary irritants—alcohol, caffeine, carbonated beverages—strictures against restricting water intake, and lessons in the need to rehydrate in order to progressively expand bladder capacity. This reeducation should be followed at home and over an extended time period. The physical therapist needs to guide the patient through progressive timed voiding, which will help decrease frequency as well as delay false bladder urges. Some studies have shown that Kegels help inhibit bladder reflex, but again, increasing contractile activity with already overactive pelvic floor muscles may further shorten or tighten the pelvic floor.

Bowel Reeducation

For bowel retraining, constipation and straining must be avoided, so it is essential to make sure the patient has full awareness of and coordination in the abdominal and pelvic floor muscles, which may require muscle reeducation in patients presenting with a paradoxical contraction.[47] Soluble and insoluble fiber and a sufficient amount of water should be added to the patient's diet when appropriate to facilitate easier and softer bowel movements. Establish a set time for voiding each day, and teach a supportive posture that creates optimal pelvic floor relaxation. For example, squatting or placing a stool under the patient's feet may increase hip flexion and thereby increase the anorectal angle.[48,49] In addition, such techniques as breathing with voiding and colon massage may further facilitate bowel movements. In cases of bowel frequency and urgency, it is important to educate the patient on urge-delay and progressive timed voiding.

Restoration of Sexual Function

When pelvic pain is a factor in sexual dysfunction, pelvic floor muscles and connective tissues often exhibit hypersensitivity, tenderness, and overactivity. Internal and external massage may help reduce tender points, ameliorate any tissue restrictions, and relax and lengthen these muscles. As part of the at-home program, dilators and internal massage tools may help normalize the tone of the muscles and desensitize hypersensitive tissue. Physical therapists typically instruct a patient in the use of a dilator along with instruction in relaxation techniques and using biofeedback to teach the muscles not to tense. Hip, trunk, and pelvic floor stretching can also assist in alleviating pelvic pain affecting sexual activity.

Behavioral training techniques incorporated into the at-home program can help relax the pelvic floor muscles at set times throughout the day and especially during sexual activity. Other strategies, such as using ice after sexual activity or taking a hot bath, may also be suggested. If the patient has experienced changes in bladder and bowel function, assigning the appropriate exercises and techniques to restore those functions to normalcy is also recommended. Research has shown a significant improvement in sexual function through physical therapy treatment in as many as 87% of women suffering from vulvodynia and similar disorders,[3] while 70% of male patients with sexual dysfunction experienced a significant improvement in symptoms.[50]

ADDRESSING CENTRAL SENSITIZATION

Both central and peripheral sensitization is common in patients suffering from chronic pelvic pain; simply put, the patient feels more pain with less provocation. Central sensitization involves changes in the central nervous system, specifically in the brain and spinal cord, due to increases in nociceptive sensitivity. As seen through imaging techniques and electrophysiology, central sensitization constitutes an increase in excitability in the synaptic neurons in the central nociceptive pathways; the increase results in hypersensitivity, allodynia, and hyperalgesia.[51]

Peripheral sensitization, an increase in sensitivity of peripheral nerve endings, represents a form of functional plasticity of the nociceptor. The nociceptor can change from being simply a noxious stimulus detector to a detector of non-noxious stimuli; it thus becomes hypersensitive. The action potential in the impaired or surrounding nerve endings is decreased; thus, a smaller stimulus sets off the action potential.

The heart of the matter, according to Hilton, is that "the pain response operates within the entire system of nociceptive input, peripheral neurogenic sensitization, and central sensitization. Intervention and treatment options are guided by the estimation of the relative contribution of each dynamic system."[52] The nociceptive input is driven by afferent fibers that travel to the spinal cord and cross the synapse to the dorsal horn. These fibers use either glutamate or substance P as neurotransmitters, which travel via pathways to the thalamus; it is there that the pain is registered. Nociceptor neuron sensitivity is modulated by a large variety of mediators in the extracellular space.

This sensitization issue needs to be addressed along with the dysfunction itself; the aim is to "reorganize" and "reeducate" the neuromatrix in chronic pelvic pain patients. This can be achieved with the guidance of a trained physical therapist addressing the issue through education on pain. It may include such techniques as relaxation training, guided imagery, mindfulness meditation, and yoga. This multipronged approach to addressing central and peripheral sensitivities, in combination with tissue and biomechanical dysfunctions, has proven to be an effective strategy for the pelvic pain patient.[52]

THERAPEUTIC EXERCISES

Both stretching and cardiovascular exercises are recommended therapies for patients with pelvic pain.

Stretching

Exercises are helpful in stretching and lengthening the tight or shortened muscles found in many pelvic pain patients. A couple examples of stretches are demonstrated in Figures 18.5 and 18.6. Care must be taken to avoid overstretching any soft tissues or tissues with trigger points or connective tissue restrictions. Skeletal muscle responds to passive mechanical stretching through sarcomerogenesis, which is the creation and serial deposition of new sarcomere units. Sarcomerogenesis is critical to muscle function, because it gradually restores the muscle to a position of optimal operating mechanics. Recent studies suggest that a restoration of normal architecture and physiological function might be possible through a gradual lengthening of the musculotendinous unit when stretched at a rate of 1 mm per day.[53]

Cardiovascular Exercise

Cardiovascular fitness has been proven to increase endorphins and enhance mental health and overall well-being. It is a boon to conditioning and flexibility and is essential to increasing blood flow and thus for the healing process. A cardio fitness regimen should therefore be incorporated into a pelvic pain patient's weekly

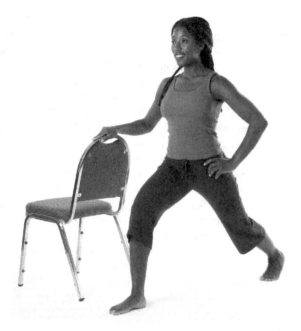

FIGURE 18.5: Hip Flexor Stretch.

Heal Pelvic Pain by Amy Stein, DPT

routine. As recommended by the American Heart Association (AHA), that regimen should consist of cardio exercise five days a week for 20 minutes per day, or four days per week for 30 minutes per day. For the more severe cases, the patient may have to do the cardio routine in intervals throughout the day, until they can work up to the AHA-recommended guidelines.

Core Stabilization Exercises

The stability of the body's core—the spine, pelvis, hip, and shoulder girdle that the muscles and fascia of the trunk, pelvis, and abdomen support—is what maintains an individual's mobility, facilitating movement from the center of the body out to the extremities. The relationships among the muscles of the pelvic floor,

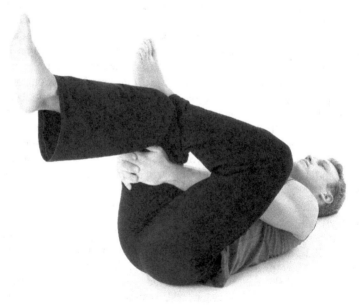

FIGURE 18.6: Hip External Rotation Stretch.

Heal Pelvic Pain by Amy Stein, DPT

deep back, diaphragm, and abdomen play an important role in this function; they also play a significant role in pelvic floor disorders. The connection among them can be seen in the co-contraction of the pelvic floor and abdominal muscles that occurs in coughing, sneezing, or laughing. This co-contraction is normal—unless there are active trigger points that further irritate the abdominal/pelvic musculature (including scarring, injury, or inflammation).[23]

Weakness in the core muscles or an imbalance in the musculoskeletal system can therefore create a slew of different dysfunctions in the back, pelvis, sacroiliac joint, ligaments, discs, and hip joints, which can result in pain in and around these areas. These dysfunctions may eventually lead to such other disorders as osteoarthritis, degenerative disk disease, incontinence, and prolapsed pelvic organs. Exercises that strengthen and balance the core muscles, which are listed in Box 18.1, may therefore also prevent pelvic floor disorders or mitigate them once they occur.

But if trigger points, fascial restrictions, hypertonicity in the muscles, skeletal malalignment, or acute injury have been identified in the patient, core strengthening exercises in these specific areas are not advised—at least not until the dysfunction is resolved. And at all times, caution should be taken lest strengthening exercises increase any pelvic, abdominal, or back pain.

Examples of some core exercises may include transverse abdominus and abdominal oblique isometric contractions, pelvic tilt, "bridge," (as shown in Figure 18.7) quadruped with opposite arm and leg raise (as shown in Figure 18.3), hip external and internal rotation exercises, squats, Kegel pelvic floor exercises (if appropriate and only after the hypertonicity of the pelvic floor and the pain have subsided), the plank and side plank. While Kegel exercises are effective in strengthening the pelvic floor, they have been overemphasized in the past;

it is important to remember that they may actually worsen symptoms in a patient experiencing pain or with hypertonic or shortened pelvic floor muscles.[7]

Patients with *diastasis recti* should also not perform any abdominal exercises until the separation of the right and left rectus abdominus muscles has been corrected, either through specific abdominal exercises or, in more extreme cases, through surgery.

Core strengthening exercises may also be appropriate for correcting the faulty postures so common in patients suffering pelvic pain. Indeed, such postures are a "contributing cause of weak, deconditioned muscles allowing for imbalances in the pelvis with formation of trigger points and hypertonicity, and as a result, pelvic pain."[54] In order to correct these faulty postures and resulting dysfunctions, certain muscles and tissues may need lengthening, while others need strengthening. A healthcare provider with extensive training in the musculoskeletal system can determine the specific lengthening or strengthening needs for each individual patient, and once the pain symptoms have subsided, exercises can further address core stability.

TREATMENT MODALITIES

A range of mechanistic modalities may effectively augment the physical therapy approach to pelvic floor dysfunction and pelvic pain, with varying and often highly individual and subjective results. Some of these modalities promote healing through both a physiological improvement and a placebo effect, and research has shown that they can positively impact pain conditions.[21] Until the evidence shows otherwise, some physical therapists will continue to use modalities as an adjunct to treatment, depending on the patient's needs.

Used as an evaluation tool to assess muscle activity, *visual/auditory biofeedback* provides instantaneous, performance-dependent, visual

---

BOX 18.1
THE CORE MUSCLES

- All of the abdominal muscles: rectus abdominus, external and internal obliques, transverse abdominus, diaphragm
- Back muscles: erector spinae, multifidus, quadratus lumborum
- Gluteal muscles: maximus, medius and minimus
- Hip flexors, external rotators, adductors, quadriceps and hamstrings
- Pelvic floor muscles

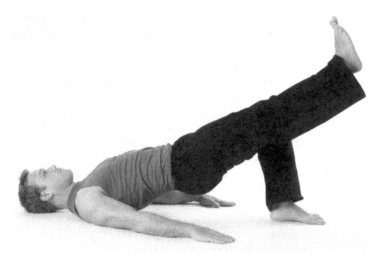

FIGURE 18.7: One-legged Bridge.

Heal Pelvic Pain by Amy Stein, DPT

and/or auditory information regarding the function of muscles; by increasing the patient's awareness, such information can also assist the patient in controlling and self-regulating that muscle activity. It is therefore an excellent treatment modality for reeducating patients in how to use their pelvic floor and abdominal muscles appropriately, thereby reducing pelvic pain and restoring proper bladder and bowel function.[55,56,57] In cases of pelvic floor dyssynergia, biofeedback has been proven to be more effective than laxatives.[58]

For pelvic floor muscle dysfunction, either electrodes are placed perianally or an internal vaginal or rectal sensor is used to detect muscle activity and transmit the information to a monitor. On the monitor, the patient can see what the muscles are doing during rest, activity, and while the patient is experiencing his or her pain symptoms. This visual feedback offers the kind of body awareness that enables patients to "teach" their overactive muscles to relax, which in turn reduces pain, thus reinforcing the "lesson." If the muscles are shortened, however, the biofeedback may not show any abnormal muscle activity, even though the patient may be experiencing pain and other symptoms of overactive pelvic floor muscles.

There are no set measurements of strength, coordination, and muscle control. It is believed, however, that if it proves difficult for the patient to contract and relax the pelvic floor muscles, incoordination may be an issue, preventing the muscles from fully relaxing, and contributing to pelvic pain and to bladder and bowel dysfunction.[13,23,24]

Low-level laser therapy (LLLT) emits photon light without heat, causing bio-stimulation at the cellular level to eliminate trigger points; the increased local microcirculation of the blood brings more oxygen to the cells and helps reduce inflammation. As distinct from other forms of laser therapy used for cutting or cauterizing tissues, LLLT uses power densities lower than those needed to heat tissue and emits low-intensity wave lengths either in scanning or spot form. It has been shown to relieve minor muscle and joint aches temporarily, to reduce pain and stiffness, relax muscles, decrease muscle spasms, break up scar adhesions, and increase lymph flow.

Real-time ultrasound can be used as a biofeedback tool for muscle reeducation. For example, the same information the examiner found in evaluating the firing pattern of muscles in a patient performing the Active Straight Leg Raise (see Evaluation Chap 17) becomes a cueing tool for the patient. By "feeling" which muscle is overactive or which muscle is not activated enough during the task, the patient is able to work on recruiting the correct muscles, redirecting the muscles, and normalizing the pattern.

Therapeutic ultrasound transmits low-intensity and low-frequency sound waves, warming the tissues and thus dilating the blood vessels to deliver more oxygen to the affected area. It has been used for acute and local inflammation, as well as for vestibular tenderness, showing most clinical benefits.

There is very little evidence to date that *electrical stimulation* itself alleviates chronic pelvic pain. One limited study, conducted among women suffering pelvic pain due to levator ani spasm, found pain reduction through vaginal electrical stimulation,[59] while studies from decades ago showed that electrogalvanic stimulation to the levator ani muscle produced some relief; such stimulation has also been shown clinically to *increase* pain in many patients. But no long-term studies on this subject have been conducted.[60,61,62]

Transcutaneous electrical nerve stimulation (TENS) is the application of mild electrical stimulation using skin electrodes near to or distant from an area of pain; it acts by interfering with the transmission of painful stimuli—the "pain gate" theory. It is an effective way to relieve pain in the abdominal, spinal, and sacral regions as well as on areas of the pelvic floor. Studies have shown that high-frequency TENS is more effective than placebo TENS, while low-frequency TENS is no more effective in reducing pain than placebo TENS.[63]

There is some evidence that therapies using *heat and cold* can produce a temporary reduction in pain.[64,65] *Moist heat* helps relax tight muscles and thus decrease pain caused by muscle tension or spasms; they also dilate the blood vessels, thus increasing circulation to the area, which helps promote healing. *Cold therapy*, by contrast, constricts the blood vessels, decreasing the inflammation in the area and thus also the pain.

CONCLUSION

Pelvic floor physical therapy is a key component of the biopsychosocial management of pelvic pain. Through weekly or biweekly hour-long treatment sessions,[45] physical therapists can help men, women, and children regain their physical and psychological balance, strengthen trusting relationships, and live a life of well-being. Treatment should be multidisciplinary and holistic, embracing stress management, pain management, nutritional counseling, support groups, and psychological services.

REFERENCES

1. Bergeron S, Lord M-J. The integration of pelvi-perineal re-education and cognitive-behavioural therapy in the multidisciplinary treatment of the sexual pain disorders. *Sex Relation Ther.* 2003;18(2):135–141.
2. Bergeron S, Binik YM, Khalife S, Pagidas K. Vulvar vestibulitis syndrome: a critical review. *Clin J Pain.* 1997;13(1):27–42.
3. Hartmann D, Strauhal MJ, Nelson CA. Treatment of women in the United States with localized, provoked vulvodynia: practice survey of women's health physical therapists. *J Reprod Med.* 2007;52(1):48–52.
4. Pukall CF, Smith KB, Chamberlain SM. Provoked vestibulodynia. *Women Health.* 2007;3(5):583–592.
5. Fenton BW. Limbic associated pelvic pain: a hypothesis to explain the diagnostic relationships and features of patients with chronic pelvic pain. *Med Hypotheses.* 2007;69(2):282–286.
6. Goetsch MF. Surgery combined with muscle therapy for dyspareunia from vulvar vestibulitis: an observational study. *J Reprod Med.* 2007;52(7):597–603.
7. Rosenbaum TY. Pelvic floor involvement in male and female sexual dysfunction and the role of pelvic floor rehabilitation in treatment: a literature review. *J Sex Med.* 2007;4(1):4–13.
8. Rosenbaum TY, Owens A. The role of pelvic floor physical therapy in the treatment of pelvic and genital pain-related sexual dysfunction (CME). *J Sex Med.* 2008;5(3):513–525.
9. Verit FF, Verit A, Yeni E. The prevalence of sexual dysfunction and associated risk factors in women with chronic pelvic pain: a cross-sectional study. *Arch Gynecol Obstet.* 2006;274(5):297–302.
10. Bergeron S, Brown C, Lord MJ, Oala M, Binik YM, Khalife S. Physical therapy for vulvar vestibulitis syndrome: a retrospective study. *J Sex Marital Ther.* 2002;28(3):183–192.
11. Peters KM, Carrico DJ. Frequency, urgency, and pelvic pain: treating the pelvic floor versus the epithelium. *Curr Urol Rep.* 2006;7(6):450–455.
12. Peters KM, Carrico DJ, Kalinowski SE, Ibrahim IA, Diokno AC. Prevalence of pelvic floor dysfunction in patients with interstitial cystitis. *Urology.* 2007;70(1):16–18.
13. Weiss JM. Pelvic floor myofascial trigger points: manual therapy for interstitial cystitis and the urgency-frequency syndrome. *J Urol.* 2001;166(6):2226–2231.
14. Rehman I, Oyama IA, Rejba A, Lukban JC, Fletcher E. Modified Thiele massage as therapeutic intervention for female patients with interstitial cystitis and high-tone pelvic floor dysfunction. *Urology.* 2004;64(5):862–865.
15. Dumoulin C, Hay-Smith J. Pelvic floor muscle training versus no treatment for urinary incontinence in women: a Cochrane systematic review. *Eur J Phys Rehabil Med.* 2008;44(1):47–63.
16. Hay-Smith EJ. Therapeutic ultrasound for post-partum perineal pain and dyspareunia. *Cochrane Database Syst Rev.* 2000;(2):CD000495.
17. Dannecker C, Wolf V, Raab R, Hepp H, Anthuber C. EMG-biofeedback assisted pelvic floor muscle

training is an effective therapy of stress urinary or mixed incontinence: a 7-year experience with 390 patients. *Arch Gynecol Obstet.* 2005;273(2):93–97.

18. Wall LL, DeLancey JO. The politics of prolapse: a revisionist approach to disorders of the pelvic floor in women. *Perspect Biol Med.* 1991;34(4):486–496.

19. Bump RC, Mattiasson A, Bo K, et al. The standardization of terminology of female pelvic organ prolapse and pelvic floor dysfunction. *Am J Obstet Gynecol.* Jul 1996;175(1):10–17.

20. Messelink B, Benson T, Berghmans B, et al. Standardization of terminology of pelvic floor muscle function and dysfunction: report from the Pelvic Floor Clinical Assessment Group of the International Continence Society. *Neurourol Urodyn.* 2005;24(4):374–380.

21. Bo K, Berghmans B, Morkved S, Van Kampen M. *Evidence-Based Physical Therapy for the Pelvic Floor.* 1st ed. Philadelphia, PA: Churchill Livingstone Elsevier; 2007.

22. Haefner HK, Collins ME, Davis GD, et al. The vulvodynia guideline. *J Low Genit Tract Dis.* 2005;9(1):40–51.

23. FitzGerald MP, Kotarinos R. Rehabilitation of the short pelvic floor. I: Background and patient evaluation. *Int Urogynecol J Pelvic Floor Dysfunct.* 2003;14(4):261–268.

24. FitzGerald MP, Kotarinos R. Rehabilitation of the short pelvic floor. II: Treatment of the patient with the short pelvic floor. *Int Urogynecol J Pelvic Floor Dysfunct.* 2003;14(4):269–275.

25. Weiss JM. Chronic pelvic pain and myofascial trigger points. *Pain Clin.* 2000;2(6):13–18.

26. Carlsson AM. Assessment of chronic pain, I: aspects of the reliability and validity of the Visual Analogue Scale. *Pain.* 1983;16(1):87–101.

27. Weijmar Schultz W, Basson R, Binik Y, Eschenbach D, Wesselmann U, Van Lankveld J. Women's sexual pain and its management. *J Sex Med.* 2005; 2(3):301–316.

28. Jantos M. Understanding chronic pelvic pain. *Pelviperineology.* 2007;26:66–69.

29. Travell JG, David G. Simons. *Myofascial Pain and Dysfunction: The Trigger Point Manual.* Baltimore, MD: Williams & Wilkins; 1983.

30. Bernstein AM, Philips HC, Linden W, Fenster H. A psychophysiological evaluation of female urethral syndrome: evidence for a muscular abnormality. *J Behav Med.* 1992;15(3):299–312.

31. FitzGerald MP, Payne CK, Lukacz ES, et al. Randomized multicenter clinical trial of myofascial physical therapy in women with interstitial cystitis/painful bladder syndrome and pelvic floor tenderness. *J Urol.* 2012;187(6):2113–2118.

32. Arung W, Meurisse M, Detry O. Pathophysiology and prevention of postoperative peritoneal adhesions. *World J Gastroenterol.* 2011;17(41): 4545–4553.

33. Barral JP, Mercier P. *Visceral Manipulation.* Seattle, WA: Eastland Press; 2005.

34. Wang SM, Kain ZN, White P. Acupuncture analgesia: I. The scientific basis. *Anesth Analg.* 2008;106(2):602–610.

35. Han JS, Tang J, Ren MF, Zhou ZF, Fan SG, Qiu XC. Central neurotransmitters and acupuncture analgesia. *Am J Chin Med.* 1980;8(4):331–348.

36. Shen J. Research on the neurophysiological mechanisms of acupuncture: review of selected studies and methodological issues. *J Altern Complement Med.* 2001;7(Suppl 1):S121–S127.

37. Butler D. *The Sensitive Nervous System.* Adelaide, Australia: Noigroup Publications; 2000.

38. Baker PK. Musculoskeletal origins of chronic pelvic pain. Diagnosis and treatment. *Obstet Gynecol Clin North Am.* 1993;20(4):719–742.

39. Laycock J, Haslam J. Therapeutic management of incontinence and pelvic pain: pelvic organ disorders. London: Springer; 2002.

40. Hadley EC. Bladder training and related therapies for urinary incontinence in older people. *JAMA.* 1986;256(3):372–379.

41. Fantl JA, Wyman JF, Harkins SW, Hadley EC. Bladder training in the management of lower urinary tract dysfunction in women. A review. *J Am Geriatr Soc.* 1990;38(3):329–332.

42. Fletcher E. Differential diagnosis of high-tone and low-tone pelvic floor muscle dysfunction. *J Wound Ostomy Continence Nurs.* 2005;32: S10–S11.

43. Reissing ED, Brown C, Lord MJ, Binik YM, Khalife S. Pelvic floor muscle functioning in women with vulvar vestibulitis syndrome. *J Psychosom Obstet Gynaecol.* 2005;26(2):107–113.

44. Glazer HI, Jantos M, Hartmann EH, Swencionis C. Electromyographic comparisons of the pelvic floor in women with dysesthetic vulvodynia and asymptomatic women. *J Reprod Med.* 1998;43(11):959–962.

45. Fisher KA. Management of dyspareunia and associated levator ani muscle overactivity. *Phys Ther.* 2007;87(7):935–941.

46. Lubowski DZ, Swash M, Nicholls RJ, Henry MM. Increase in pudendal nerve terminal motor latency with defacation straining. *Br J Surg.* 1988;75(11):1095–1097.

47. Anderson RU, Wise D, Sawyer T, Chan C. Integration of myofascial trigger point release and paradoxical relaxation training treatment of chronic pelvic pain in men. *J Urol.* 2005;174(1):155–160.

48. Tagart RE. The anal canal and rectum: their varying relationship and its effect on anal continence. *Dis Colon Rectum.* 1966;9(6):449–452.

49. Rasmussen OO. Anorectal function. *Dis Colon Rectum.* 1994;37(4):386–403.

50. Anderson RU, Wise D, Sawyer T, Chan C. Sexual dysfunction in men with chronic prostatitis/chronic pelvic pain syndrome: improvement after trigger point release and paradoxical relaxation training. *J Urol.* 2006;176(4):1538–1539.

51. Woolf CJ. Central sensitization: implications for the diagnosis and treatment of pain. *Pain.* 2011; 152(3 Suppl):S2–S15.

52. Hilton S, Vandyken C. The puzzle of pelvic pain—a rehabilitation framework for balancing tissue dysfunction and central sensitization, I: pain physiology and evaluation for the physical therapist. *J Women Health Phys Ther.* 2011;35(3): 103–113.

53. Zollner AM, Abilez OJ, Bol M, Kuhl E. Stretching skeletal muscle: chronic muscle lengthening through sarcomerogenesis. *PLoS One.* 2012;7(10): e45661.

54. Howard FM. *Pelvic Pain: Diagnosis and Management.* Philadelphia, PA: Lippincott Williams & Wilkins; 2000.

55. Battaglia E, Serra AM, Buonafede G, et al. Long-term study on the effects of visual biofeedback and muscle training as a therapeutic modality in pelvic floor dyssynergia and slow-transit constipation. *Dis Colon Rectum.* 2004;47(1):90–95.

56. Heymen S, Scarlett Y, Jones K, Ringel Y, Drossman D, Whitehead WE. Randomized, controlled trial shows biofeedback to be superior to alternative treatments for patients with pelvic floor dyssynergia-type constipation. *Dis Colon Rectum.* 2007;50(4):428–441.

57. Rao SS, Seaton K, Miller M, et al. Randomized controlled trial of biofeedback, sham feedback, and standard therapy for dyssynergic defecation. *Clin Gastroenterol Hepatol.* 2007;5(3):331–338.

58. Chiarioni G, Whitehead WE, Pezza V, Morelli A, Bassotti G. Biofeedback is superior to laxatives for normal transit constipation due to pelvic floor dyssynergia. *Gastroenterology.* 2006;130(3):657–664.

59. Fitzwater JB, Kuehl TJ, Schrier JJ. Electrical stimulation in the treatment of pelvic pain due to levator ani spasm. *J Reprod Med.* 2003;48(8):573–577.

60. Oliver GC, Rubin RJ, Salvati EP, Eisenstat TE. Electrogalvanic stimulation in the treatment of levator syndrome. *Dis Colon Rectum.* 1985;28(9): 662–663.

61. Sohn N, Weinstein MA, Robbins RD. The levator syndrome and its treatment with high-voltage electrogalvanic stimulation. *Am J Surg.* 1982;144(5): 580–582.

62. Nicosia JF, Abcarian H. Levator syndrome. A treatment that works. *Dis Colon Rectum.* 1985;28(6): 406–408.

63. Proctor ML, Smith CA, Farquhar CM, Stones RW. Transcutaneous electrical nerve stimulation and acupuncture for primary dysmenorrhoea. *Cochrane Database Syst Rev.* 2002(1):CD002123.

64. French SD, Cameron M, Walker BF, Reggars JW. Superficial heat or cold for low back pain. *Cochrane Database Syst Rev.* 2006;31(9):998–1006.

65. Rakel B, Barr JO. Physical modalities in chronic pain management. *Nurs Clin North Am.* 2003; 38(3):477–494.

19

Implantable Devices for the Treatment of Pelvic Pain

CHRIS R. ABRECHT, ALISON M. WEISHEIPL,
AND ASSIA T. VALOVSKA

Chronic pelvic pain (CPP) is an intermittent or constant pain in the lower abdomen or pelvis of at least six months' duration causing significant functional disability and affects an estimated 2.1–24% of the worldwide female population.[1] Dysfunction in myriad organ systems (e.g., endometriosis, inflammatory bowel syndrome, pudendal neuralgia, interstitial cystitis) can contribute to CPP; yet in most cases, the precise etiology is not known.[2] Given that CPP can be nociceptive, neuropathic, or occur in the absence of an actual injury (similar to complex regional pain syndrome), patients may improve with stimulation of the central nervous system or centrally acting medications.[3] This chapter will address various stimulation modalities as well as intrathecal delivery of opioids for patients with CPP.

SACRAL NERVE STIMULATION (SNS) FOR TREATMENT OF CPP

History and Contemporary Use of SNS

Electrotherapy for pain management dates back to antiquity, when, in AD 46, the court physician of Roman emperor Claudius documented in his *Compositiones* the treatment of headaches using electric eels (40–100V, 100Hz).[4] The first documentation of sacral nerve stimulation came a few millennia later, when Brindley et al. in 1976 successfully used implanted sacral neuromodulators to treat urinary incontinence in paraplegic patients.[5] Later, in 1995, came the description of sacral nerve stimulation (SNS) for the treatment of fecal incontinence.[6]

Current Food and Drug Administration (FDA)–approved uses of SNS include urinary urge incontinence, urgency-frequency, non-obstructive urinary retention, and fecal incontinence. Implantation of SNS has increased significantly recently, with more than half of the estimated 125,000 implants occurring in the last 3.5 years.[7] SNS implantation for CPP remains an off-label intervention.

Unfortunately, there are no high-quality (i.e., large, prospective, multi-center, randomized, controlled) trials that evaluate SNS specifically for the treatment of CPP. A systematic review in 2012 by Tirlapur et al. found that the few studies that did assess neuromodulation as an intervention for CPP did not include a control, thus significantly limiting the inferences that could be drawn. Additional issues included a wide variation in the definition of CPP, the outcome measurements (e.g., the pain scores via the McGill questionnaire vs. the Visual Analog Scale (VAS) vs. SF-36 quality-of-life questionnaire), as well as the short follow-up duration, usually limited to 12 weeks.[8] In the interim, until high-quality studies arrive, neuromodulation continues to be used to effectively treat women with intractable chronic pelvic pain.

Proposed Mechanisms of Action of Neuromodulation

Understanding how SNS works requires an understanding of pelvic neuroanatomy and pain physiology. This complex region receives sympathetic innervation from the T1–L2 nerve roots via the superior hypogastric plexus, parasympathetic innervation from the S2–S4 nerve roots via the pelvic splanchnic nerves, and somatic innervation from S2–S4 via the pudendal nerve. In CPP, injury to lower abdominal or pelvic organs, manifesting as somatic or visceral pain, may ultimately develop into injury to the nervous system itself, manifesting as neuropathic pain.

The exact mechanism by which SNS and other well-established modalities of neuromodulation such as spinal cord stimulation work is not completely understood, but it is thought to hinge on the "gate theory" of analgesia proposed by Melzack and Wall in 1965. This theory suggests that the activation of large-diameter non-pain Aβ fibers is able to inhibit the transmission of smaller-diameter pain Aδ and C fibers.[9] The electric current delivered by the sacral nerve stimulator may, therefore, cause depolarization of pelvic non-nociceptive fibers and inhibition of the pelvic nociceptive or neuropathic afferent signals responsible for the patient's pain.

This prevailing explanation, however, is probably an oversimplification. Recent studies, for instance, have shown that some patients with CPP receive relief with neuromodulation leads placed as high as T6/7, perhaps due to sympathetic and visceral pain fibers following an atypical path.[10]

Patient Selection
for SNS Implantation

SNS is an effective, yet off-label, treatment for patients with chronic pelvic pain. The appropriate patient has already tried other interventions, including but not limited to medical management, pelvic floor physical therapy, and nerve blocks using local anesthetics or steroids (e.g., pudendal nerve blocks). There are no known evidence-based prognostic factors for successful neuromodulation, but patients appear anecdotally to have better results if they lack severe neurological deficits such as spinal cord injury preventing ambulation.[11] Prior to a SNS trial, patients should also undergo a psychological evaluation to determine if the patient has addiction, depression, or anxiety disorders contributing to the patient's pain syndrome. If present, these disorders should be psychologically and, if needed, pharmacologically treated prior to the trial. Moreover, this assessment should determine if the patient has the cognitive ability to operate the neurostimulatory device as well as whether the patient has history of sexual abuse, a negative predictor of successful stimulation.[11]

Therapeutic Trial of SNS Prior
to Implantation

Prior to the trial, the clinician should emphasize the goal of increased functionality and improvement, but probably not complete resolution, of pain episodes. These sacral nerve stimulator trials performed at our institution, Brigham and Women's Hospital, are done in the clinic, with local anesthesia and minimal sedation. There is, however, geographic variation in the depth of sedation used during these procedures; in many European countries, deep sedation or general anesthesia are also employed.[12] In either way, using fluoroscopic guidance, the electrode is maneuvered into the sacral foramen and linked to an external stimulator that the patient carries during the duration of the trial, usually lasting a week. During this period, the patient keeps a diary documenting VAS recordings, functional status, analgesic use, and any other relevant findings. If at the end of this period the patient reports a greater than 50% relief, the therapeutic trial is considered a success. The temporary lead is then removed, and the patient is scheduled for permanent lead placement in the operating room at a later date. If the patient experiences less than 50% relief, the placement of the leads should be checked, as in an estimated 11–18% of therapeutic trials, lead migration occurs and may call for a repeat trial after correction of the placement.[11]

Surgical Technique
for SNS Implantation

The following is a brief description of the surgical practice at our institution, representative of the national standard practice for these procedures.

First, the prone position is employed, with the patient resting on an abdominal pillow to reduce lumbar lordosis. Chlorhexidine prep is applied along the sacrum, including the buttocks. Sterile towels are then positioned at the border of the disinfected area and a half sheet onto the patient's legs. Ioban is then applied over the prepared skin. Antibiotic prophylaxis is administered prior to incision according to institutional guidelines. At our institution, cefazolin 2 g is administered to patients without a beta-lactam allergy.

We use the sacral transforaminal technique, wherein the leads are directly inserted into the sacral foramina (S3 and S4). The basic steps for this procedure are usually as follows: Place the electrodes, create an impulse pulse generator (IPG) pocket, and tunnel the leads to the IPG. To place the electrodes, we align x-rays, infiltrate local anesthetic to the superficial skin, and insert an introducer at the sacral foramina. We then place the electrodes through the introducer. The electrodes are tined, which allows them to stay in the correct position without using an anchor. After the electrodes are placed, we then create an IPG pocket (usually along the buttock), taking care to not make the pocket too deep so that recharging the IPG is not inhibited by deep tissue. Finally, we tunnel the stimulating leads from sacral roots to buttock and connect the leads to the IPG. After irrigating with antibiotic solution and ensuring adequate hemostasis, the wound is closed. Potential risks of this technique include lead migration because no anchors are used. Other surgical options include the retrograde technique, wherein the epidural needle and the leads are inserted in a cranial-to-caudal direction to the S2, S3, and S4 levels. These procedures are done in the operating room, with an anesthesiologist providing sedation so that the patient is comfortable, yet aware enough to alert the interventionalist to paresthesias, indicating correct placement.

Additional Targets for Peripheral Neuromodulation

Peripheral neuromodulation using targets other than the sacral nerve is also available to treat pain in the pelvic territory. One such example is ilioinguinal neuralgia, usually manifesting as neuropathic pain with hyperesthesia in the upper medial thigh, inguinal region, and genitals. The known causes of this condition include nerve injury from lower abdominal and pelvic surgery or trauma; in many instances, however, the exact cause is not clear. In patients for whom pharmacological management and physical therapy are not effective, peripheral nerve stimulation targeting the ilioinguinal nerve is an alternative to surgical techniques such as inguinal neurectomy, which is not effective in all patients and may cause problematic paresthesias.[13] After a patient-selection process similar to the one described for SNS, patients with ilioinguinal neuralgia may undergo implantation of a permanent stimulator with leads placed along the affected dermatome in the area of greatest pain. Targeting the ilioinguinal nerve at L1 has been shown to provide significant and long-lasting relief for patients with ilioinguinal neuralgia following lower abdominal surgery[13] and trauma.[14]

Peripheral neuromodulation is also a possible treatment for coccygodynia, which manifests as pain around the coccyx. The etiology of this condition is often unclear, but known causes include osteoarthritis of the sacrococcygeal joint, injury from delivery, and spasm of the pelvic floor.[15] Pain relief may be achieved by placing stimulating electrodes over the course of the peripheral nerve corresponding to the painful dermatome.[16] In cases of coccygodynia with non-dermatomal distribution of pain, placement of the stimulating electrode directly at the site of pain may be more effective. [15]

SPINAL CORD STIMULATION (SCS) FOR TREATMENT OF CPP

History and Contemporary Use of SCS

As described in the previous section, neuromodulation sprang from Melzack and Wall's gate control theory of pain in the 1960s; the first published use of spinal cord stimulation (SCS) for the treatment of pain was in 1967, when a platinum electrode placed in the subarachnoid space was used to treat a patient with chronic pain. The first commercially available stimulators sent radio frequency messages to stimulator electrodes placed directly on the dorsal columns.[17] In the modern system, multi-lead electrodes placed in the epidural space either percutaneously with fluoroscopic guidance or surgically with direct visualization connect with subcutaneously located impulse pulse generators via tunneled wires. Multiple studies have demonstrated this modality's efficacy in treating a variety of chronic pain conditions, with minimal morbidity and relatively decreased healthcare costs. The PROCESS RCT in 2007, for instance, provided Class I evidence of efficacy in the treatment of failed back surgery syndrome (FBSS).[18] SCS has FDA approval for the treatment of chronic pain of the trunk or extremities, with most implants occurring to treat FBSS and chronic regional pain syndrome (CRPS). Other off-label uses include peripheral vascular disease, refractory angina pectoralis, and CPP.

Multiple reports have supported the use of SCS to treat CPP. A case series in 2006 described six female patients with chronic pelvic pain, each treated for over a decade with multiple medications and nonsurgical interventions, who experienced a sustained and greater than 50% reduction in their pain after an SCS was placed at either T11 or L1.[19] Another case report describes a woman with debilitating vulvodynia and pelvic pain for over a decade on high doses of methadone and other opioids who was able to wean herself off all opioids several months after SCS at L3.[20] More recently, a multicenter prospective study followed 27 patients with chronic pelvic pain with pudendal neuralgia not relieved by pudendal nerve compression surgery. Of the 20 of these patients with a positive test phase who underwent permanent implantation of the SCS at the level of the conus medullaris, all experienced greater than 50% reduction in their pain and a statistically significant doubling of their mean sitting time at a mean follow-up of 15 months.[21] Also noteworthy, the complications from these procedures were mild, mostly post-surgical pain, superficial infections, and lead migration requiring reprogramming. Similarly, a review of 707 SCS cases at the Cleveland Clinic from 2000–2005 revealed a 22.6% incidence of lead migration and a 6% incidence of lead breakage requiring re-implantation. These rates have probably decreased with improvements in the SCS hardware. Infection incidence was 4.5%, with roughly two-thirds of those cases requiring re-implantation due to a deep infection. Of note, though, only about 15% of these implants were performed due to "visceral pain" or "neuropathic pain," the categories into which CPP would fit. Most of the implants studied in this trial were for CRPS-related extremity pain, perhaps explaining the relatively high rate of lead migration.[22]

The established use of neuromodulation in the treatment of chronic pain targets the dorsal columns of the spinal cord. Growing evidence suggests, however, that ventral spinal cord stimulation may also provide pain relief. For instance, a retrospective case series of 26 patients with chronic visceral neuropathic pain in the abdomen showed a statistically significant reduction in visual analog pain scores and opioid consumption after spinal cord stimulation—regardless of whether the target was dorsal or ventral.[23] The spinal cord targets in this study were T9/10 for upper abdominal pain and T10/11 or T11/12 for lower abdominal pain. While the rest of this chapter will address the standard SCS approach targeting the dorsal columns, this recent study suggesting an anterior approach is important to mention because it emphasizes the need for additional research in neuromodulation. Without a doubt, new advances in neuromodulation in the coming years will translate into a higher quality of life for patients with CPP.

Patient Selection for SCS Implantation

The patient-selection process for SCS implantation is similar to that of SNS implantation, as described above. These patients with CPP should have already undergone extensive interventions, including, but not limited to, physical therapy and medical management with multiple agents. These patients should also undergo a psychological assessment to address any depression, anxiety, and other comorbidities frequently associated with chronic pelvic pain, as well as to confirm that they have the capacity to manage the SCS implant. In the patient who has met these criteria, the next step is a therapeutic trial of SCS.

Therapeutic Trial of SCS Prior to Implantation

The therapeutic trial of SCS prior to implantation is again similar to that of the SNS trial. At our institution, most patients undergo percutaneous, fluoroscopically guided placement of the electrodes in the clinic, under minimal sedation so the patient can inform the proceduralist when the distracting induced paresthesia covers the area of pain. In rare cases of severe epidural scarring, scoliosis, or spinal stenosis, this trial may require direct, surgical placement in the operating room instead of in the clinic. In either case, the patient goes home with a temporary SCS system attached to an external programmer. Prior to discharge home, the patient receives instruction on how to adjust the SCS settings. In the subsequent week or two, the patient keeps a diary documenting pain and the SCS settings that provide the most pain relief. A reduction of at least 50% in VAS pain score is again considered a successful trial.

Surgical Technique for SCS Implantation

The following is a brief description of percutaneous SCS implantation with fluoroscopic guidance, our preferred method as well as the national standard for pain physicians with a background in anesthesiology. In contrast, paddle-lead SCS implantation via direct visualization is the preferred method of neurosurgeons and is sometimes necessary if significant scarring from previous back surgeries prevents the passage of the percutaneous leads into the epidural space.

In either case, the patient is again in the prone position, resting on an abdominal pillow to reduce lumbar lordosis and thereby facilitate access to the epidural space. Chlorhexidine prep is applied broadly to the back and to the planned location of the IPG pocket, with sterile towels at the border of the disinfected area and Ioban applied over the prepared skin. For antibiotic prophylaxis, we usually give a single dose of cefazolin; in the case of a B-lactam allergy, we give clindamycin.

The basic steps are as follows: Identify the intended vertebral level using fluoroscopy (with T11 being our usual goal for these patients with CPP), infiltrate the superficial tissues with local anesthetic, and identify the epidural space using a Tuohy needle with a loss of resistance technique to air or saline. The epidural electrode leads are then threaded through the epidural space to the desired level using fluoroscopic guidance. The

leads are anchored to the fascia to decrease the risk of lead migration. The IPG pocket is made in either the buttocks, flank, or lumbar paraspinal area, based on the patient's habitus and preferences. The electrodes are then tunneled from the back incision to the IPG pocket, thereby connecting the electrodes to the IPG. The back incision and IPG pocket are closed after proper antibiotic irrigation and ensuring adequate hemostasis. Once the incisions are sutured, the IPG in turn is controlled via an external device. As with SNS implantation, these procedures are done in the operating room under the care of an anesthesiologist so that the patient can tolerate the procedure but also indicate correct lead placement to the interventionalist. (See Figure 19.1 for an overview

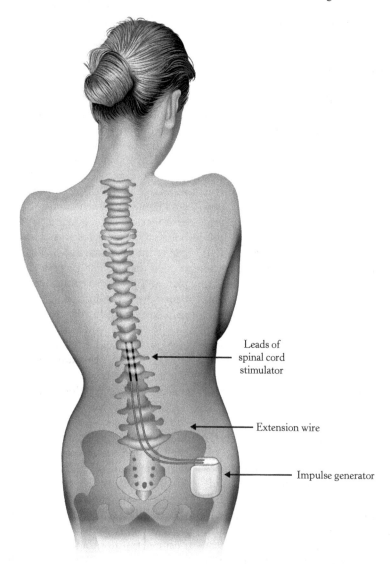

Leads of spinal cord stimulator

Extension wire

Impulse generator

FIGURE 19.1: Spinal cord stimulator overview.

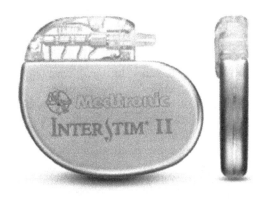

FIGURE 19.2: Medtronic InterStim II Neurostimulator.

of the implanted spinal cord stimulator. See Figure 19.2 for an image of a neurostimulator; see Figure 19.3 for an image of tined leads.)

INTRATHECAL OPIOID THERAPY FOR THE TREATMENT OF CPP

History and Contemporary Use of Intrathecal Pumps (ITPs)

The discovery in 1976 of the µ opioid at the spinal cord's dorsal horn laid the groundwork for the practice of intrathecal opioid administration, in which medications are delivered directly to their ultimate site of action. By largely bypassing the absorption, metabolism, and distribution hurdles of enteral opioid administration, intrathecal opioid administration may allow significantly lower doses of drug and may cause fewer opioid-related side effects. While a variety of medications are used in this manner to treat chronic pain—including, but not limited to, opioids, local anesthetics, α-2 agonists, and calcium channel blockers—the FDA in 1995 granted approval only for intrathecal morphine via intrathecal drug delivery systems (IDDS) in the treatment of chronic pain.[24] Since then, multiple studies have shown that IDDS can cause a statistically significant and sustained (lasting multiple years) reduction in pain, reduction in enteral analgesic intake, and improvement in functional status in patients with nociceptive, neuropathic, or mixed pain. Currently, the calcium channel ziconotide has also received approval for the treatment of chronic pain via IDDS.[25]

Most IDDS in use today treat chronic malignant pain, but an increasing number of IDDS treat chronic non-malignant pain. No studies have specifically examined IDDS in the treatment of non-malignant chronic pelvic pain, but IDDS have been shown to provide statistically significant results in patients with non-malignant visceral pain disorders, a group into which patients with chronic pelvic pain would fit.[24] A prospective three-year study of 58 patients with chronic, non-malignant pain—a cohort that did include a few patients with pelvic pain as their primary diagnosis—showed that intrathecal opioid therapy provided a statistically significant and sustained reduction in pain as well as functional improvement.[26] In our practice, IDDS are reserved for patients with chronic pelvic pain who have failed other therapies, including neuromodulation therapies and medication management, and who exhibit low-risk behaviors based on psychological evaluation.

Patient Selection for ITP Implantation

As was the case with implantable devices for neuromodulation, implantable devices for intrathecal opioid administration are not a first-line treatment for patients with CPP. The ideal patient has already undergone an extensive multidisciplinary treatment regimen and has exhibited relief from oral analgesics but has not been able to take the maximum effective dose due to side effects of the analgesic. In addition, the patient should again first undergo a psychological assessment and confirm that he or she is prepared after the initial implantation for the multiple subsequent office visits required for intrathecal pump refilling, a process that requires skin puncture.

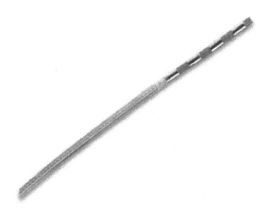

FIGURE 19.3: Medtronic tined leads prior to being deployed.

Therapeutic Trial of ITP Prior to Implantation

A therapeutic trial is again a requirement before permanent implantation. In this trial, the opioid may be administered either via a one-time intrathecal bolus, continuously via an epidural catheter, or continuously via a spinal catheter. Inpatient admission may be required to facilitate the trial, especially if epidural or intrathecal catheters are used. Some practitioners prefer a catheter over a one-time bolus injection so that the tip of the catheter can be placed at the dermatome corresponding most closely to the patient's site of pain, thus delivering medication even more specifically to the desired site of action. At a meeting of the Polyanalgesic Consensus Conference, however, catheter trials were not considered superior to single-injection trials.[27] At our institution, we generally perform trials using epidural catheters. After placement of the catheter and administration of neuraxial opioids, the patient is admitted to the hospital to be monitored for respiratory depression or other complications related to catheter placement. In the following three to four days, we attempt to wean the patient from the opioid medications and encourage the patient to use a journal to keep track of pain scores and functional status. A successful trial is considered an at least 50% reduction in pain scores.

Surgical Technique for ITP Implantation

The patient may be placed under general anesthesia, or the interventionalist may choose to use a local and inject intrathecal bupivacaine at T10 as the intrathecal catheter is threaded to achieve surgical analgesia. The patient assumes a lateral decubitus position and is then prepped and draped in the usual fashion as described for the SNS and SCS sections in this chapter. The area of interest includes the spine at the level of insertion, as well as the lower abdomen, which will be the position of the pump reservoir. Chlorhexidine and Ioban are applied to the back and to the lower abdomen, sterile towels and drapes are placed around the disinfected site, and antibiotic prophylaxis is administered prior to incision. Once the patient is put under general anesthesia, a spinal needle is introduced into the intrathecal space, and an intrathecal catheter is threaded under fluoroscopic guidance to the desired level. The ITP pocket is then created, the ITP is placed in the pocket, and the

spinal catheter is tunneled to the ITP pump. Once hemostasis is achieved, the site is irrigated with antibiotic solution and closed.

As with the neuromodulation devices, ITP complications include infection, hematoma, and device migration. Additional concerns with the placement of ITP include cerebrospinal fluid leak manifesting as a post-dural puncture headache and the formation of an intrathecal granuloma—an inflammatory, fibrous collection at the catheter tip. Loss of analgesia from an ITP may herald the presence of an intrathecal granuloma, best detected with an MRI of the spine with contrast. If the granuloma causes neurological deficits from cord compression, it may warrant neurosurgical intervention. Fortunately, though, the intrathecal granuloma is an uncommon occurrence and is usually asymptomatic.

SPECIAL CONCERNS WITH IMPLANTABLE DEVICES FOR THE TREATMENT OF CPP

Pre-operative Anesthetic Assessment and Optimization for Surgery

Just as the patient will meet with the interventionalist who will perform the implantation of the neuromodulation device to discuss the plan and expectations, patients at our institution also meet with an anesthesiologist prior to the procedure. In other institutions, this assessment may be done by an internist. In either case, the purpose of this meeting is to address any comorbidities that might affect the anesthetic, such as ischemic heart disease, chronic obstructive pulmonary disease, obstructive sleep apnea, morbid obesity, gastroesophageal reflux disease, liver and kidney disease, and anxiety. The result of this consultation may be pre-operative testing and medical interventions to optimize the patient before the procedure and to determine the best agents to use for the anesthetic.

Contraindications to Device Implantation

While neuromodulation device and ITP implantation is overall a safe intervention, it is not without risks and contraindications. First, no patient who fails to exhibit a response to therapeutic trial should undergo a permanent implantation. Other contraindications include the following: patients with sepsis or an infection at the surgical site; patients with developmental delay preventing operation of the neurostimulatory device or ITP; and patients with a life expectancy of less than six months.

Two areas of debate relate to cardiac pacemakers and MRI in patients with stimulator devices (intrathecal pumps are compatible with pacemakers and MRI). Historically, concern existed that the current produced by the sacral nerve stimulator would interfere with the functioning of cardiac pacemakers. This concern has decreased somewhat in light of case series documenting no cardiac pacemaker interference intra-operatively and 24 hours post-operatively in patients undergoing implantation of the Medtronic InterStim device.[28] Medtronic data also indicate that interference is not likely unless the pacemaker and the stimulator are within eight inches of one another.

MRI is another issue: Concern exists among clinicians that patients with a neuromodulatory implant may experience painful heating of the leads, generator movement, or generation dysfunction. Case series have shown that MRI performed in areas other than the pelvis in patients with the Medtronic InterStim device experienced no such problems.[29] The technology regarding MRI compatability has been advancing rapidly. Currently, Medtronic InterStim is MRI-conditional, with some specific recommendations against MRI with specific models. For specific guidelines regarding MRI compatibility or conditionality, we recommend contacting the support services of the particular device company for full guidelines.

SNS in the Pregnant Patient

Most clinicians who do not regularly care for pregnant women have some degree of uncertainty regarding how pregnancy will precisely affect their medical niche. There are few studies on the safety of SNS in pregnancy. A recent case report and literature review by El-Khawand et al. in 2012 concluded that women of childbearing age should use some form of contraceptive while they have an SNS in place, or should inactivate the device as soon as their pregnancy is confirmed. This recommendation is based more on a lack of evidence than evidence showing a harmful relationship. Animal studies in rats have shown no effects of spinal cord stimulation on the fetus, and a small case review of six cases showed no harmful effects, other than lead movement after pregnancy, probably from displacement by the fetal head. Of note, none of these women used SNS for CPP; most of these patients used SNS to treat urinary incontinence, as the potential benefit of avoiding of urinary tract infections was thought to outweigh any generator-related risk to the fetus. Also notable is that the case report in this review described a woman using a Medtronic InterStim device throughout her pregnancy for bladder pain syndrome whose child ultimately developed a chronic motor tic disorder.[30] Clearly, additional research on this subject is required. In the meantime, it is probably best in most cases to avoid SNS during pregnancy.

Complications of Implantation

Myriad potential post-operative complications can require prompt return to the clinic for further evaluation and treatment, so close follow-up after implantation of an SNS is a necessity. As with all surgical procedures, infection is a risk. A recent multicenter prospective observational trial examining 120 patients undergoing implantation of the Medtronic InterStim device found a 10.8% infection rate over an average 28-month period. Approximately half of these infections were successfully treated with antibiotics, and approximately half required either a surgical intervention (e.g., abscess drainage) or device explantation.[31]

Other complications include pain to the perineum or lower extremity, pain around the electrode, movement of an electrode causing loss of the desired effect, or loss of the desired effect for unclear reasons. A majority of patients will require reprogramming in the clinic for loss of effect. Moreover, patients may require reoperation for one of these complications; one review puts the range of reoperation rate at 16–54%.[12]

Similar complications are possible after implantation of the SCS. The additional complications after ITP implantation include post-dural puncture headache and intrathecal granuloma, as discussed above.

Rehabilitation Considerations for Patients with SNS and SCS Implants

Most patients who undergo implantation of a neuromodulator are admitted overnight; some of these patients may require patient controlled analgesia (PCA) to manage their post-operative pain. Dressings, consisting usually of Telfa and Tegaderm, remain in place for a week, during which time patients should not shower. The first post-op visit occurs at one week. During this visit, the dressings are removed, the incision site is checked by the interventionalist, and, if the incision is well healed, the dressings remain off and the patient is permitted to shower. At this first post-op visit, the neurostimulator is also activated. We wait one week before activating the device to minimize the likelihood that post-operative pain will interfere with the programming of the device. Further post-op visits should hopefully be distinguished by the patient happily relaying an improvement in his or her chronic pelvic pain.

FUTURE DIRECTIONS
Advances in neurostimulation and implantable drug-delivery technology, as well as improved insight into the neuropathophysiology of chronic pelvic pain, will certainly lead to even more effective implantable devices for the treatment of CPP in the coming years. As we eagerly await these advances, we will continue to use the current sacral nerve stimulators, spinal cord stimulators, and intrathecal pumps to effectively treat our patients with the debilitating disorder that is chronic pelvic pain.

REFERENCES

1. Latthe P, et al. WHO systematic review of prevalence of chronic pelvic pain: a neglected reproductive health morbidity. *BMC Public Health*. 2006 Jul 6;6:177.
2. Daniels JP, Khan KS. Chronic pelvic pain in women. *BMJ*. 2010;341:772–775.
3. Udoji, MA, Ness, TJ. New directions in the treatment of pelvic pain. *Pain Manag*. 2013 Sep; 3(5):387–394.
4. Martellucci J, Naldini G, Carriero A. Sacral nerve modulation in the treatment of chronic pelvic pain. *Int J Colorectal Dis*. 2012 27:921–926.
5. Brindley GS. Polkey CE, Rushton DN, et al. Sacral anterior root stimulators for bladder control on paraplegia: the first 50 cases. *J Neurol Neurosurg Psychiatry*. 1986;49:1104–1114.
6. Matzel KE, Stadelmaier U, Hohenfellner M, et al. Electrical stimulation of sacral spinal nerves for treatment of faecal incontinence. *Lancet*. 1995;346:1124–1127.
7. Noblett KL, Cadish LA. Sacral nerve stimulation for the treatment of refractory voiding and bowel dysfunction. *Am J Obstet Gynecol*. 2014 210(2):99–106.
8. Tirapur SA, Vlismas A, Ball E, Khan KS. Nerve stimulation for chronic pelvic pain and bladder pain syndrome: a systematic review. *Acta Obstet Gynecol Scand*. 2013 Aug;92(8):881–887.
9. Melzack R., Wall PD. Pain mechanisms: a new theory. *Science*. 1965;150:971–979.
10. Hunter C, Dave N, Diwan S, Deer T. Neuromodulation of pelvic visceral pain: review of the literature and case series of potential novel targets for treatment. *Pain Pract*. 2013;13(1):3–17.
11. Butrick, C. Patient selection for sacral nerve stimulation. *Int Urogynecol J*. 2010;21:S447–S451.
12. Norderval S, Ryningen M, Lindsetmo RO, Lein D, Vonen B. Sacral nerve stimulation. *Tidsskr Nor Legeforen*. 2011 Jun 17;131(12):1190–1193.
13. Rauchwerger JJ, Giordano J, Rozen D, Kent JL, Greenspan J, Closson CWF. On the therapeutic viability of peripheral nerve stimulation for ilioinguinal neuralgia: putative mechanisms and possible utility. *Pain Pract*. 2008;8(2):138–143.
14. Banh DPT, Moujan PM, Haque Q, Han TH. Permanent implantation of peripheral nerve stimulator for combat injury-related ilioinguinal neuralgia. *Pain Physician*. 2013;16:789–791.
15. Kothari S. Neuromodulatory approaches to chronic pelvic pain and coccygodynia. *Acta Neurochir Suppl*. 2007;97(1):365–371.
16. Slavin, K. Peripheral nerve stimulation for neuropathic pain. *Neurotherapeutics*. 2008;5:100–106.
17. Kumar, K, Rizvi, S. Historical and present state of neuromodulation in chronic pain. *Curr Pain Headache Rep*. 2014;18:387–392.
18. Kumar, K, Taylor RS, Jacques L, et. Al. Spinal cord stimulation versus conventional medical management for neuropathic pain: a multicentre randomised controlled trial in patients with failed back surgery syndrome. *Pain*. 2007;132:179–188.
19. Kapural, L, Narouze SN, Janicki TI, Mekhail N. Spinal cord stimulation is an effective treatment for chronic intractable visceral pelvic pain. *Pain Med*. 2006;7(5):440–443.
20. Nair, AR, Klapper A, Kushnerik V, Margulis I, Del Priore G. Spinal cord stimulator for the treatment of a woman with vulvovaginal burning and deep pelvic pain. *Obstet Gynecol*. 2008;111(2):545–547.
21. Buffenoir K, Rioult, B, Hamel, O, Laba JJ, Riant, T, Robert R. Spinal cord stiulation of the conus medullaris for refractory pudendal neuralgia: a prospective study of 27 consecutive cases. *Neurourology and Urodynamics*. 2015;34(2):177–182. Epub 2013 Nov 19.
22. Mekhail, N, Matthews, M, Nageeb, F, Guirguis M, Mekhail MN, Cheng, J. Retrospective review of 707 cases of spinal cord stimulation: indications and complications. *Pain Practice*. 2011;11(2): 148–153.
23. Baranidharan G, Simpson K, Dhandapani K. Spinal cord stimulation for visceral pain—a novel approach. *Neuromodulation*. 2014;17(8):753–758.
24. Atli, A, Theodore, BR, Turk DC, Loeser, JD. Intrathecal opioid treatment for chronic

non-malignant pain: a retrospective cohort study with 3-year follow-up. *Pain Med.* 2010 Jul;11(7): 1010–1016.

25. Hayek, SM, Deer, TR, Pope JE, Panchal SJ, Patel V. Intrathecal therapy for cancer and non-cancer pain. *Pain Physician.* 2011;14:219–248.

26. Hamza M, Doleys D, Wells M et al. Prospective study of 3-year follow-up of low-dose intrathecal opioids in the management of chronic non-malignant pain. *Pain Med.* 2012 Oct;13(100): 1304–1313.

27. Deer TR, Levy R, Prager J, et al. Polyanalgesic Consensus Conference 2012: Recommendations to reduce morbidity and mortality in intrathecal drug delivery in the treatment of chronic pain. *Neuromodulation.* 2012;15:467–482.

28. Wallace PA, Lane FL, Noblett KL. 2007. Sacral nerve neuromodulation in patients with cardiac pacemakers. *Am J Obstet Gynec.* 197(94): e91–e93.

29. Elkelini MS, Hassouna MM. 2006. Safety of MRI at 1.5Tesla in patients with implanted sacral nerve stimulator. *Eur Urol.* 2006;50:311–316.

30. El-Khawand D, Montogomery OC, Wehbe SA, Whitmore KE. Sacral nerve stimulation during pregnancy: case report and review of the literature. *Female Pelvic Med Reconstr Surg.* 2012 Mar–Apr; 18(2):127–129.

31. Wexner SD, Hull T, Edden Y et al. Infection rates in a large investigational trial of sacral nerve stimulation for fecal incontinence. *J Gastrointest Surg.* 2010;14:1081–1089.

20

Sample Clinical Cases

BETHANY SKINNER, NICHOLE MAHNERT, AND COURTNEY S. LIM

CASE 1

Ms. D is a 24-year-old gravida 0 who presents with complaints of daily pelvic cramping. She reports a history of dysmenorrhea that was previously controlled with nonsteroidal anti-inflammatory drugs (NSAIDs).

Are there other details of her history that are important to elicit?

As with all pelvic pain, you should elicit a timeline of her pain (When did it start worsening? Any coinciding events? Timing with menses?), as well as provocative or palliative factors. You should also inquire about her menstrual history, including the frequency, duration, and heaviness of menses. A thorough medical and surgical history should be obtained, including a history of prior surgeries performed for evaluation or treatment of pelvic pain.

Ms. D reports daily pelvic cramping, which worsens shortly before and during her menses. She has no past medical or surgical history.

What are you looking for on examination?

As with all chronic pelvic pain patients, a thorough physical exam including a back, abdominal, pelvic, and hip exam should be performed. When examining women with dysmenorrhea in whom endometriosis is suspected, the pelvic exam should evaluate the mobility of the uterus and adnexa, presence of adnexal masses, nodularity of the uterosacral ligaments, and tenderness upon palpation of these structures. A rectal exam should also be considered to assess for evidence of rectovaginal nodularity concerning for endometriosis.

Her abdominal exam is notable for diffuse tenderness in the bilateral lower quadrants. On pelvic exam, her uterus is retroverted and minimally mobile. She has thickening and tenderness of her right uterosacral ligament and fullness in her right adnexa.

Based on her exam, what should be done next?

In this patient, given the finding of adnexal fullness suggestive of a pelvic mass, a pelvic ultrasound should be considered. Additional imaging is rarely indicated in women with chronic pelvic pain, and should only be performed if patients have a concerning history of dyschezia, hematochezia, hematuria, or an exam suggestive of a pelvic mass.

What management options does this patient have for her pain?

When endometriosis is suspected, the patient has the option of medical or surgical management. First-line medical therapy often consists of NSAIDs and hormonal suppression (Table 20.1).

It is important to remember that improvement of pain on Lupron is not diagnostic of endometriosis. A randomized controlled trial by Ling in 1999 randomized 95 women with pelvic pain to Lupron or placebo. At three months, 81% of women in the Lupron group had pain relief, versus 39% in the placebo group. However, improvement in pain with Lupron therapy was experienced by 82% of women with endometriosis and 73% of women without endometriosis.

All methods of hormonal suppression are equally effective in head-to-head clinical trials. On average, 70–85% of users report improvement in their symptoms with medical management with hormonal suppression. Therefore,

TABLE 20.1 HORMONAL SUPPRESSION OF ENDOMETRIOSIS

First-line therapy	
Combined oral contraceptive (estrogen + progestin)	Pill, patch, vaginal ring; may be given cyclically or continuously used
Norethindrone 5 mg/day	Continuous pill
Levonorgestrel IUD	
Second-line therapy	
Depo GnRH analogues + add back	
Medroxyprogesterone	Oral, intramuscular, subcutaneous
Letrozole (off label) + ovarian suppression	2.5 mg daily
Third-line therapy	
Low-dose danazol	e.g., 200 mg/day; oral, intravaginal

Adapted from Vercellini P. et al. Endometriosis: current and future medical therapies. Best Pract Res Clin Obstet Gynaecol. 2008;22:275–306.

treatment should be selected based on patient preference, costs, and side effects.

Ms. D undergoes an ultrasound that demonstrates a 4 cm complex ovarian cyst suggestive of an endometrioma. She ultimately decides to proceed with surgical management.

Surgery for endometriosis should be considered for the following reasons:

- To establish a diagnosis
- To improve or relieve symptoms (refractory to empirical medical therapy)
- To normalize anatomy for sub-fertility
- To investigate a suspected and persistent endometrioma over 3 cm in size

How should the diagnosis of endometriosis be made?

When endometriosis is suspected, a biopsy should be taken for histological diagnosis. The positive predictive value for visual inspection is approximately 45% (with the literature showing a range of 32–85%, depending on appearance and location). In one study by Fernando et al. in 2013, the accuracy of visual diagnosis of endometriosis was substantially influenced by the American Society of Reproductive Medicine stage, the depth and volume of the lesion, and to a lesser extent the location of the lesion.

Post-operatively, what is her expected symptomatic improvement?

In Sutton et al., a double-blinded, randomized, controlled trial was conducted to evaluate the effect of surgical management with laser ablation for the treatment of pelvic pain in patients with stage I–III endometriosis. Women were randomized to surgical management with laparoscopic laser ablation and uterine nerve ablation or diagnostic laparoscopy. There was no difference in pain between the two groups at three months, with 48% of the diagnostic laparoscopy group reporting improved pain. However, at six months, 77% of patients who had diagnostic laparoscopy had recurrence of their pain, compared to only 37% of patients who had operative laparoscopy ($p < 0.01$).

Vercellini et al. also examined the extent and duration of the therapeutic benefit of surgical management of endometriosis. Upon review of three randomized control trials looking at the effectiveness of laparoscopic surgery for symptomatic stage I–IV endometriosis, the absolute benefit compared to diagnostic laparoscopy appears to be between 30–40% after short follow-up periods.

Ms. D. wonders if there is anything she can do to reduce the risk of recurrent post-operative pelvic pain.

A Cochrane review was conducted in 2004 to assess the utility of medical therapy after conservative surgery for endometriosis. This included eight randomized controlled trials examining the use of GnRH agonists, medroxyprogesterone, danazol, and combined oral contraceptive pills. There was no statistically significant difference in pain, recurrence of endometriosis, or pregnancy rates; however, medical management following surgery may delay recurrence of pain, with a trend towards decreased pain at 24 months (95% confidence interval [C.I.] 0.47–1.03, $p = 0.15$).

Key Points

- History and physical for suspected endometriosis should focus on timeline of pain and association with menses. Physical exam should assess for mobility of the pelvic organs, presence or absence of adnexal masses, and nodules suggestive of rectovaginal endometriosis on rectovaginal exam.

- Use of imaging should be based on pertinent findings on history and physical exam.
- Both medical and surgical management of endometriosis result in symptom improvement in approximately 70% of women.
- All methods of hormonal suppression are equally effective for management of endometriosis-associated pain. On average, 70–85% of users report improvement in their symptoms with medical management with hormonal suppression.
- After the first surgery for endometriosis, approximately 25% of patients have recurrence of pain within a year.

FURTHER READING

Fernando S, Soh PQ, Cooper M, Evans S, Reid G, Tsaltas J, Rombauts L. Reliability of visual diagnosis of endometriosis. *J Minim Invasive Gynecol.* 2013 Nov–Dec;20(6):783–789.

Ling FW. Randomized controlled trial of depot luprolide in patients with chronic pain and clinically suspected endometriosis. *Obstet Gynecol.* 1999 Jan; 93(1):51–58.

Sutton CJ, Ewen SP, Whitelaw N, Haines P. Prospective, randomized, double-blind, controlled trial of laser laparoscopy in the treatment of pelvic pain associated with minimal, mild and moderate endometriosis. *Fertil Steril.* 1994;62(4):696–700.

Vercellini P, Crosignani PG, Abbiati A, Somigliana E, Viganò P, Fedele L. The effect of surgery for symptomatic endometriosis: the other side of the story. *Hum Reprod Update.* 2009;15:177–188.

Vercellini P, Somigliana E, Viganò P, Abbiati A, Daguati R, Crosignani PG. Endometriosis: current and future medical therapies. *Best Pract Res Clin Obstet Gynaecol.* 2008;22:275–306.

Yap C, Furness S, Farquhar C. Pre and postoperative medical therapy for endometriosis surgery. *Cochrane Database Syst Rev.* 2004;(3):CD003678.

CASE 2

Ms. S is a 28-year-old gravida 3, para 2 who presents with complaints of chronic daily pelvic pain and dyspareunia. Her symptoms are worse around the time of her menses. She complains of urinary frequency, urgency, and incomplete bladder emptying. She has a history of recurrent urinary tract infection. She also had a recent laparoscopy that demonstrated normal pelvic anatomy and no evidence of endometriosis.

Regarding her urinary symptoms, what focused questions should you ask on history?

"Interstitial cystitis, or bladder pain syndrome" (IC/BPS), refers to chronic pain related to the bladder, in the absence of infection or other identifiable causes. It is a clinical diagnosis made by patient history, physical, and relevant testing. Questions regarding symptom characteristics, duration, relationship to full bladder or voiding, urinary frequency, as well as association with certain foods should be asked. As defined by the American Urological Association (AUA), symptoms should be present for longer than six weeks with no other identifiable cause.

Use of a voiding diary to quantify the degree of urinary frequency and oral fluid intake should be considered. The Pelvic pain, Urgency, Frequency (PUF) questionnaire is a simple screening test for IC/BPS that was validated by Parsons (Figure 20.1). It assesses the symptoms of IC/BPS, including urgency, frequency, pain, and dyspareunia, and the extent to which the patient is affected by these symptoms. The PUF is self-administered and takes about five minutes to complete.

What should you look for on examination?

Exam findings can contribute to clinical suspicion of, but are not diagnostic for, IC/BPS. These findings can include tenderness on palpation of the abdominal wall, as well as pain with palpation of the bladder and urethra. Other conditions that may be contributing to symptoms should be ruled out, including vaginal infection, pelvic mass, or pelvic organ prolapse.

On Ms. S's abdominal exam, she has suprapubic tenderness. On bimanual exam, she has moderate anterior vaginal wall tenderness without any palpable masses. She has a tender uterus on bimanual exam.

What do you recommend next to aid in your diagnosis?

A urinalysis with microscopy should be performed in all patients with suspected interstitial cystitis to exclude infection and hematuria. If infection is suspected, a urine culture should be performed. If hematuria is present, urine cytology and cystoscopy are generally required to exclude other pathologies, including urinary tract malignancy. Post-void residual volume

Please circle the answer that best describes how you feel for each question.

		0	1	2	3	4	SYMPTOM SCORE	BOTHER SCORE
1	How many times do you go to the bathroom during the day?	3–6	7–10	11–14	15–19	20+		
2	a. How many times do you go to the bathroom at night?	0	1	2	3	4+		
	b. If you get up at night to go to the bathroom, does it bother you?	Never Bothers	Occasionally	Usually	Always			
3	a. Do you now or have you ever had pain or symptoms during or after sexual intercourse?	Never	Occasionally	Usually	Always			
	b. Has pain or urgency evermade you avoid sexual intercourse?	Never	Occasionally	Usually	Always			
4	Do you have pain associated with your bladder or in your pelvis (vagina, labia, lower abdomen, urethra, perineum, testes, or scrotum)?	Never	Occasionally	Usually	Always			
5	a. If you have pain, is it usually		Mild	Moderate	Severe			
	b. Does your pain bother you?	Never	Occasionally	Usually	Always			
6	Do you still have urgency after going to the bathroom?	Never	Occasionally	Usually	Always			
7	a. If you have urgency, is it usually		Mild	Moderate	Severe			
	b. Does your urgency bother you?	Never	Occasionally	Usually	Always			
8	Are you sexually active? Yes ———— No ————							

SYMPTOM SCORE = (1, 2a, 3a, 4, 5a, 6, 7a)	
BOTHER SCORE = (2b, 3b, 5b, 7b)	
TOTAL SCORE (Symptom Score + Bother Score) =	

Total score ranges from 1 to 35.

A total score of 10–14 = 74% likelihood of positive potassium sensitivity test (PST); 15–19 = 76%

likelihood of positive PST; 20 or above = 91% likelihood of positive PST.

FIGURE 20.1: The PUF (Pelvic pain, Urgency, Frequency) questionnaire.

2000 C. Lowell Parsons, MD

should also be measured to rule out urinary retention as a cause of bladder pain.

Potassium sensitivity tests, lidocaine instillation, and urodynamic tests have a limited role in the diagnosis of IC/BPS. Further imaging should only be ordered if other anatomical abnormalities, such as kidney stones, are suspected. Cystoscopy with hydrodistension and presence of Hunner's lesions is no longer required for diagnosis.

What treatment options are available?

The treatment options are outlined in Figure 20.2 from the AUA:

Treatment modalities for IC/BPS (briefly) include:

1. Behavior modification: fluid modification and timed voiding

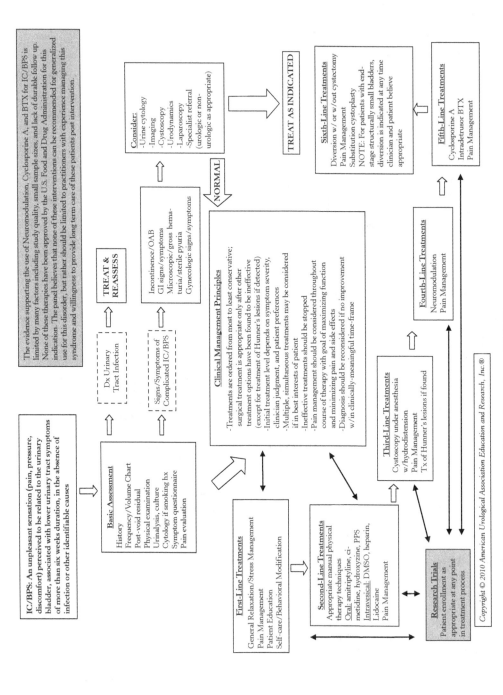

FIGURE 20.2: Treatment options for interstitial cystitis, or bladder pain syndrome (IC/BPS).

Adapted from the American Urological Association.

2. Dietary modification: avoidance of foods that may irritate the bladder, including alcohol, carbonated drinks, spicy foods, monosodium glutamate, aspartame, saccharin, and foods with preservatives or artificial ingredients and colors
3. Pharmacological treatments: oral pentosan polysulfate sodium, neuropathic pain medications
4. Intravesicular instillations: dimethyl sulfoxide (DMSO), buffered xylocaine + heparin
5. Pelvic floor physical therapy

Key Points

- "Interstitial cystitis/bladder pain syndrome" refers to chronic pain related to the bladder for more than six weeks with no other identifiable cause.
- It is a clinical diagnosis made by history, physical, and relevant testing. Cystoscopy, potassium sensitivity tests, lidocaine instillations, and urodynamics are not needed for the diagnosis.
- Like many other chronic pain disorders, management is often multimodal, including medical, procedural, and psychological therapies.

FURTHER READING

Hanno PM, Burks DA, Clemens JQ, et al. AUA guideline for the diagnosis and treatment of interstitial cystitis/bladder pain syndrome. *J Urol.* 2011;185(6):2162–2170.

CASE 3

Ms. R is a 36-year-old gravida 2, para 2 with a long-standing history of pelvic pain, beginning with painful menstrual cycles. Additionally, she complains of painful intercourse, especially with deep penetration. She describes her pain as cramping pain radiating to her lower back, with aching and a feeling of heaviness in her pelvis. She has tried various methods of menstrual suppression, including combined oral contraceptive pills, the etonorgestrel/ethinyl estradiol ring and depo medroxyprogesterone acetate, and stopped each secondary to unwanted side effects.

Are there any other details of her history that are important to elicit?

Myofascial pain syndrome is often one component of chronic pelvic pain, which commonly has multiple contributing etiologies. Muscular pain can both exacerbate and be exacerbated by other sources of pain. For example, pelvic floor spasm can lead to voiding difficulties and pain, thereby leading to straining maneuvers that worsen muscular spasms. Additionally, emotional and physical stressors may negatively influence the pain cycle. Other exacerbating factors include diet, irritable bowel syndrome, interstitial cystitis, dyspareunia, and constipation. Therefore, it is important to elicit a complete history to identify other contributors to pain such as bowel or bladder symptoms as well as mood disorders and emotional stressors.

Myofascial pelvic pain may be a result of both subtle chronic and traumatic acute injury involving the pelvis or trunk. Asking about a history of acute injury such as a car accident or sports injury as well as a history of low back pain may help guide diagnosis and treatment. It is also relevant to identify other potential sources of injury such as pelvic or abdominal surgery and pregnancy and deliveries.

What exam components are helpful?

"Myofascial pain syndrome" or pelvic floor tension myalgia is associated with muscular tightness, tenderness, and spasticity caused by trigger points in the muscle or the muscular fascia. Trigger points develop secondary to acute or chronic muscular injury and are hyper-irritable focal points or bands of skeletal muscular tissue that are tender when compressed. The associated pelvic floor muscles include the pubococcygeus, obturator internus, and piriformis. Symptoms can include referred pain, hyperalgesia, or motor dysfunction.

Key components of the physical exam include assessing for muscular function and tenderness at the lower back and the pelvic floor. Start with an assessment of the patient's gait and lumbar spine and hip range of motion as well as examining the pubic symphysis and the sacroiliac joint. The lower back should be palpated at the paraspinal muscles and the coccyx.

A detailed pelvic exam paying close attention to the pelvic floor musculature is crucial. After a visual inspection of the external genitalia, attention should turn toward palpation of the transverse perineal muscles, followed by bilateral palpation of the pubococcygeus at 7–9 o'clock on the right and 3–5 o'clock on the left, the obturator internus at 9 o'clock and 3 o'clock, and lastly, the piriformis muscles deeper in the pelvis at 10 o'clock and 2 o'clock. Each muscle area should be assessed for tightness, spasticity, and elicited pain. It is helpful to ask the patient if the exam recreates the same type of pain she typically feels.

Ms. R's exam showed tenderness of the coccyx on back exam, and no tenderness on palpation of the abdomen. On palpation of the pelvic floor musculature, tenderness was demonstrated, as described in the accompanying table (see Table 20.2).

Is any other evaluation indicated?
Rarely is any other evaluation indicated, unless suspicion for another disease process arises based on the history and physical examination.

What management options can be offered?
Directed pelvic *physical therapy* geared toward relaxing and retraining the dysfunctional muscles has proven to be beneficial for women with myofascial pelvic pain. The physical therapist typically completes an initial assessment of the patient to identify imbalances in specific muscle strength and length, and joint dysfunction. Therapies aimed at improving function and reducing pain are then employed. These therapies include manual techniques ranging from trigger-point and scar release to joint mobilization. Breathing exercises are helpful supportive therapy to aid in performance of therapeutic exercises as well as daily activities. Biofeedback and transcutaneous electrical nerve stimulation (TENS) have also been employed as adjuvants to physical therapy.

Medications for the treatment of pelvic floor myofascial pain include oral or intravaginal muscle relaxants. A common first-line medication is cyclobenzaprine, a centrally acting skeletal muscle relaxant, which can help reduce muscle tone and also act as a sleep aid when taken at night.

Compounded medications used vaginally such as baclofen and diazepam are effective adjuncts in treating myofascial pelvic pain. Baclofen and diazepam vaginal suppositories may be initiated once daily and up-titrated as tolerated. Lastly, if a neuropathic pain component is evident, neuromodulating medications may be of benefit. (Please see Case 5 for further discussion of this management option.)

When other treatments are unsuccessful, *trigger-point injections* may be used to help alleviate pain. Different formulations have been described and may include a combination of local anesthetic and steroid. The injection is typically given locally at the trigger point or specific area of tenderness. The duration of pain relief varies and may last anywhere from hours to several days. If significant pain relief is experienced, these injections may be repeated every one to two weeks. In the setting of refractory pain, recent attention has been directed toward injecting botulinum toxin in spastic or tense pelvic floor muscles. Although data are limited, preliminary studies have suggested its success in reducing muscle spasm and pain. Unfortunately, the expense of this therapy may be prohibitive for many patients.

As previously mentioned, myofascial pelvic pain is often only one component of chronic pelvic pain. As part of multimodal management, it is also essential to identify and treat mood disorders such as anxiety and depression. Women with dyspareunia often have associated difficulties with partner relationships. In this situation, it can be helpful to refer women to sexual health counselors. Other contributing conditions such as dysmenorrhea, irritable bowel syndrome, interstitial cystitis, and fibromyalgia should be treated as well. Lastly, healthy sleep habits, regular exercise, and stress coping mechanisms should be promoted, as these factors play a vital role in the pain cycle.

Key Points

- Assess for pelvic floor muscle spasticity and tenderness as part of a complete pelvic examination.
- Women with pelvic floor myofascial pain should be referred to physical therapists knowledgeable in specific pelvic floor treatment techniques.
- Additional treatment options include oral and intravaginal muscle relaxants and trigger-point injections.

TABLE 20.2 PELVIC EXAM FINDINGS

Pelvic floor muscles	Right	Left
Pubococcygeus	6/10	6/10
Obturator internus	6/10	6/10
Piriformis	8/10	8/10

FURTHER READING

George SE, Clinton SC, Borello-France DF. Physical therapy management of female chronic pelvic pain: anatomic considerations. *Clin Anat.* 2013; 26:77–88.

Kozasa EH, Tanaka LH, Monson C, Little S, Leao FC, Peres MP. The effects of meditation-based interventions on the treatment of fibromyalgia. *Curr Pain Headache Rep.* 2012;16:383–387.

Lavelle ED, Lavelle W, Smith HS. Myofascial trigger points. *Anesthesiol Clin.* 2007;25:841–851.

Montenegro MLLS, Vasconcelos ECLM, Candido Dos Reis FJ, Nogueira A, Poli-Neto OB. Physical therapy in the management of women with chronic pelvic pain. *Int J Clin Pract.* 2008;62:263–269.

Prather H, Dugan S, Fitzgerald C, Hunt D. Review of anatomy, evaluation, and treatment of musculoskeletal pelvic floor pain in women. *PM&R.* 2009;1: 346–58.

CASE 4

Ms. M is a 43-year-old gravida 2, para 1 with chronic pelvic pain that started when she was 25 years old, after the birth of her child. She describes the pain as a sharp, stabbing pain, with a heavy feeling in her pelvis at times. She took oral contraceptive pills for several years and ultimately underwent an uncomplicated total laparoscopic hysterectomy five years ago. Her pain improved for a brief time, but returned eight months later. She was referred to a pelvic pain specialist and tried a variety of neuropathic pain medications, including cyclobenzaprine, amitriptyline, and duloxetine, which she discontinued due to significant side effects. She subsequently tried pregabalin, which improved her pain by about 50%. She also completed a course of pelvic physical therapy with mild pain improvement. She has seen a therapist for her depression and anxiety in the past, and her mood is stable on sertraline. In addition, she has a history of migraine, chronic low back pain, and irritable bowel syndrome managed by her primary care physician. Currently, she complains of "flares" of pain and requests further management, as she desires her pain level to be 0/10. She is interested in alternative treatments for pain.

Are there any other details of her history that are important to elicit?

This patient has a long history of chronic pelvic pain with appropriate evaluation and treatment in the past. It is still important to obtain a detailed history of her pain, including the questions outlined in Box 20.1.

As part of a comprehensive history, new patients are provided a detailed questionnaire regarding their medical and surgical history, pain history and description, and a complete review of systems with special attention given to bowel and bladder symptoms, sleep assessment, and sexual health. A pain map is included in this packet and is an ideal way for patients to localize their pain, which can be helpful in formulating a differential diagnosis (see Figure 20.3).

For this patient, it is important to elicit and document all prior treatments and medications used. It would be useful to assess her understanding of her diagnosis as well as her expectations. She states a goal of 0/10 pain, which is likely to be unachievable in the setting of long-standing chronic pelvic pain.

What examination components are helpful?

The abdominal exam should begin with visual inspection and notation of scars related to surgery or injury. Palpation of the abdominal wall with increasing pressure in all four quadrants is performed, paying special attention to any areas of tenderness. The Carnett test is useful in differentiating visceral pain versus abdominal wall muscular pain. A localized area of tenderness is palpated while the patient simultaneously elevates her head to contract her abdominal wall muscles. Abdominal wall pain is worsened with this maneuver, while visceral pain is alleviated. In this setting, the patient's facial cues and response to any elicited pain should be observed.

A thorough pelvic examination should be performed, with attention given to the pelvic floor musculature, as she has previously indicated treatment with pelvic physical therapy.

Ms. M's exam is significant for diffuse tenderness in her bilateral lower quadrants, rated 5/10 on the right and 7/10 on the left. No trigger points are identified. On pelvic exam, visual inspection is normal, with a surgically absent uterus and cervix. She has pelvic floor tenderness as demonstrated on pelvic exam in the following table (see Table 20.3).

Is any other evaluation indicated?

No specific testing is usually required beyond a complete history and physical examination unless prompted by abnormalities noted during

BOX 20.1
PELVIC PAIN: QUESTIONS TO ASK DURING INITIAL PELVIC PAIN HISTORY

CHARACTERISTICS OF PAIN SYMPTOMS
- ☐ Where does it hurt?
- ☐ How did your pain start, and has it changed since then?
- ☐ Is your pain constant or intermittent?
- ☐ On average, how many days of pain do you have per month?
- ☐ What is your average, least, and maximum pain level (0–10)?
- ☐ What is the quality or character of your pain? (e.g., cramping, stabbing, pulling, burning?)
- ☐ Does your pain change before, during, or after your menstrual period?
- ☐ What makes your pain better or worse?

ASSOCIATED SYMPTOMS
- ☐ Do you have any urinary symptoms such as pain with urination, pain with a full bladder, frequent urge to urinate, blood in your urine, or urine leakage?
- ☐ Do you have any bowel symptoms such as pain associated with constipation, diarrhea, blood or mucus in your stool, or abdominal bloating?
- ☐ Do you have any associated weakness, numbness or tingling in your pelvis, buttocks, vulva, or legs?
- ☐ Do you have pain during sexual intercourse? If so, it is with initial entry, with deep penetration, or both? Does it continue afterwards?

ASSOCIATED MEDICAL CONDITIONS AND PRIOR TREATMENTS
- ☐ Have you ever used any form of birth control? If so, have any been helpful for your pelvic pain?
- ☐ Do you have any other pain symptoms? (e.g., headaches, back pain, etc.)
- ☐ What other medical problems do you have?
- ☐ Have you ever been diagnosed with or treated for a sexually transmitted disease or pelvic inflammatory disease?
- ☐ Have you undergone any surgeries? Were any of these for the evaluation or treatment of pain?
- ☐ What prior evaluations or treatment have you had for your pain? Have any of these treatments been helpful, and if so, how much?

MENTAL HEALTH AND SOCIAL STRESSORS
- ☐ Have you been, or are you now being, abused verbally, physically, or sexually? Are you now safe?
- ☐ How has the pain affected your quality of life?
- ☐ Do you feel depressed or anxious?
- ☐ Do you have trouble falling or staying asleep? Do you feel well rested in the morning?
- ☐ Are you taking any non-prescription drugs?

PATIENT-CENTERED GOALS
- ☐ What are your goals for this visit? What are your long-term goals?
- ☐ What do you believe is the cause of your pain?
- ☐ What are *you* worried about?

As-Sanie S, Hoffman M, Shuchman D. Managing Pain: Essentials of Diagnosis and Treatment. Ed. Brummett C, Cohen S. Oxford, UK: Oxford University Press; 2013:412–413, Table 18.2.

1. Place an X on the point of your <u>worst</u> pain
2. Shade in all other painful areas, including <u>all other areas in your body that hurt</u>

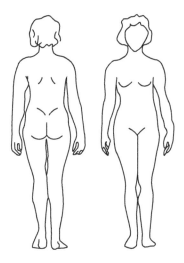

3. Place mark the box next to the one picture that *best describes the course* of your pelvic pain over the <u>past month</u>. *(check one only)*

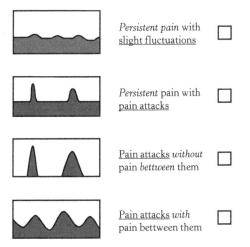

Persistent pain with <u>slight fluctuations</u>   ☐

Persistent pain with <u>pain attacks</u>   ☐

Pain attacks *without* pain *between* them   ☐

<u>Pain attacks</u> *with* pain bettween them   ☐

FIGURE 20.3: Patient pain map.

assessment. Depending on the presence of new pain symptoms, pelvic ultrasound for adnexal evaluation may be warranted.

What management options can be offered?

This patient has previously undergone formal evaluation and treatment for her chronic pelvic pain with relief from both *pelvic physical therapy* and *neuropathic medications*. She should continue pregabalin, as it has proven beneficial. She may

TABLE 20.3 PELVIC FLOOR EXAM FINDINGS		
Pelvic floor muscles	Right	Left
Pubococcygeus	3/10	3/10
Obturator internus	4/10	4/10
Piriformis	4/10	4/10

also benefit from another course of physical therapy with a new physical therapist. Given her long history of pain with accompanying mood disorders, referral to a counselor or psychiatrist who specializes in chronic pain should also be offered.

Alternative modalities can be employed at any point in the patient's treatment plan, and this patient is specifically asking for guidance regarding these therapies. It is not uncommon for patients to actively seek out alternative treatment modalities for chronic pain syndromes. A study of patients with functional bowel disorders found that as many as 35% used complementary and alternative medicine. Although data are limited, evidence suggests that acupuncture, Chinese herbal medicine, and yoga may be beneficial in alleviating chronic pelvic pain.

There are few studies that specifically address *acupuncture* as a treatment for chronic pelvic pain. A 2011 Cochrane review suggests improved endometriosis-related pain with acupuncture treatment. Similarly, a Cochrane review from 2012 reports pain improvement with acupuncture when used for dysmenorrhea. A randomized controlled trial evaluating acupuncture for the treatment of dysmenorrhea demonstrated improved pain intensity and quality of life, at an increased financial cost compared to the control group.

Chinese herbal medicine has also been investigated as a treatment for dysmenorrhea. The evidence is varied, but trends toward improvement in pain were found when compared to NSAIDs, oral contraceptive pills, acupuncture, and heat. Caution must be used, as these medications are not regulated by the FDA, and the number of qualified Chinese herbal practitioners in the community may be limited.

Lastly, *yoga therapy* has been employed as an adjunct treatment for multiple pain syndromes. Research in this area is largely limited to treatment for low back pain, and these studies suggest an improvement in pain and a decrease in use of pain medications. A pilot study evaluating women with fibromyalgia who completed a tailored yoga program found improvements in pain, coping, energy, and mood. Similarly, a review examining the effects of meditation found beneficial outcomes among women with fibromyalgia. It must be noted that these studies are difficult to interpret; likewise, it is difficult to make a specific recommendation regarding the most useful style of yoga. In general, the gentlest forms of yoga that incorporate mindfulness or meditation appear to be successful at improving pain and quality of life.

Key Points

- A detailed history, including pain mapping, and a thorough physical exam are important components of the evaluation of all patients with chronic pelvic pain.
- It is important to discuss the expectations of treatment for chronic pelvic pain.
- Addressing mood disturbances is important in the treatment of chronic pain disorders.
- Alternative forms of treatment such as acupuncture, Chinese herbs, and yoga therapy may provide some benefit in treatment of chronic pain, but solid data are lacking.

FURTHER READING

As-Sanie S, Hoffman M, Shuchman D. *Managing Pain: Essentials of Diagnosis and Treatment*. Ed. Brummett C, Cohen S. Oxford, UK: Oxford University Press; 2013:412–413.

Carson JW, Carson KM, Jones KD, Mist SD, Bennett RM. Follow-up of yoga of awareness for fibromyalgia: results at 3 months and replication in the wait-list group. *Clin J Pain*. 2012;28:804–813.

Smith CA, Zhu X, He L, Song J. *Acupuncture for Primary Dysmenorrhoea*. The Cochrane Collaboration. 2011.

Van Tilburg O, Palsson R, Levy R, et al. Complementary and alternative medicine use and cost in functional bowel disorders: a six-month prospective study in a large HMO. *BMC Complement Alt Med*. 2008;8:46–52.

Witt CM, Reinhold T, Brinkhaus B, Roll S, Jena S, Willich SN. Acupuncture in patients with dysmenorrhea: a randomized study on clinical effectiveness and cost-effectiveness in usual care. *Am J Obstet Gynecol*. 2008;198:166.e1–e8.

Wren A, Wright M, Carson JW, Keefe FJ. Yoga for persistent pain: new findings and directions for an ancient practice. *Pain*. 2011;152:477–480.

Zhu X, Hamilton KD, McNicol ED. *Acupuncture for Pain in Endometriosis*. The Cochrane Collaboration. 2011.

Zhu X, Proctor M, Bensoussan A, Wu E, Smith CA. *Chinese Herbal Medicine for Primary Dysmenorrhoea*. The Cochrane Collaboration. 2011.

CASE 5

Ms. R is a 30-year-old gravida 3, para 2-0-1-2, who presents for evaluation of a 15-year history of chronic pelvic and lower abdominal pain. She always had painful periods, and her pain gradually increased from cyclical to constant daily pain over the years. She has had two diagnostic laparoscopies, which showed normal pelvic anatomy. Two years ago, she underwent total laparoscopic hysterectomy with ovarian preservation, and no identifiable abnormalities were present on pathological examination of her uterus. This surgery did not provide relief of her pain, and she notes her pain has continued to increase over time. Prior to hysterectomy, she used NSAIDs, narcotics, and multiple forms of hormonal suppression, and completed a course of physical therapy, all of which failed to relieve her pain.

Are there any other details of her history that are important to elicit?

Approximately 20–40% of women will experience persistent pelvic pain following hysterectomy. Risk factors for persistent pelvic pain following hysterectomy include age less than 30 with pelvic pain as an indication for surgery, pain in other locations, and negative pathological findings. Because of the shared visceral innervation of the pelvic organs, pelvic pain may not be relieved with hysterectomy alone. This patient's pain may be the result of multiple etiologies, many of which are non-gynecological. Urological, gastrointestinal, and musculoskeletal pain can be important contributors, so it is important to screen for symptoms related to these systems. The description and distribution of the pain can help identify possible sources of pain. For example, neuropathic pain arises as a consequence of a lesion or disease that affects the central nervous system, and is often described as electric, burning, itching, and/or dull. Mononeuropathies can result from direct nerve compression or entrapment, and may be present in the distribution of a nerve injured intraoperatively, including ilioinguinal, iliohypogastric, and pudendal nerves, among others. It is important to obtain a detailed pain history, as neuropathic pain is generally identified by history and exam alone.

Ms. R's pain is located diffusely throughout her lower abdomen and pelvis. She has constant dull pain punctuated by sudden unpredictable "attacks" of incapacitating pain. She is unable to identify any triggers for these exacerbations. She has been seen in the local emergency department numerous times, with repeated negative evaluations including multiple imaging studies.

Mechanisms of chronic pain include central pain amplification and changes in the central nervous system that lead to persistence of pain when no pathological abnormality is present. There are various chronic pain conditions that are likely to involve central pain amplification. (See Box 20.2.) It is important to identify these disorders, as many respond to similar medical and behavioral management methods. In addition, assessment of comorbid pain conditions and mood also provides useful information about quality of life and the impact of chronic pelvic pain on overall well-being. Compared to women without pelvic pain or depression, the subset of women with both of these characteristics preoperatively was found to be 3–5 times more likely to have continued pelvic pain and

dyspareunia, and decreased quality of life following hysterectomy.

Ms. R stays in bed at least 20 days per month due to pain and has lost her job as a result of absenteeism. She sleeps poorly. Her medical history is pertinent for fibromyalgia, depression, anxiety, and irritable bowel syndrome.

What examination components are helpful?

Women with chronic pain often show evidence of hyperalgesia or allodynia on exam. Begin by performing a light touch exam of the abdomen to map painful areas. It is important to start away from areas the patient identifies as painful, as palpating these sites can trigger pain in surrounding areas. Pain that is localized to the region of a single sensory nerve can be evidence of post-surgical nerve injury or entrapment; however, most pain symptoms are not limited to an identifiable nerve distribution. Single-digit exam of the low back, abdominal wall, and pelvic floor to evaluate for areas of tenderness and spasticity consistent with myofascial pain is a useful component of the exam. Light-touch exam of the vulva using a cotton swab can be used to evaluate for vulvar pain. (See Case 6 for further review of evaluating vulvar pain.) Visual

---

BOX 20.2

CLINICAL ENTITIES CURRENTLY CONSIDERED PARTS OF THE SPECTRUM OF CENTRAL SENSITIVITY SYNDROME (CSS)

CLINICAL SYNDROMES

Myofascial pain syndrome/regional soft tissue pain syndrome

Fibromyalgia

Chronic fatigue syndrome (CFS)

Irritable bowel syndrome (IBS) and other functional GI disorders

Temporomandibular joint disorder (TMJD)

Restless leg syndrome (RLS) and periodic limb movements in sleep (PLMS)

Idiopathic low back pain (LBP)

Multiple chemical sensitivity (MCS)

Primary dysmenorrhea

Headache (tension > migraine, mixed)

Migraine

Interstitial cystitis/chronic prostatitis/painful bladder syndrome

Chronic pelvic pain and endometriosis

Reprinted with permission from Phillips K, et al. Central pain mechanisms in chronic pain states—maybe it is all in their head. Best Pract Res Clin Rheumatol. April 2011;25(2):141–154.

inspection of the vagina as well as palpation of the vaginal cuff with a cotton swab and with digital exam should be performed to assess for focal sites of pain and/or masses. The ovaries should be examined if possible, but are often difficult to palpate following hysterectomy due to their lateral location in the pelvis.

Is any other evaluation indicated?

As noted above, sources of persistent pain after hysterectomy are often identified based on history and exam, and additional studies are not required unless a pelvic mass or other focal area of concern is identified on exam.

What management options can be offered?

Multimodal therapy is recommended for the management of central pain and pain after hysterectomy. Options for treatment of neuropathic pain include medical management, nerve blocks, nerve decompression if a mononeuropathy is present, and physical therapy with or without use of TENS. Physical therapy is also useful for treatment of myofascial pain, which may persist following hysterectomy. (See Case 3 for further review of management of myofascial pain.)

Several medications have been used to manage central and neuropathic pain, including tricyclic antidepressants, selective serotonin and mixed reuptake inhibitors, and anticonvulsants. Topical options include lidocaine and capsaicin patches. These medications achieve their effect by modulating neuronal hypersensitivity. For oral medications, patients should be instructed to start at a low dose and up-titrate slowly until a stable treatment dose is reached, determined by a balance of maximal pain relief and limited side effects. They should be counseled that it may take several weeks to achieve maximum benefit. They should also be informed of possible side effects, and care should be taken to avoid interactions with other medications. A second medication from a different class can be added if needed. (See Table 20.4 for details on neuropathic medications, dosing protocols, and side effects.)

Finally, it is important to note that up to 70% of pelvic pain is of non-gynecological etiology, and coexisting conditions such as irritable bowel syndrome, interstitial cystitis, fibromyalgia, mood disorders, and sleep disorders should be treated in order to improve pain and quality of life. Cognitive behavioral therapy provided by pain psychologists can be a useful component of the treatment regimen.

Key Points

- Central pain amplification can lead to persistence of pain when no pathological abnormality exists.
- Chronic pain and persistent pain following hysterectomy are often multifactorial. It is important to enquire about gastrointestinal, urological, musculoskeletal, and mood symptoms, and to screen for comorbid pain conditions.
- A detailed history and physical exam can identify contributors to chronic pain. Additional evaluation with laboratory and imaging studies is often unnecessary, unless focal findings on exam warrant these studies.
- Multimodal management of chronic pain is recommended, including medical therapy, injections, physical therapy, and cognitive behavioral therapy, as well as treatment of comorbid pain conditions.

FURTHER READING

Brandsborg B, Nikolajsen L, Hansen CT, Kehlet H, Jensen TS. Risk factors for chronic pain after hysterectomy: a nationwide questionnaire and database study. *Anesthesiology.* 2007 May;106(5): 1003–1012.

Butrick CW. Chronic pelvic pain: how many surgeries are enough? *Clin Obstet Gynecol.* 2007 Jun;50(2): 412–424.

Hartmann KE, Ma C, Lamvu GM, Langenberg PW, Steege JF, Kjerulff KH. Quality of life and sexual function after hysterectomy in women with preoperative pain and depression. *Obstet Gynecol.* 2004 Oct;104(4):701–709.

Hillis SD, Marchbanks PA, Peterson HB. The effectiveness of hysterectomy for chronic pelvic pain. *Obstet Gynecol.* 1995 Dec;86(6):941–945.

Lamvu G. Role of hysterectomy in the treatment of chronic pelvic pain. *Obstet Gynecol.* 2011 May;117(5):1175–1178.

Phillips K, Clauw DJ. Central pain mechanisms in chronic pain states—maybe it is all in their head. *Best Pract Res Clin Rheumatol.* 2011 Apr;25(2): 141–154.

Stovall TG, Ling FW, Crawford DA. Hysterectomy for chronic pelvic pain of presumed uterine etiology. *Obstet Gynecol.* 1990 Apr;75(4):676–679.

Tu FF, Hellman KM, Backonja MM. Gynecologic management of neuropathic pain. *Am J Obstet Gynecol.* 2011 Nov;205(5):435–443.

TABLE 20.4 DOSING RECOMMENDATIONS FOR REPRESENTATIVE AGENTS THAT HAVE BEEN USED IN NEUROPATHIC PAIN

Class	Suggested dosing guidelines	Side-effects
Tricyclic antidepressants (nortryptiline, desipramine, amitryptiline, imipramine)	Start 10–25 mg at night; can increase by 10–25 mg every 4–7 d as tolerated to effect, or maximum dosage of 150 mg; selected patients may tolerate higher doses (suggest obtain pharmacological consult); some patients will tolerate divided dosing morning/evening better	Dry mouth, somnolence, dizziness, blurry vision, constipation, arrhythmia (check pretreatment electrocardiogram in patients above age 40)
Selective serotonin/norepinephrine reuptake inhibitors		
Duloxetine	Start 30 mg once daily; increase to 60 mg once daily after 7 d to a maximum of 60 mg twice daily	Dizziness, fatigue, nausea, somnolence, dry mouth, serotonin syndrome, constipation
Venlafaxine	Start 37.5 mg once daily or twice daily; increase by 75 mg weekly to effect or a maximum 225 mg once daily	Sweating, weight loss, reduced appetite, nausea, dry mouth, dizziness, somnolence, elevated blood pressure, arrhythmias
Anticonvulsants		
Gabapentin	Start 300 mg at night; increase by 300 mg every 4–7 d until effective or up to 600–900 mg 3 times daily; in older patients or drug-sensitive patients, consider starting/increasing by 100 mg; some patients may find twice-daily dosing better, with the majority of the dosing at night	Dizziness, somnolence, blurry vision, fever, hostile behavior
Pregabalin	Start 75 mg twice daily; increase by 75 mg twice daily every 4–7 d up to effect or to 300 mg twice daily	Weight gain, somnolence, dizziness, blurry vision, impaired thinking
Topiramate	Start 50 mg twice daily; increase weekly by 50–100 mg up to 200–400 mg/d in 2 divided doses	Gastrointestinal discomfort, diarrhea, loss of appetite, nausea, weight loss, dizziness, paresthesia, impaired concentration, somnolence, blurred vision, fatigue
Topical agents		
8% capsaicin patch	Single 60-min application of up to 4 patches every 3 mo as needed; must be limited to area identified by physician as hyperalgesic; do not apply more frequently than every 3 mo; wear gloves while handling	Pain during treatment, skin rash, blood pressure elevation during treatment
5% lidocaine patch	Apply patch (cut to appropriate size) to affected skin up to 12-/24-h period	Local skin irritation, rare systemic lidocaine toxicity (light-headedness, dizziness, drowsiness, tinnitus, blurred or double vision, bradycardia, hypotension)

Reprinted with permission from Tu FF, et al. Gynecologic management of neuropathic pain. *Am J Obstet Gynecol.* 2011;205(5):435–443.

Zondervan KT, Yudkin PL, Vessey MP, Dawes MG, Barlow DH, Kennedy SH. Prevalence and incidence of chronic pelvic pain in primary care: evidence from a national general practice database. *Br J Obstet Gynaecol.* 1999 Nov;106(11):1149–1155.

CASE 6

Ms. L is a 27-year-old gravida 0 who presents to clinic complaining of vulvar pain. She describes it as burning and stinging. Her pain started about five years ago and has been gradually increasing. Now it is present nearly all of the time, and she has been unable to have intercourse for the past two years due to severe entry dyspareunia. She uses cold compresses and over-the-counter oral analgesics without relief.

Are there any other details of her history that are important to elicit?

It is notable that women with vulvodynia often describe their vulvar pain as burning, stinging, irritated, raw, swollen, and throbbing. The presence and intensity of symptoms can change over time, and many women experience "flares" of pain. Vulvodynia can be localized or generalized, and provoked, unprovoked, or mixed, so it is important to elicit the pain's timing, location, and provocative or palliative factors. In addition to obtaining a detailed pain history, inquiring about medical, surgical, sexual, and allergy histories can provide useful information regarding other possible contributors to pain, as vulvodynia is a diagnosis of exclusion. Pertinent historical elements include a history of focal vulvar lesions, skin changes suggestive of vulvar dermatoses, infections such as genital herpes or *Candida vulvovaginitis*, entry or deep dyspareunia, and local reactions to various substances that may have come in contact with the vulva such as clothing, soaps, and topical therapies. It is also useful to ask about typical vulvar care practices and prior treatments for vulvar complaints. Eliciting the effect of a woman's pain on her quality of life, functional ability, and sexual relationships can provide insight into the negative impact of vulvar pain on overall well-being and highlight the need for multimodal therapy.

What examination components are helpful?

Start with inspection of the vulva and note any focal lesions or skin changes. Evaluate the distribution and intensity of pain by performing a cotton swab test. Beginning on the medial thighs, systematically palpate the structures of the vulva gently with a cotton swab, including the labia majora, interlabial sulcus, labia minora, and vestibule at 2, 4, 6, 8, and 10 o'clock positions. The patient is asked to rate pain as absent, mild, moderate, or severe. A speculum exam is performed if tolerated to assess for evidence of vaginitis or lichen planus of the vagina. The oral mucosa should be examined for Wickham's striae, fine white lines that are an oral manifestation of lichen planus. Finally, the pelvic floor musculature should be examined with a single digit to assess tone and tenderness, as myofascial pain is a common contributor to pelvic pain. Lower abdominal, back, and hip exams are performed for similar reasons.

Is any other evaluation indicated?

The need for other studies is at the discretion of the clinician. Vaginal wet preparation, vulvovaginal yeast culture, herpes simplex swab, vulvar biopsy, and skin patch testing for allergies can be performed on an individualized basis if the patient's history and exam findings warrant these additional tests.

What management options can be offered?

Vulvodynia is a chronic condition. A comprehensive treatment plan involving multimodal therapy can help improve her symptoms and quality of life. (See Figure 20.4.) Many treatment options are available, but studies regarding these therapies are limited by small sample size and lack of randomization or placebo control. It is useful to begin by providing education about vulva care, including avoiding irritants such as soaps and topical agents, washing with water alone, applying emollients such as plain petrolatum, wearing cotton underwear, and using cool gel packs as needed.

Topical therapies can be irritants themselves, so consideration should be given to stopping prior treatments and observing for symptom improvement before initiating new therapies. Ointments are generally better tolerated than creams. Some topical therapies may need to be obtained through a compounding pharmacy. Options include 5% lidocaine ointment and compounded gabapentin/amitriptyline/baclofen. Topical corticosteroids, testosterone, and antifungals have been found to be of no benefit for the treatment of vulvodynia.

Oral medications such as antidepressants (tricyclics, selective serotonin reuptake inhibitors

Physical examination

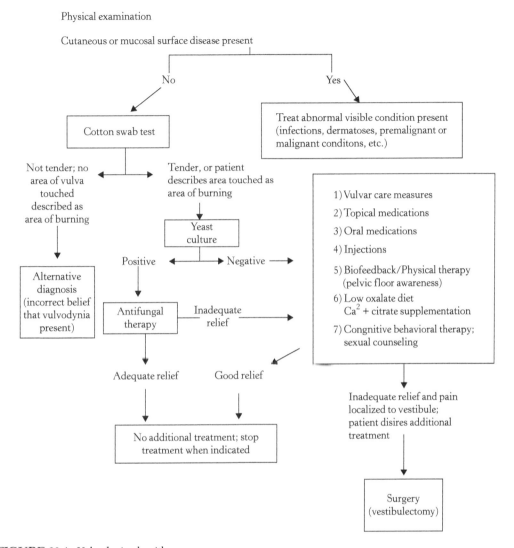

FIGURE 20.4: Vulvodynia algorithm.

Reprinted with permission from Haefner HK. The vulvodynia guideline. *J Low Genit Tract Dis.* 2005 Jan;9(1):40–51.

[SSRIs], venlafaxine) and anticonvulsants (gabapentin, carbamazepine, topiramate) can be used to treat vulvar pain. These are initiated at a low dose and up-titrated slowly to achieve benefit. Several weeks may be needed at a stable dose to see treatment effect. Patients should be cautioned regarding side effects, which commonly include drowsiness, and care should be taken to avoid interactions with other medications.

Injections are often targeted at concurrent pelvic floor myofascial pain, but may be beneficial for some women with vulvodynia. Options include use of bupivicaine for trigger-point injections or pudendal block, as well as Botox injections of hypertonic pelvic floor musculature.

Surgical management with vestibulectomy is an option for women with provoked or secondary vestibulodynia; however, women with unprovoked or primary vestibulodynia are less likely to receive benefit from this intervention. In vestibulectomy, the epithelium of the vestibule including the hymen is excised in a U-shaped manner, and the vaginal epithelium is advanced to close the defect. Surgical management is generally reserved for women who have localized pain and have failed multiple other methods of management. It is important to emphasize that other sources of pain, such as pelvic floor myofascial pain, will continue to require treatment in order to achieve symptom improvement.

Multimodal therapy including physical therapy with possible use of biofeedback and TENS, sex therapy, and cognitive behavioral therapy provided by pain psychologists are important components of the comprehensive treatment regimen for many women with vulvodynia. These therapies can provide support to women and couples, address relationship problems that arise in conjunction with pelvic pain, facilitate return to sexual activity, and help women develop strategies to manage pain.

Key Points

- Vulvodynia is a diagnosis of exclusion, and can be made with careful history, exam, and limited laboratory studies as indicated based on exam findings.
- Gentle vulva care and medical therapies are used for initial management of vulvodynia.

- Additional treatment options including injections, physical therapy, sex therapy, and cognitive behavioral therapy are important components of multimodal care.
- Surgical management has a limited role in treatment of vulvodynia, and is more useful in women with localized and provoked pain.

FURTHER READING

Haefner HK, Collins ME, Davis GD, et al. The vulvodynia guideline. *J Low Genit Tract Dis.* 2005 Jan;9(1):40–51.

Nunns D, Murphy R. Assessment and management of vulval pain. *BMJ.* 2012 Mar 28;344:e1723.

Stockdale CK, Lawson HW. 2013 Vulvodynia Guideline update. *J Low Genit Tract Dis.* 2014 Apr;18(2):93–100.

INDEX